Dysphagia Post Trauma

Clinical Dysphagia Series

John C. Rosenbek and Harrison N. Jones
Series Editors

Dysphagia Following Stroke by Stephanie K. Daniels and Maggie-Lee Huckabee

Dysphagia in Movement Disorders by John C. Rosenbek and Harrison N. Jones

Dysphagia Post Trauma by Elizabeth C. Ward and Angela T. Morgan

Dysphagia Post Trauma

A Volume in the Clinical Dysphagia Series

Elizabeth C. Ward, PhD
Angela T. Morgan, PhD

PLURAL PUBLISHING
INC.
SAN DIEGO
OXFORD
BRISBANE

PLURAL PUBLISHING
INC.

5521 Ruffin Road
San Diego, CA 92123

e-mail: info@pluralpublishing.com
Web site: http://www.pluralpublishing.com

49 Bath Street
Abingdon, Oxfordshire OX14 1EA
United Kingdom

FSC
Mixed Sources
Product group from well-managed forests and other controlled sources

Cert no. SW-COC-002283
www.fsc.org
© 1996 Forest Stewardship Council

Typeset in 10½/13 Garamond by Flanagan's Publishing Services, Inc.
Printed in the United States of America by McNaughton and Gunn

Cover image courtesy of Andrew Davidhazy, Professor, School of Photo Arts and Sciences, Rochester Institute of Technology, Rochester, New York.

Library of Congress Cataloging-in-Publication Data:

Ward, Elizabeth C., Dr.
Dysphagia post trauma / Elizabeth C. Ward and Angela T. Morgan.
p. ; cm. – (Clinical dysphagia series)
Includes bibliographical references and index.
ISBN-13: 978-1-59756-236-2 (alk. paper)
ISBN-10: 1-59756-236-X (alk. paper)
1. Deglutition disorders. 2. Wounds and injuries–Complications. 3. Wounds and injuries–Nursing. I. Morgan, Angela. II. Title. III. Series: Clinical dysphagia series.
[DNLM: 1. Deglutition Disorders–etiology. 2. Deglutition Disorders–therapy. 3. Wounds and Injuries–complications. WI 250 W257d 2009]
RC815.2.W37 2009
616.3'23–dc22

2008054874

Contents

Foreword

Dysphagia Post Trauma, edited by Elizabeth C. Ward and Angela T. Morgan, joins *Dysphagia Following Stroke* by Stephanie K. Daniels and Maggie-Lee Huckabee and *Dysphagia in Movement Disorders* by John C. Rosenbek and Harrison N. Jones in the Clinical Dysphagia Series. Plural's Clinical Dysphagia Series was created because we realized that the modern management of swallowing disorders is so vast as to threaten the binding of a single book. A single practitioner's feelings of competence are similarly stretched by the expanse that has become dysphagia evaluation and treatment. Thus, as Ward and Morgan themselves observe, special conditions such as dysphagia following a variety of traumatic events require special expertise. No area of dysphagia practice is faster growing or more challenging and no group of practitioners is more up to the task of offering sound, practical guidance than the authors of this book.

Chapter 1, titled "Dysphagia Assessment and Intervention: Basic Principles for Trauma Management" and written by Morgan and Ward, provides an overview of neural control of swallowing, normal physiologic swallow function, current assessment approaches, and dysphagia management approaches. Chapter 2, also by Morgan and Ward, covers the more specific topic of traumatic brain injury (TBI). Major topics on TBI covered include incidence and epidemiology, pathophysiology, classification and diagnostic tools, medical management, dysphagia, and associated disorders of speech and language. Chapter 3, by Solley and Ward, is an exhaustive appraisal of dysphagia in individuals with traumatic spinal cord injury, including review of mechanisms, classification, incidence, and epidemiology; clinical management including respiratory, nonsurgical, and surgical interventions; swallowing disorders; and associated speech and communication impairments. Chapter 4, by Rumbach, Ward, McKinnon DuBose, and Clayton, is concerned with swallowing disorders in the setting of burn injury. As noted by the authors, this is an emerging area for dysphagia assessment and treatment due to medical and surgical advances, which result in decreasing mortality following burn injury, as well as the increasing recognition of the need for such survivors to receive multidisciplinary evaluation and treatment. Chapter 5 is titled, "Multitrauma and Iatrogenic Trauma," and is authored by Crombie, Spurgin, and Ward. Topics covered under multitrauma include mechanisms, classification, and impact of management; neurological trauma; structural trauma including hard and soft tissue injuries; and thoracic trauma. Iatrogenic trauma topics include neurosurgery, anterior cervical spine surgery, carotid endarterectomy, cardiac surgery, thyroidectomy, and parotidectomy.

This book is, of course, not the whole solution to the challenges of specialized practice of treating dysphagia after traumatic injury, but it provides an excellent foundation for clinicians. Additional requirements include vast experience working as part of a multidisciplinary team, continuing education, keen intellect, courage, humility, and tolerance for ambiguity. We believe this is a special book written by gifted individuals. Read it for the joy that comes with discovering new, useful ideas elegantly presented.

John C. Rosenbek
Harrison N. Jones

Preface

The term *trauma* is commonly defined as a severe injury to any body structure by an outside agent or force that has the potential to be life threatening. In the United States, trauma is one of the leading causes of critical illness and death. Similarly, traumatic injury is a major public health issue in Australia, representing a significant proportion of all hospital, emergency care, and rehabilitation costs.

Management of the critically ill trauma patient is highly complex and is best achieved within designated trauma centers by trauma teams with specialist skills in critical care management. Survivorship for critically ill patients has markedly increased over the past few decades due to advances in medical care and the growth of specialized trauma centers. This increase in survival has in turn focused efforts towards improving clinical rehabilitation management and optimizing outcomes for this patient group. Acute care for this population is particularly complex, and is often characterized by extensive and protracted ventilation, surgical, and pharmacological management prior to achieving medical stability or commencing recovery. Safe and early re-establishment of oral intake is an important area for recovery, and dysphagia management for the patient with severe trauma requires an advanced level of clinical skill. To this end, there has been a gradual increase in the involvement of speech-language pathologists (SLPs) with the critically ill trauma population over recent times.

The SLP must take multiple factors into consideration for successful management of dysphagia in patients with trauma, including: the immediate and long-term anatomical and physiological damage caused by the traumatic injury; the potential influence of various aspects of critical care management (e.g., tracheostomy); the various stages of trauma recovery; as well as the potential impact of comorbid states or conditions that can adversely influence patient outcome. Although Chapter 1 of the current textbook provides the reader with a basic orientation to dysphagia and its management, the remaining content of the textbook focuses on advanced clinical practice specific to the trauma population. Our contributing authors have attempted to cover core information for each of the specific trauma populations discussed in this text, but it is highly recommended that any clinician working with the trauma population seek additional reading and training. Establishing clinical mentors and links with larger trauma centers is also strongly advised. As for most populations with dysphagia, the importance of working closely with other members of the multidisciplinary team cannot be overemphasized for this group.

The nature and extent of traumatic injury that may befall an individual is immensely varied. Consequently, the current textbook has been designed to provide the SLP with clinically relevant information specific to types of traumatic injury that have an increased potential to impact on swallow function. To this end, Chapters 2 and 3 cover the most common types of neurotrauma, that is, traumatic brain injury and spinal cord injury, and their impact on the swallow. Chapter 4 details the complex medical and physiological impact of burn injury, whereas the final chapter covers the complex issues of multitrauma and iatrogenic trauma. The content of each chapter has been designed to provide the reader with a basic orientation to the medical condition and associated issues that result from the physical trauma, and to then discuss specific issues regarding dysphagia assessment and management that are particular to these trauma populations.

On behalf of all the contributing authors, we hope you find this text a useful clinical resource for managing dysphagia post-traumatic injury. We wish your patients the best of outcomes.

Liz Ward and Angela Morgan

Acknowledgments

First, we wish to thank our team of contributing authors. Maura, Anna, Nicola, Cynthia, Jane, and Ann-Louise, your extensive clinical expertise with these patient populations has greatly enhanced the content of this text. As editors we are mindful of how much additional work was required to complete this project beyond already significant clinical workloads and important family commitments. We sincerely thank you for your dedication to this project. Thanks are also extended to your families who supported you through this extra workload. Special mention goes to the little league who were there through it all: Liam, Hugh, and Jean Solley; and also to baby Benjamin Spurgin—welcome to the world!

We are also grateful to a number of people who assisted with the images in this textbook. To those patients who consented to the photography in this text: thank you for allowing us to share your images here with our readers. We also give our sincere thanks to Chris Edghill, who tirelessly produced multiple versions of the illustrations; thank you for your infinite patience for correcting little things! Thanks also go to the commercial companies referenced throughout the text who provided us with images to illustrate key points.

Finally, we wish to thank our personal support team. *From Liz to her husband Adam:* Despite promising "no more textbooks" after the last one, you supported me again through a second one. Sorry again for all the lost time together. As usual, your unwavering support and uncanny understanding of when to leave me to write and when I need to be dragged away from the computer are deeply cherished. Love you. I also need to extend a special thank you to Brad and Simone Bennett for access to their "writers retreat"; it's always easier to work when looking at the sea! *From Angela to her husband Adam:* Thank you for your unconditional love and support.

Liz Ward and Angela Morgan

Contributors

Nicola A. Clayton, BAppSc (Speech Pathology), MScMed
Senior Speech Pathologist-Burns Unit
Concord Repatriation General Hospital
Sydney, New South Wales
Australia
Chapter 4

Jane Crombie, BSpPath, Grad Cert Management
Senior Speech Pathologist
Royal Brisbane & Women's Hospital
Brisbane, Queensland
Australia
Chapter 5

Cynthia McKinnon DuBose, MA CC-SLP
Clinical Coordinator
Shands at University of Florida
Gainesville, Florida
Chapter 4

Angela T. Morgan, BSpPath (Aud Hons), PhD
Postdoctoral Research Fellow, Language & Literacy Group
Healthy Development Theme
Murdoch Children's Research Institute
Melbourne, Victoria
Australia
Chapters 1 and 2

Anna F. Rumbach, BSc, MSpPathSt
Speech Pathologist and PhD Candidate
Division of Speech Pathology
The University of Queensland
and
Royal Brisbane & Women's Hospital
Brisbane, Queensland
Australia
Chapter 4

Maura Solley, BSpThy
Speech Pathologist
Brisbane, Queensland
Australia
Chapter 3

Ann-Louise Spurgin, BSpPath(Hons), Grad Cert Management
Senior Speech Pathologist
Royal Brisbane & Women's Hospital
Brisbane, Queensland
Australia
Chapter 5

Elizabeth C. Ward, BSpThy(Hons), Grad Cert Ed., PhD
Associate Professor
Division of Speech Pathology
The University of Queensland
Brisbane, Queensland
Australia
Chapters 1–5

1 Dysphagia Assessment and Intervention

Basic Principles for Trauma Management

ANGELA T. MORGAN AND ELIZABETH C. WARD

INTRODUCTION

The oropharyngeal phase of normal swallowing is a highly coordinated, rapid process that is typically completed in less than 1.5 seconds. Given the apparent ease of this process in healthy individuals, the complexity of the neurological control or physiological function of swallowing is commonly underestimated. Any form of trauma to the brain or to the physical structures involved in swallowing may significantly disrupt this normally effortless process, with potential deleterious effects on a patient's respiration, nutrition, and quality of life.

As previously acknowledged in the preface to this textbook, the assessment and management of dysphagia in the trauma population requires an advanced level of clinical skill. In order to accurately assess and manage these patients, the speech-language pathologist (SLP) must have a sound understanding of the normal swallowing process and an understanding of the nature of the traumatic injury that has been incurred. The current chapter has therefore been included to provide the reader with a brief review of (a) the neuroanatomical control of swallowing, (b) physiological functioning of the normal swallowing mechanism, (c) current approaches to assessment of swallowing, and (d) dysphagia management techniques. Within the subsequent chapters, the impact of the specific type of trauma on the normal swallowing process, and clinical insights into how assessment and management may vary depending on the impact of trauma, will be discussed in greater detail. Readers seeking more comprehensive information on the normal swallowing process or on the assessment and treatment of dysphagia are referred to the many textbooks dedicated solely to this topic (see the Further Reading section at the end of this chapter).

NEURAL CONTROL OF THE NORMAL SWALLOW

Early theory regarding the neural control of swallowing was derived largely from studies of animal models. Recent developments in magnetic resonance imaging

(MRI) data acquisition and analysis techniques, however, have led to expanded research on the neural control of swallowing in human subjects. Consequently, there have been significant advances in our understanding of the relative contribution of neural networks subserving swallowing function. Further research is required in this area however: in particular in relation to understanding the white matter pathways that connect specific neural regions thought to subserve specific swallowing functions (e.g., involvement of the supplementary motor area in the initiation of swallowing).

Neural damage is most commonly widespread following traumatic brain injury. This widespread damage commonly manifests from diffuse axonal injury, as is typically associated with the acceleration-deceleration forces exerted on the brain subsequent to motor vehicle accident. Focal lesions are less common, but may arise due to gunshot wounds or blunt trauma to the head. As a result, dysphagia post trauma may result from either "direct" damage to a specific cortical region or nerve pathway, or "indirectly" through disruption at any level of the white matter ascending or descending pathways. It is clear that with such expansive neurological control being required for efficient and accurate execution of the swallowing process, the likelihood of dysphagia occurring following traumatic disruption of the neural control of swallowing is high, and the nature of its presentation diverse. Understanding the neural network subserving the normal swallowing mechanism assists the clinician to comprehend the nature of dysphagia that may result following trauma to specific areas of the brain. Although swallowing is subserved by a complex neural network, for ease of understanding this network may be divided into the areas of cortical control, brainstem control, and peripheral sensory factors and will be discussed under these headings in the sections below. Damage at each of these regions can have a differential impact on the swallow as highlighted in Table 1 1.

Cortical Control of Swallowing

The cortex has higher order control over the swallowing mechanism, including a primary role in the voluntary initiation of swallowing. Swallowing is reported as being largely under bilateral cortical control, with specific neural substrates including the somatosensory and somatomotor cortex, supplementary motor area, the insular cortex, and the anterior cingulate cortex (see Humbert & Robbins, 2007, for review). Both bilateral and unilateral cortical lesions have been reported to disrupt the oropharyngeal initiation of swallowing. In addition to controlling voluntary swallowing, cortical projections also synapse in the lower brainstem centers that integrate sensory information and transmit and modify motor information for mastication and swallowing.

Brainstem Control of Swallowing

The swallowing process is thought to come under involuntary or automatic control at the end of the oral phase at the point of the swallow being "triggered." These involuntary aspects of swallowing are reported to be largely mediated by the lower brainstem, or specifically, the medulla oblongata. This region houses swallowing-related neurons that form the central swallowing pattern generator (SPG). Findings from both animal and

Table 1–1. Dysphagia Outcomes Associated with Trauma to Neural Regions

Neural region	***Mediates***	***Dysphagia outcomes associated with trauma to neural region***
Cortical	Pre-oral anticipatory/cognitive aspects of swallowing	Lack of response to food Lack of awareness of dysphagia and failure to modify behavior to compensate for physiological deficit
	Voluntary initiation of swallow	Delayed oropharyngeal swallow initiation
	Modulation of swallow	Disrupted coordination of oropharyngeal swallow
Subcortical region	Integration of eating behavior and visceral responses	Loss of internal regulation of appetite May result in hyperphagia or hypophagia
Brainstem	Bilateral coordination and execution of swallow	Disrupted coordination of any aspect of oropharyngeal swallow
	Coordination of breathing and deglutition	Disrupted respiration-deglutition cycle and increased aspiration risk Lack of breathing cessation and glottal closure during pharyngeal phase with increased aspiration risk
Peripheral sensory receptors	Permits modification of oral and pharyngeal stages of the swallow in response to sensory feedback regarding the bolus Modifies swallow and feedback for mastication	Reduced sensory feedback associated with poor continual modification and adjustment of the swallow, resulting in reduced coordination of oropharyngeal swallow/disrupted masticatory pattern

human clinical studies affirm the existence of the SPG (see Jean & Dallaporta, 2006, for review).

The SPG consists of a dorsal and ventral group of neurons. The dorsal group is situated in the primary sensory relay area of the medulla oblongata: the nucleus tractus solitarii (NTS). The dorsal group may be thought of as "generator" neurons that initiate and modify or organize the swallow (Jean & Dallaporta, 2006). The ventral group of neurons is connected to the motor neurons involved in swallowing, associated with cranial nerve nuclei V, VII, IX, X, and XII (Table 1–2) and the ansa cervicalis (c1–c3), which joins to run with the hypoglossal nerve (XII). It is believed that the ventral group of neurons distributes and coordinates the drive already generated in the dorsal neurons to modify the swallowing process. Both the dorsal and ventral group of swallowing-related neurons receive sensory inputs (see Table 1–2) regarding taste and sensation from the tongue and oral-pharyngeal mucosa, and proprioceptive

Table 1–2. Cranial Nerves Associated with Swallowing

Nerve	*Sensory*	*Motor*
V—Trigeminal	Sensation from nasal mucosa, tongue, teeth, gums, palate, lip, cheek; proprioception of muscles of mastication	Muscles of mastication, keeping mouth closed for oral preparation, and palatal movement
VII—Facial	Sensation from tastebuds on anterior ⅔ tongue, nose, and palate; proprioception of muscles of facial expression	Muscles of facial expression, secretion of saliva (submandibular, sublingual glands)
IX—Glossopharyngeal	Sensation from tastebuds on posterior ⅓ tongue, pharynx; proprioception of pharynx	Motor impulses to muscles of pharynx; secretion of saliva (parotid gland)
X—Vagus	Sensation from tastebuds on rear of tongue; proprioception of pharynx and larynx	Motor contraction of muscles of pharynx and larynx
IX—Accessory	Priopriоception for muscles controlling head and neck	Laryngeal movement and muscles for movement of head and neck
XII—Hypoglossal	Priopriоception of muscles of the tongue	Motor control of intrinsic and extrinsic muscles of the tongue and infrahyoid

information from swallowing-related musculature. Sensory input is also received from higher-level cortical centers, ventral brainstem centers, the cerebellum, and basal ganglia. This information is integrated and used to mediate the swallow to ensure that the generated movements are appropriate for the particular bolus being ingested (Jean & Dellaporta, 2006).

The brainstem is also primarily responsible for the control of swallowing and respiration. The close proximity of the SPG to the respiratory control centers in the medulla oblongata facilitates the critical, highly coordinated interaction between the initiation of swallowing, glottal approximation, and the cessation of respiration during the pharyngeal phase of swallowing (Ichord, 1994). Given the critical role of the brainstem in controlling swallowing, it is not surprising that direct or indirect trauma to this neural region can have a deleterious effect on swallowing outcome, including an increased risk for aspiration.

Peripheral Sensory Factors

As summarized in Table 1–1, sensory feedback and afferent pathways carrying this information play a critical role in mastication (Bakke, Møller, Thomsen, Dalager, & Werdelin, 2007; Tsuboi, Kolta, Chen, & Lund, 2003) and in stimulating and modifying a swallow (Plant, 1998). The oral cavity, pharynx, and larynx are all lined with a variety of different types of sensory cells. Within the oral cavity, the largest concentration and most widespread coverage are provided by the mechanoreceptive cells, which are most numerous at the tip of the tongue and along the midline of the palate (Plant, 1998). The dorsal surface of the tongue, faucial pillars, pharynx, and posterior larynx are thought to be the origins of the major sensory stimuli needed to elicit swallowing (Miller, 1986), with the tonsillar or faucial pillars being the most sensitive to light touch (Dodds, Stewart, & Logemann, 1990; Shinghai & Shimada, 1976; Storey, 1968). Following initiation of the swallow, local sensory input variables including bolus volume and consistency are then believed to modulate or alter the swallow (Dodds et al., 1990). Ascending sensory tracts therefore evoke motor programs via the SPG and provide ongoing feedback to monitor the descending motor systems.

Loss of sensation in the oral cavity, pharynx, or larynx may disrupt afferent or sensory signals being sent to the swallowing centers, thereby resulting in swallowing deficits, and perhaps even aspiration. For example, disrupted sensation to the laryngeal region may lead to suppression or elimination of the cough reflex, resulting in asymptomatic or *silent aspiration*. A recent study examined the impact that applying topical anesthesia (i.e., disrupting functional sensory input) to the oropharyngeal region had on swallowing function (Teismann et al., 2007). Results demonstrated that healthy control participants experienced swallowing difficulties and reduced swallowing speed and volume of amount swallowed when oropharyngeal input was impaired (Teismann et al., 2007). In turn, abnormal patterns of neural activation were also associated with the disrupted oropharyngeal sensation. Although normal swallowing was associated with bilateral activation of the midlateral primary sensorimotor cortex, anesthesia of the oropharyngeal mechanism resulted in reduced cortical activation of both sensory and motor regions (as revealed via magnetoencephalogram analysis; Teismann et al. 2007). This evidence highlights the importance of sensory input and the crucial interplay between sensory and motor systems for producing a normal functional swallow.

PHYSIOLOGICAL FUNCTION OF SWALLOWING

Trauma may lead not only to brain and spinal cord injuries that can affect the neural control of swallowing, but damage to the physical structures involved in swallowing (e.g., fractured jaw) at the time of trauma, and interventions undertaken during the post-trauma management (e.g., intubation, spinal stabilization) have the potential to further disrupt swallow physiology. Due to the extensive and diverse nature of traumatic injury and its management, it is anticipated that there may be disruption to at least one or more phases of the swallowing mechanism following trauma.

The normal swallow consists of four key phases, including the (a) oral preparatory phase, (b) oral phase, (c) pharyngeal phase, and (d) esophageal phase. There is also an additional phase preceding this sequence, referred to as the pre-oral anticipatory stage, which is especially relevant for the trauma population who suffer diffuse brain injury (see Chapter 2). The critical processes performed at each of the phases in a healthy swallow are summarized in Table 1-3. Understanding the role of each phase and the physiological processes involved is critical for

Table 1–3. The Stages of Swallowing

Stage	***Primary role***	***Key characteristics***
I. Pre-oral anticipatory	Interaction of pre-oral motor, cognitive, psychosocial, and somatoesthetic elements	• Sensory acknowledgement that food is present and appropriate responses (e.g., visual: anticipatory mouth opening to spoon; somatoesthetic: judging temperature of food that is approaching; sensory: smelling of food, etc).
II. Oral preparatory	Preparation of food and fluid for oral transit and initiation of the pharyngeal swallow	• The duration and nature of this stage vary; influenced by factors such as the characteristics of the bolus (size, texture, taste, temperature) and cognitive/emotive factors (appetite, pleasure, fatigue, etc). • Once bolus enters the mouth, the lips are compressed together and pressed against the incisors, sealing the oral cavity anteriorly. • Liquids: Lip seal and buccal tone assist oral control and manipulation of the liquid bolus and prevention of anterior spillage. For liquid boluses, the soft palate is often "draped" or contacting the posterior tongue, which assists with oral containment and allows continued respiration during oral preparatory stage. • Solids: Both tongue and buccal contractions work to manipulate the bolus, exposing it to the teeth for mastication. The velum is less likely to be fully lowered against posterior aspect of the tongue for a solid bolus, though it remains relaxed to allow ongoing respiration during mastication. • During the process of mastication, the bolus is mixed with saliva from the salivary glands (parotid, submandibular, sublingual) and broken down into particle sizes appropriate for swallowing. • Post-mastication, food particles are gathered to form a cohesive bolus of appropriate size and consistency ready for initiation of the swallow. • Bolus is held near front or center of the palate in preparation for the oral phase.
III. Oral	Posterior propulsion of the bolus from the oral cavity into the pharynx within 1 second	• Anterior tongue is elevated and pressed against the hard palate to seal the oral cavity anteriorly and contain the bolus. • Velum begins to elevate. • Sequential lingual stripping action creates posterior propulsion of bolus past anterior tonsillar pillars into the pharynx to trigger the "reflex" swallow.

Table 1–3. *continued*		
Stage	***Primary role***	***Key characteristics***
III. Oral *continued*		• Due to the combined effects of lip seal, buccal contraction, and lingual contraction/propulsion, interoral pressure is increased.
IV. Pharyngeal	Propulsion of the bolus through the pharynx and into the esophageal sphincter, and simultaneous protection of the airway, all within 1 second	• The soft palate is elevated against the posterior pharyngeal wall to seal the nasopharynx. • The respiratory cycle is suspended creating a temporary apneic period. • The bolus is propelled posteriorly into the pharynx by contractions of the intrinsic and extrinsic muscles of the tongue. • As the bolus moves into the oropharynx, a liquid bolus is typically divided in half at the epiglottis, with each half travelling either side of the larynx down through the lateral channels and pyriform sinus, at which point they rejoin behind the cricoid cartilage at the upper esophageal sphincter (UES). Solid boluses do not divide and travel unilaterally. • Contractions of the submental, superhyoid, and infrahyoid muscles assist the superior and anterior movements of the hyoid and reposition the larynx superiorly to a position under the base of the tongue. • Laryngeal closure is achieved through adduction of the true vocal folds (arytenoids medialize and tilt anteriorly). Additional airway protection is achieved through adduction of the false cords, inversion of the epiglottis, and approximation of the aryepiglottic folds, which help to close the laryngeal vestibule. • The base of tongue connects with the posterior pharyngeal wall behind the tail of the bolus to propel it though the pharynx. • The combined effects of laryngeal elevation and pharyngeal contraction help to shorten the pharynx to assist movement of the bolus through into the esophagus. • Opening of the UES (which normally remains actively contracted) is achieved through the combined actions of relaxation of the cricopharyngeus muscle and the superior and anterior movement of the hyoid and larynx.

continues

Table 1–3. *continued*

Stage	*Primary role*	*Key characteristics*
V. Esophageal	Transit of the bolus from the esophageal sphincter to the stomach	• This stage begins with entry of the bolus through the UES. • Bolus transport through esophagus is achieved via esophageal peristalsis, which typically occurs every 2 to 4 seconds, with each wave traversing the length of the esophagus to the lower esophageal sphincter (LES) at the entrance to the stomach in 6 to 10 seconds.

diagnosing the physiological bases of dysphagic impairments, identifying targets for treatment, and selecting appropriate treatment strategies. The following text and the contents of Table 1-3 outline the physiological components of each stage of the swallow process and are provided as a summary guide for practical use, until internalized by the clinician. More detailed discussions of the phases of the swallow can be found in dedicated dysphagia textbooks (see Further Reading section at end of chapter).

Pre-oral Anticipatory Stage

The Pre-oral anticipatory stage encompasses the interaction of pre-oral motor, cognitive, psychosocial, and somatoesthetic elements involved during mealtimes (Leopold & Kagel, 1983; 1997); see Table 1-3 for a summary of key components of this phase. Disruption of the pre-oral phase is of particular relevance to patients with traumatic brain injury, where cognitive deficits may be a substantial factor affecting feeding and swallowing (detailed further in Chapter 2).

Oral Preparatory Phase

The oral preparatory phase is a voluntary process, involving the manipulation of food or liquid in order to form a cohesive bolus ready for swallowing. Key elements to ensure successful oral preparation include: lip closure to seal the oral cavity; rotary and lateral motion of the mandible to aid mastication; symmetrical and functionally intact buccal or facial tone to aid in manipulation of the food around the oral cavity and to avoid oral spillage; and rotary tongue movement to assist in moving the food and fluid around in the oral cavity and for repositioning food back onto the teeth for chewing (see Table 1-3).

Oral Phase

The oral phase is a further voluntary stage of the swallowing process. In healthy individuals, this phase should take less than 1 second. It begins with the posterior propulsion of the food bolus by the tongue and ends with the trigger or production of a "reflex" swallow (see Table 1-3).

Pharyngeal Phase

The pharyngeal phase also takes less than 1 second, and involves both pharyngeal bolus transit and protection of the airway (see Table 1–3). Three main functions of this phase include (a) sealing the nasopharynx, larynx, and oral cavity to aid direction of the bolus and to avoid spillage of food/fluid; (b) opening of the upper esophageal sphincter (UES); and (c) creation of a pharyngeal pressure gradient to assist transportation of the bolus from the oral cavity to the superior opening of the esophagus (Kennedy & Kent, 1988).

Esophageal Stage

The esophageal phase begins at the end of the pharyngeal phase of the swallow when the cricopharyngeal sphincter relaxes to allow a bolus of food or liquid to pass from the pharynx into the cervical esophagus. The primary function of this phase is the passage of the bolus through the esophagus to the stomach via an automatic peristaltic wave (see Table 1–3). The peristaltic wave and contraction of the cricopharyngeus muscle help to prevent food or fluid reentering the pharynx from the esophagus [i.e., gastroesophageal reflux (GER)].

DYSPHAGIA ASSESSMENT POST-TRAUMA

Dysphagia post-trauma is typically complex, with multiple factors potentially contributing to its severity and nature of presentation. A strategic and detailed assessment is therefore critical to provide a sensitive diagnosis of the symptoms and underlying cause(s) of the problem in order to guide optimal dysphagia management. For these reasons, a thorough swallowing assessment following trauma typically involves both a clinical swallow examination (CSE), followed by the most appropriate instrumental evaluation of swallowing. In the following sections the main aspects of clinical and instrumental assessments will be outlined. Further practical considerations relevant to conducting these assessments with each of the different trauma populations discussed in this text (traumatic brain injury, spinal cord injury, burns injury, multitrauma and iatrogenic trauma) are provided in more detail in Chapter 2 through Chapter 5.

Dysphagia Screening Tools

Dysphagia screening tools are quick and simple assessments designed to determine whether dysphagia is present. They provide very little or no information about swallowing physiology. Screening tools are most often designed to be implemented by other health professionals (e.g., nursing) in order to identify patients at risk of dysphagia who require referral to speech-language pathology for detailed assessment. Each health setting seems to have its own form of dysphagia screening assessment in place. However, despite subtle differences, the majority include some version of a water swallow test. The 3-oz. water swallow test (DePippo, Holas, & Reding, 1992) is possibly the most common dysphagia screening assessment for adult individuals with neurological disease. Although some research groups have presented slight modifications to the standard assessment (e.g., encouraging the patient to take one single sip before continuing with the full amount), the actual 3-oz. water test involves a person drinking 3 oz. (90 cc) of water without interruption. Patients are referred for further assessment if they are unable to complete the task or if there is coughing, choking, or a wet, hoarse voice quality exhibited either during or within 1 minute of completing the test (DePippo et al., 1992).

Although initial exploration of validity and reliability of the water swallow test was conducted predominantly in the stroke population, a recent paper by Suiter and Leder (2008) examined the use of this test with a very large (n = 3000) heterogeneous population. They found passing the test was a good predictor of the ability to tolerate thin liquids. However, it was also noted that failure on the test did not necessarily indicate the inability to tolerate thin liquids (low specificity and high false positive rate): so the patient who fails this test requires further investigation prior to final oral intake decisions—as is the normal process following failure on any screening assessment.

Clinical Swallow Examination

The clinical swallow examination (CSE) is the first stage of conducting a more detailed assessment of the presenting dysphagia. Multiple components make up the CSE, including taking a detailed case history, observing the general presentation and cognitive-behavioral state of the patient, examining oromotor, laryngeal, and respiratory status, and determining aspiration risk during trials of foods and fluids (+/− compensatory strategies). The CSE enables the speech-language pathologist (SLP) to make preliminary decisions about aspiration risk, and on the basis of structured observations, provide some initial insight into the physiological basis of the presenting dysphagia. In particular, the CSE results will inform (a) the severity of the presenting dysphagia, (b) potential physiological factors contributing to the dysphagia determined through direct observation (oral stage), palpation (laryngeal elevation), or deduction (coughing immediately post-swallow suggests penetration/aspiration), (c) impact of postural or compensatory strategies to reduce aspiration risk, (d) if further instrumental assessment is required for a particular patient, and (e) which instrumental procedure will be most appropriate. The CSE, however, cannot provide a comprehensive picture of the nature of pharyngeal stage deficits or confirm the presence of penetration or aspiration.

Feeding and Swallowing History

Information regarding general medical, psychosocial, and swallowing history is compiled in order to identify any factors contributing to the presenting dysphagia. Special attention should be paid to neurological, respiratory, and gastrointestinal status given the interrelationship between these functions and swallowing. This is particularly true for the patient with dysphagia post-traumatic injury, for whom a number of existing comorbidities may impact swallow function

General Observations

General observation and consideration of a range of factors that may influence swallowing are then conducted prior to progressing further with the CSE. For the trauma patient, this will involve consideration of generic factors that are considered for all dysphagic patients (e.g., level of alertness) as well as other trauma-specific factors. Examples of some relevant observations have been outlined in Table 1-4. Further details regarding specific observations for each of the different trauma populations covered in this text are outlined in Chapter 2 through Chapter 5.

Oropharyngeal Examination

Following general observations, the CSE then involves careful examination of oral structure and symmetry, and motor and sensory function of the oropharyngeal and laryngeal structures (Table 1-5). This oropharyngeal examination is initially performed in the absence of food and/or fluid. The anatomical structure is initially observed at rest, and then during movement. Any obvious abnormalities in the oral cavity or oropharynx are recorded (e.g., cuts, tears, or abrasions of the lips, tongue, or buccal cavity; broken jaw, etc.). This is most important for the trauma population who often may present with compromised bony or soft tissue integrity, or may have restriction of oromotor movements due to altered positioning (such as following spinal cord injury) or use of external devices (like neck braces).

Following this, performance of oral motor movements to command provides information on the level of voluntary control over the oropharyngeal musculature in the absence of food and fluid.

Table 1–4. Examples of Key Factors to Consider During Observation of the Trauma Patient

Variable	*Potential complicating factors*
Level of alertness	Reduced level of alertness/lethargic: patient requires verbal/tactile stimulation to remain alert
Location and extent of injury	Fractures or injuries to the upper body/face; multitrauma
Positioning	Specialized full body positioning due to nature of injury (e.g., supine for spinal injury; special positioning for burn wound management and contracture management)
Upper body function and tone	Asymmetry of upper body tone; abnormal resting tone (e.g., writhing movements, etc.)
Presence of potentially limiting medical devices	Nasogastric tubes, orogastric tubes; tracheostomy tubes; neck braces for spinal stabilization; wires and plating for management of maxillofacial fractures
Respiratory function	Shallow/rapid breathing; ventilation/respiratory support
Secretion management	Level of awareness and management of secretions (e.g., presence of drooling)
Communication	Absence of appropriate communication and pragmatics
Cognitive-behavioral attributes	Agitated/uncooperative: patient verbally/physically refuses to complete task; distractible: patient requires constant verbal or tactile prompts to remain on task

Table 1–5. Oropharyngeal Examination Checklist

Area	*Component*	*CN*	*Observation/criterion/task*
Orofacial region (facial, buccal, labial, lingual, uvula)	Tone	V, VII, XII, IX, X, XI, XII	Resting tonal state (e.g., asymmetry; fasciculations/tremor at rest) Tone during movement (e.g., disordered, uncoordinated movement)
	Structure	V, VII, XII, IX, X, XI, XII	Oral structural deficits: physical trauma (e.g., lip/buccal tear; severed tongue) or congenital anomalies (e.g., bifid uvula; cleft lip; ankyloglossia)
	Oral motor function	V, VII, XII	Range, rate, accuracy, and strength of voluntary and involuntary movements
Orofacial region (including gums, floor of mouth, hard palate)	Oral sensitivity	V, VII, IX, X, XI, XII	Aversive response (e.g., verbal refusal, head turning) to touch of these regions
Orofacial reflexes	Lip reflexes	VII	Abnormal reflex patterns noted (e.g., lip retraction, lip pursing)
	Jaw reflexes	V, VII	Patient demonstrates abnormal reflex patterns of the jaw (e.g., jaw clenching, jaw extension)
	Tongue reflexes	X, XII	Patient demonstrates abnormal reflex patterns of the tongue (e.g., tongue thrust)
Vocal quality	Wet voice post-feeding	X, XI	Gurgly voice quality indicates possible presence of food/fluid on the vocal folds
	Hoarse/harsh/ extremely weak and breathy voice	X, XI	May indicate vocal pathology such as unilateral vocal fold palsy and the need for further instrumental examination (e.g., stroboscopy)
Management of secretions	Excessive drooling/reduced spontaneous swallowing	VII, IX, X, XII	Lack of oral-sensory awareness/ ability to control secretions
Respiratory control	Breath support for speech	X	Indicative of breath support and coordination of voicing and breath support
Cough	Voluntary cough	X	Present/absent, strong/weak

The oropharyngeal musculature may respond differently during a functional task of eating and drinking, and little is currently understood about the relationship between oral motor movements and functional eating/drinking ability. Performance on the oral motor tasks will be rated in relation to the range, rate, accuracy, and speed of voluntary movements of the facial, lingual, labial, and palatal musculature. This assessment is sometimes also known as the cranial nerve assessment, where poor performance on specific tasks is assumed to relate to motor impairment of a particular cranial nerve (e.g., poor jaw function may be due to impairment of the trigeminal nerve or perhaps the brainstem motor neurons subserving the cranial nerve).

An oropharyngeal evaluation should also involve an assessment of oral sensation where the SLP touches the lips, tongue, inner cheeks, and floor of the patient's mouth with an object such as a tongue depressor or laryngeal mirror. Particular attention should be paid to the presence of any inappropriate oral (e.g., tonic bite reflex) and pharyngeal reflexes (such as hyperactive gag reflex) upon touch. Any inappropriate reflexes may result in disruption of the swallowing sequence.

Laryngeal functioning must be assessed during the CSE as vocal quality is an important indicator of possible underlying laryngeal deficits. A harsh, hoarse, or breathy vocal quality may indicate the need for laryngological investigation to define the presence of any laryngeal pathology or neuromuscular abnormality with vocal fold adduction. Vowel prolongation of /a/, or conversational speech, is often used to assess vocal quality. Asking the patient to increase loudness levels from soft to loud while counting to 5 is another common task used to assess vocal and respiratory control.

The ability of patients to cough voluntarily may be assessed to determine potential capacity to clear the airway; however, it is important to note that the sensitivity and specificity of a voluntary versus a reflexive cough in screening patients for dysphagia is variable (see Smith-Hammond, 2008, for review). Although a reflexive cough should be initiated when food or fluid enters the laryngeal area (Smith-Hammond, 2008), it is well established that a high proportion of patients with neurological impairment do not have a reflexive cough, and are likely to be silent aspirators. In addition, long-term intubation (+/– ventilation) may affect or suppress the cough reflex, potentially increasing the risk for silent aspiration.

Evaluations of how the patient handles his own secretions in the oral cavity and pharynx should also be made during this stage of the CSE, as this skill may indicate the patient's ability to control food. Evidence of spontaneous swallowing, occurrence of drooling, pooling of secretions in the oral cavity, and the patient's reactions to these secretions should be noted (Logemann, 1997). Direct observation and palpation during a dry swallow of saliva only should also be performed prior to any oral trials.

Oral Trials

Swallowing involves a number of reflexively mediated processes that occur only in response to certain food stimuli. Following the evaluation of a patient's oral and structural anatomy and physiology in the absence of food or fluid, a feeding trial normally follows to assess the patient's true level of functional swallowing. However, this stage of the assessment is not completed if the prior steps of the CSE have identified factors contraindicating oral intake.

Observation of a feeding trial provides information on the level of competency of demonstrated oral skills, general coordination of the oropharyngeal stages of swallowing, and any associated behavioral issues that may affect feeding such as muscular weakness/fatigue or cognitive-behavioral deficits. Often in direct response to anticipated aspiration risk, bolus modifications will be implemented for initial fluid and food trials. A variety of food textures is generally trialed during an initial assessment to evaluate how the patient handles specific food and fluid consistencies. The consistency of foods to be trialed is dependent upon cognitive and medical status, in addition to oromotor functioning. Typically for the trauma patient, the trial begins with introduction of a thickened liquid as many patients tend to cope well with the more viscous material, which holds together and results in a slower flow of the bolus, allowing more time to coordinate the swallowing sequence. Progressive trials of thinner consistencies will follow, ceasing once there is clinical indication of aspiration (e.g., coughing). Various food consistency trials will then follow, progressing from puree through to softened and then normal consistencies, depending on aspiration risk and mastication capabilities (for example, trials of normal food for the edentulous patient are typically not undertaken). Once a "safe" (i.e., no clinical signs of aspiration) fluid and food consistency has been identified, the clinician should then implement trials of other strategies (such as sensory modifications, compensatory techniques, swallow maneuvers, etc., discussed further below), to determine if multiple strategies can allow intake of other consistencies; for example, a patient who coughs on initial trials of thin fluids may show no clinical signs of aspiration if he takes small sips of thin fluids while maintaining a chin tuck posture. Unfortunately, in the early stages of swallow management with the trauma patient, cognition and levels of alertness often prohibit the patient from actively implementing additional strategies, and hence texture modification may be the only technique available to the clinician to minimize aspiration risk. However, as soon as cognitively and medically feasible, such additional strategies should be explored in order to facilitate non-texture-modified intake.

Instrumental Assessment

The greatest weakness of the CSE is the inability to objectively diagnose impairment in the pharyngeal or esophageal phases of swallowing. Objective measurement therefore requires utilization of instrumental diagnostic imaging techniques. The instrumental assessment provides objective information on specific areas of the anatomy and physiology of the swallowing process. Instrumental methods are of special importance to the SLP for the evaluation of the pharyngeal phase of swallowing, and for determining the presence of aspiration. A further advantage of instrumental assessment is the ability to objectively evaluate the effect of various swallow rehabilitation techniques. During instrumental assessments, most clinicians evaluate aspiration risk, and then explore the effect of implementing various techniques to minimize that aspiration risk (e.g., chin tuck maneuver, supraglottic swallow). This information provides insight into the potential of various techniques for rehabilitation. Consequently, instrumental assessment is of paramount importance to the clinician for both diagnosis and rehabilitation planning.

Although a number of different instrumental techniques can provide information about the swallow process, the procedures most commonly used internationally include the endoscopic swallowing examination (ESE) and the videofluoroscopic swallow examination (VFSE; also referred to as the modified barium swallow [MBS]). Other techniques such as ultrasonography, manometry, scintography, high-speed MRI, electromyography, and electroglottography are used primarily in research applications and so will not be detailed further in the current text. The following discussion outlines briefly the main strengths and weaknesses of both the ESE and VFSE instrumental procedures. However, it is important to state that these assessments should be viewed as complementary, with the procedure of choice (VFSE or ESE) determined not by personal bias but by the clinical question, particular deficits, and medical considerations applicable to each individual patient.

Endoscopic Swallow Examination

Endoscopic swallow examination is the technique of fiberoptic endoscopy that has been modified to examine aspiration and laryngeal function during swallowing (Sonies, 1991). The ESE procedure involves the use of a flexible scope fitted with a videocamera and a light source, which is passed via a patent nasal passage through the nasopharynx and hypopharynx, and positioned above the false vocal folds, superior to the epiglottis. The use of the flexible scope allows the clinician to visualize the status and function of the physical structures of the velopharynx, oropharynx, and pharynx and larynx. It also provides the clinician with particularly useful information regarding the extent and consistency of any secretions. At this stage sensory testing can also be completed (see Aviv & Murry, 2005, for further details). This can involve the delivery of small calibrated puffs of air onto the vocal folds (often specifically the arytenoids), or in a more crude manner, physical contact with the tip of the scope on the laryngeal tissue. Although there is currently debate as to the lack of standardization of sensory testing, it can provide valuable information especially for those patients with severely reduced laryngeal and pharyngeal sensation.

Following the examination of the physical structures and secretions, a series of food and fluid trials are conducted to determine their suitability dependent on the capacity of the patient. For this component of the assessment, the consistencies are commonly dyed a contrast color from surrounding tissues (e.g., green or blue) to assist in tracking the bolus movement and in visualization of any residue in the laryngeal area and pharyngeal sinuses. Although the larynx is entirely obscured when the vocal folds adduct and the epiglottis descends, laryngeal anatomy is visible before the swallow, providing information on the presence or absence of supraglottic laryngeal penetration (i.e., premature spillage into the hypopharynx and laryngeal vestibule); the presence of pharyngeal dysphagia and clinical symptoms including excess residue and aspiration can be examined using this technique (Langmore, Schatz, & Olson, 1991; Sonies, 1991). In most clinical settings systematic protocols have been developed to assist the assessment process. An example of specific assessment tasks can be seen in Langmore et al. (1991).

ESE has become a particularly valuable assessment tool for the trauma population.

This is largely due to the ability to conduct ESE at the bedside of the trauma patient. This is desirable for patients who are either too medically unstable to be moved to radiology for the VFSE procedure, or for patients who cannot be seated upright. In addition, the procedure is quick and easy to perform. This means ESE is frequently performed, allowing for close monitoring of changes in swallowing physiology. ESE has further clinical utility in this group because the trauma patient may already undergo repeated endoscopic examination as part of his general respiratory and medical management during the early stages of critical care. It is possible to add a brief assessment of the swallow at these times, thereby reducing patient burden by addressing a number of clinical questions (i.e., regarding respiration and swallowing) during the one endoscopic procedure.

Recently, the application of ESE with patients with a tracheostomy in the intensive care unit (ICU) has been reported. Patients with a cuffed tracheostomy tube are often reported to complain of thirst in the ICU, but they are unable to tolerate cuff deflation and therefore may not be able to experience oral fluid intake (McGowan, Hirsch, Shuldman, Gleeson, & Smith, 2007). A recent study evaluated the use of ESE for the evaluation of swallowing in four patients with neurological impairment in an intensive care setting (McGowan et al., 2007). The authors reported that ESE was used successfully in all four patients in the study, and concluded that ESE is feasible for use with patients with cuffed tracheostomy tubes in the ICU setting, facilitating early recommencement of safe oral intake (McGowan et al., 2007).

Early reports of endoscopic assessments of swallowing cautioned about possible contraindications or side effects of the procedure, including hypotension, bradycardia, or cardiac dysrhythmia due to stimulation of the nose, pharynx, or larynx (Kidder, Langmore, & Martin, 1994). However, previous studies were largely based on small numbers of participants, and thus the generalization of these study findings to multiple patient populations was limited. More recently, Aviv and Murry (2005) studied patient characteristics and complications in 1340 consecutive cases that underwent ESE and reported that it was a safe and comprehensive assessment of the sensory and motor aspects of the swallow. The reader is referred to Aviv and Murry (2005) for further reading about specific contraindications noted in individual patients.

Videofluoroscopic Swallow Examination

In the wider dysphagic population, the videofluoroscopic swallow examination currently remains the most extensively used instrumental procedure largely due to its ability to provide information about the physiology of both the oral and pharyngeal phases of the swallow. In the trauma population, although ESE has become a valuable diagnostic tool, particularly for those patients within the critical care setting, a VFSE is seen as providing both complementary and unique information (e.g., oral stage function). Consequently in many settings, once the trauma patient is sufficiently stable and able to be transported to the radiology suite, a VFSE assessment is often completed.

The VFSE is also referred to as the modified barium swallow (MBS) in reference to the fact that it is derived from the barium swallow study of esophageal motility performed by radiologists that was modified by Logemann (1983) for inclusion of the oropharyngeal phase of swallowing. Similar to the ESE, VFSE is used to determine not only *whether* a patient is aspirating, but also the *reason* for the aspiration, so that appropriate treatment can be initiated (Groher, 1997). A wide range of features, not observable during a clinical examination, can be visualized during VFSE including oral control of the bolus; oropharyngeal function and coordination; velopharyngeal function; hyoid movement; laryngeal elevation and closure; pharyngeal constriction; pharyngeal transit time; presence, amount, and location of residue; number of swallows to clear material; and the presence and timing of penetration/aspiration in relation to the swallow (Jones & Donner, 1988; Sorin, Somers, Austin, & Bester, 1988). In addition under videofluoroscopy, clinicians also have the capacity to observe positioning of any metal screws or plates that have been used in post-trauma stabilization and repair, and determine any potential impact these may have on swallow physiology.

Despite its many strengths, however, radiation exposure is a time limiting factor for the VFSE. During a VFSE procedure, swallow physiology and aspiration risk are evaluated during limited trials of barium-impregnated foods or fluids. Once again, the food and fluid trials conducted are determined by the capacity of the patient. Most typically, assessment begins at the thicker fluid consistencies and progresses to thinner consistencies. Food trials are typically performed after the fluid trials. Dynamic radiographic tracking of the food bolus occurs as it moves through the upper aerodigestive tract, subsequently monitoring the structure and function of the oral, pharyngeal, and potentially esophageal phases of swallowing. Trialing of possible compensatory (e.g., postural) or rehabilitation (e.g., maneuvers) strategies is advocated during the VFSE procedure (Logemann, 2007; Logemann et al., 2008) to evaluate the effects of these strategies on the swallowing physiology for an individual. Those readers unfamiliar with the VFSE assessment protocol and analysis processes are referred to Logemann (1993).

The disadvantages of the VFSE procedure include exposure to radiation (as mentioned previously), the expense of the system, the inability to directly and adequately assess laryngeal sensation, and the inability to repeat the procedure frequently (Bastian, 1998). Radiation exposure can be controlled by limiting the number of repeat procedures over time and reducing the amount of "on" time during the assessment, in order to meet national health standards. In light of this, the clinician should plan in advance the consistencies and swallowing strategies they wish to examine under videofluoroscopy so that exposure levels are minimized. A further disadvantage of the VFSE procedure, especially for the trauma population, is that it requires the patient to move to the radiology suite for the VFSE to be performed and thus may be inappropriate for a highly immobile patient.

MANAGEMENT OF DYSPHAGIA

Due to the typically complex nature of the comorbid deficits of patients with traumatic injury, the management of the presenting dysphagia is challenging and typically requires individualized intervention programs that reflect the extent of the unique comorbid issues of the patient (e.g., structural/physiological/cognitive deficits) and that are responsive to the changes in the medical state of the patient. Due to the complexity of the medical condition, a multidisciplinary or interdisciplinary team approach is advocated for achieving optimal patient outcomes.

As discussed in previous sections, the fluctuant and complex medical status of patients with trauma requires a coordinated multidisciplinary team approach. Patients must be carefully monitored for changes across all aspects of their medical status from the critical care phase in ICU, through surgical management, into the post-acute recovery phase and the long-term rehabilitation phase. Teamwork (e.g., across neurology, rehabilitative consultants, gastroenterology, radiology, ear nose and throat surgery, allied health disciplines, nursing) is critical for managing this population.

Non-Oral Supplementation

Dysphagia management typically begins while the trauma patient is still in the critical care unit and continues during the ongoing, long-term rehabilitation period. In the early stages of care, the patient may still be experiencing periods of fluctuating alertness, may have a tracheostomy in situ, and/or be in the final stages of weaning from the ventilator. During this initial period of recovery, the majority of patients will require periods of non-oral supplementation. Then, once they are medically stable and able to be assessed for oral intake, non-oral supplementation is often continued until the point at which either the severity of the dysphagia or the nutritional demands of their medical condition (for example, the hypermetabolic state post-burn injury; see Chapter 4) enable all nutritional needs to be met orally.

Aside from the maintenance of good general medical status (especially respiratory function), the maintenance of adequate nutrition is an essential foundation for maximizing recovery from traumatic injury. It is the aim of the rehabilitation team to identify those patients at risk of aspiration, lessen the impact of the dysphagia, and assist in the provision of adequate nutrition and hydration (Groher, 1997). When determining the optimal method of nutritional support, early evaluation of swallowing ability and aspiration risk is of paramount importance, along with a multidisciplinary approach involving the physician, dietitian, respiratory therapist, and SLP (Logemann, Pepe, & Mackay, 1994). The degree of swallowing impairment and the nature of the traumatic injury (e.g., high metabolic needs of a burn injury) in particular will help to guide the medical team in its determination of how nutritional support can safely be provided, and whether non-oral nutritional support or supplementary feeds are required in the short or long term.

There are three common forms of nutritional support provided for the trauma patient. These include parenteral nutrition (PN) and the two main forms of enteral nutrition: nasogastric (NG) and percutaneous endoscopic gastrostomy (PEG) feeding. No specific type of alternative nutritional support method is without complications. Depending upon the individual presentation of the patient, both enteral and parenteral methods of support are necessary at certain times, in order to be compatible with the gastric functions and heightened energy needs of the patient. Each of these main types is discussed further below.

Parenteral Nutrition

Parenteral nutrition (also referred to as total parenteral nutrition [TPN]) is the process of feeding a person intravenously, typically to a vein with a high blood flow rate, such as via the superior vena cava. Access is provided via either a central line (this line is inserted through the upper chest region and flows into a large vein) or a peripherally inserted central catheter line (PICC, a line that is inserted into a vein in the arm, ending up in a large vein in the chest). PN is often used in the short term (typically no longer than 1 week) for patients in a coma or with severe structural damage (e.g., burns) where they are unable to eat by the normal oral process, or when intestinal failure inhibits absorption of nutrients via the gastrointestinal tract. PN feeding delivers liquid nutrition containing water, energy, fats, vitamins, and amino acids. PN feeding may be extended in severe cases of trauma where oral and/or nasogastric feeding or food absorption is precluded for long periods of time. Feeding schedules may include continuous feeding, or patients may be fed in a regimen so as to simulate a pattern of regular mealtimes with the hope to maintain the patient's hunger-satiation cycles. Given the presence of a central venous catheter, the most typical complication from PN is bacterial infection.

Enteral Feeding: Nasogastric Feeding

Although TPN is recommended for patients with gastric feeding intolerance, for the majority of trauma patients enteral nutrition administered via nasogastric (NG) tube is the predominant mode of non-oral supplementation in the early stages post-injury. NG feeding or intubation involves the insertion of an NG tube via the nose and pharynx through to the stomach. NG feeding utilizes a liquid formula with added fiber and vitamins and a calorie density dependent on the patient's age, size, and required calorie intake. The NG tube is typically inserted by nursing staff who must ensure that (a) the tube is passed to an appropriate level in the patient's stomach and (b) the tube is passed into the esophagus and not into the trachea. Tube placement is commonly checked by removing some fluid from the tube with a syringe and testing it for acidity with pH paper (if the pH ≤5.5 then the tube is in the correct position). NG tube feeding is frequently used for nutritional support for patients on admission to the ICU, and its use is often prolonged throughout the rehabilitation period as it is well tolerated by many patients (Annoni, Hubert, Frischknecht, & Uebelhart, 1998).

Given the fact the tube is inserted through the nose (and often secured to the patient's face with tape), NG feeding is not advised for patients with facial trauma (discussed further in Chapter 5). In some cases an orogastric tube will be used instead, in which case the tube is inserted via the mouth and into the stomach. NG feeding may also be contraindicated for patients with severely impaired cognition or behavior who may not understand the purpose of the tube, and who may attempt to remove the tube with obvious potential negative consequences. Other common complications of NG feeding include sinus infections, bleeding from the nose, and a sore throat. The presence of an NG tube has also been reported to delay therapy and aggravate swallowing dysfunction (Ciocon, Silverstone, Graver, & Foley, 1988). Negative impacts on laryngeal and pharyngeal function have been reported, specifically vocal cord paralysis, muscle lesions, laryngeal inflammations, and granulations (Har-El & Balwally, 1995; Ibuki, Ando, & Tanaka, 1994).

Aspiration pneumonia is an additional side effect from NG tube feedings (Norton et al., 1988), although incompetence of the lower esophageal sphincter in patients with brain injury also appears to contribute to this risk (Norton et al., 1988). From their review of the literature, Akkersdijk et al. (1998) found that the risk of aspiration, frequently associated with NG feeding, has not been eliminated by the application of PEG in place of NG feeding.

Enteral Feeding: Percutaneous Endoscopic Gastrostomy

PEG, often referred to simply as gastrostomy, is a procedure for the insertion of a feeding tube into the stomach via the abdominal wall. PEG is advocated for patients who are unable to take food orally or via a NG tube or for patients requiring supplemental feeding for a prolonged period of time.

If oral feeding is not possible or effective for longer periods of time, a PEG is often used to avoid the potential deleterious effects of prolonged NG tube use. Annoni et al. (1998) examined the outcomes of replacing NG tube feeding with PEG in six patients with severe neurological impairment who required hospitalization for rehabilitation or supportive care for at least 1 year. The patients in the study had been receiving enteral feeding via NG for between 15 months and 4 years post-impairment. Annoni et al. (1998) stated that the PEG was performed in these patients for two reasons: to achieve full energy intake in the absence or ineffectiveness of oral feeding, and to allow better rehabilitation of oropharyngeal functions. The study revealed that three of the patients demonstrated improved swallowing/voicing following PEG placement (Annoni et al., 1998).

Aside from the fact that PEG feeding does not interfere with the swallowing mechanism, further advantages of the PEG procedure include allowing bolus feeds (allowing greater freedom for therapeutic rehabilitation), and the cosmetic advantage of the PEG, which can be worn invisibly underneath clothes (Akkersdijk et al., 1998). Akkersdijk et al. (1998) advocated a liberal use of PEG for patients with severe cerebral injury who do not recover within 14 days.

Despite its advantages, however, PEG has been associated with a number of risks including: 1 to 3% mortality rate; 2.4 to 9% major complication rate; and 5 to 45% minor complication rate (Akkersdijk, Roukema, & van der Werken, 1995; Bussone, Lalo, Piette, Hirsch, & Senecal, 1992; Figueiredo et al., 2007; Larson, Burton, Schroeder, & DiMagno, 1987; Miller, Castlemain, Lacqua, & Kotler, 1989; Steffes, Weaver, & Bouwman, 1989; Stiegmann et al., 1990).

For those patients who have stomach or esophageal complications (e.g., surgery) a percutaneous endoscopic jejunostomy (PEJ) tube is used. Similar in concept to a PEG, the difference lies in the insertion of the tube via an opening in the abdomen directly into the jejunum (small intestine). With PEJ, feeding is typically delivered over 24 hours at a slow rate to assist absorption.

Swallow Rehabilitation Principles

The nature of dysphagia intervention changes as the patient progresses from a passive to an active role in rehabilitation. Typically in the early stages of post-trauma recovery, the patient is unable to actively participate in swallow rehabilitation due to his impaired medical state and altered cognitive levels. At this stage compensatory techniques such as bolus modification and some simple postural adjustments (discussed further below) are commonly implemented to minimize aspiration risk as they require little active effort from the patient. However, once medical and cognitive status has improved (perhaps following emergence from post-traumatic amnesia [PTA]) and the patient has reached an understanding of swallowing difficulties, he is able to fulfil a more active role in his own rehabilitation. At this stage, active rehabilitation involving the motor rehabilitation of the swallow commences (i.e., oral motor tasks and swallowing maneuvers).

Implementing effective swallow rehabilitation involves an understanding of the mechanisms causing injury, the effects of brain damage that may impact on relearning, and the processes of relearning. To this end there has recently been increased discussion in the literature regarding fundamental principles of *neural plasticity*: the ability of the brain to change (Kleim & Jones, 2008). These principles of neural plasticity govern learning in both the intact and damaged brain and may be used to help guide the optimization of both speech and swallow rehabilitation (Gonzalez Rothi, Musson, Rosenbek, & Sapienza, 2008; Ludlow et al., 2008; Robbins et al., 2008).

Although the principles of neural plasticity have yet to be studied in any systematic form in relation to swallow rehabilitation, "the relevance of [applying] established principles of learning to the recovery of swallowing function appears clinically intuitive and evident in an emerging body of literature" (Robbins et al., 2008, p. S291). For this reason Table 1-6 has been included here to outline some of the key principles of experience-dependent neural plasticity as outlined by Kleim and Jones (2008). Future research into improving efficacy of swallowing rehabilitation needs to explore these principles to determine how they may help formulate improved rehabilitation tasks and treatment programs. For example, although principles such as "repetition matters" and "intensity matters" (see Table 1-6) are potentially central to the success of rehabilitation, as yet we do not know how intensive and how much repetition is necessary to effect and sustain change for our dysphagic patients. Similarly, although many embrace the principle of early intervention ("time matters," see Table 1-6), the issue of the optimal time for swallowing rehabilitation is yet to be established. These and many other questions are important directions to explore in future research into swallow rehabilitation for neurological populations, such as the trauma population. As an initial starting point for further reading in this emerging and important area in swallow rehabilitation, the reader is directed to Robbins et al. (2008).

Table 1–6. Principles of Experience Dependent Plasticity as They Relate to Issues of Swallow Rehabilitation

Principle	*Issue for trauma rehabilitation*
Use it or lose it	Functional degradation may be a consequence of the failure to use specific functions
Use it and improve it	Training leads to enhanced function
Specificity	Changing certain behaviors requires rehabilitation strategies that target that specific behavior
Repetition matters	Extensive and prolonged practice is necessary to effect change
Intensity matters	The intensity of a behavioral intervention effects the potential for change
Time matters	Timing of behavioral treatments post-injury may be critical—neural recovery and relearning occur in different phases post-injury
Salience matters	Where rehabilitation treatments are purposeful and related to the behavior being trained, the training experience is enhanced
Age matters	With advanced age, training induced plasticity occurs less readily than in the younger brain
Transference	Change, evoked by training in one area, can *facilitate* acquisition of other related behaviors
Interference	Change, evoked by training in one area of function, may interfere with the acquisition of other behaviors

Note. Adapted from "Principles of Experience-Dependent Neural Plasticity: Implications for Rehabilitation after Brain Damage," by J. A. Kleim & T. A. Jones, 2008, *Journal of Speech, Language and Hearing Research*, 51(1), pp. S225–S239, and "Swallowing and Dysphagia Rehabilitation: Translating Principles of Neural Plasticity into Clinically Oriented Evidence," by J. Robbins, S. G. Butler, S. K. Daniels, R. D. Gross, S. Langmore, C. L. Lazarus, et al., 2008, *Journal of Speech, Language and Hearing Research*, 51(1), pp. S276–S300.

Swallow Rehabilitation Strategies

There are numerous behavioral techniques and treatments than can be implemented to assist swallow safety and improve swallow physiology. A summary of these behavioral techniques is outlined below, supported by information in Table 1-7 through Table 1-10. For those readers seeking further information, we refer you to any one of the numerous textbooks dedicated to the topic of dysphagia (see references in Further Reading section at end of chapter), where these techniques have been discussed in more detail.

In the numerous publications dedicated to discussing the techniques used in dysphagia management and rehabilitation, authors have grouped the behavioral strategies under various headings, such as postural techniques, compensatory adjustments, and so on. Following the Promoting Neuroplasticity in Speech Language Swallowing (PNSLS) meeting held in the USA (Gonzalez Rothi et al., 2008), the workgroup designated to target and explore issues relating to dysphagia recently regrouped behavioral swallow treatments into the four categories of (a) sensory, (b) compensatory, (c) motor without swallow, and (d) motor with swallow (Robbins et al., 2008). Although this most recent conceptualization or classification of treatment techniques is not perfect (e.g., altering bolus viscosity is discussed under both the sensory and compensatory subgroups outlined by Robbins et al., 2008), it represents the most recent consensus regarding grouping our behavioral management techniques, and as such these groupings will be used in the current chapter.

Sensory

The dynamics of the oropharyngeal swallow alters with changes to sensory input. It is the body's physiological adjustment to these changes that can be used to benefit swallow safety. The main types of sensory manipulation include altering the characteristics of the bolus itself (e.g., volume, viscosity, taste, or temperature of the bolus), modifications to the presentation of the bolus, and stimulation of the swallow mechanism (Table 1-7).

Compensatory

As in the case of sensory modifications, the effects of postural change on the swallow are indirect and may not alter swallowing physiology; that is, the effects are likely to be immediate but transient. Postural adjustments of the head, neck, and body are designed to alter the dimensions of the pharynx and the direction of the flow of the bolus. Examples of the main forms of postural adjustment (such as chin tuck, head rotation, head tilt, head back, and side lying) and their effects on bolus flow are outlined in Table 1-8.

Table 1–7. Sensory Adjustments

Approach	*Specific techniques*
Bolus modification	• Modification to consistency of food and fluids: altering texture (smooth, lumpy), altering viscosity (thickening liquids, moistening foods with sauces/gravy) • Increasing bolus taste/flavor, volume, temperature (e.g., sour bolus; Logemann et al., 1995)
Changes in the feeding process	• Increased downward pressure with spoon when placing food in mouth • Reducing speed of presentation of bolus • Presenting food differently in the mouth; e.g., using different pressure, different location • Self-feeding (increases awareness) rather than fed
Stimulation	• Manual thermal tactile stimulation (cold, pressure) • Instrumental techniques: deep brain stimulation, electrical stimulation

Table 1–8. Postural Changes to Alter Bolus Flow

Posture	*Rationale*
Head back	• Utilizes gravity to clear oral cavity
Chin down	• Pushes tongue base posteriorly towards posterior pharyngeal wall • Puts epiglottis in more protective position, narrows the laryngeal entrance • Widens valleculae, narrows airway entrance
Head rotated to damaged side	• Eliminates damaged side path • Places extrinsic pressure on thyroid cartilage, assisting vocal fold closure • Pulls cricoid cartilage away from posterior pharyngeal wall, facilitating opening of upper esophageal sphincter
Lying down on one side (unoperated/stronger side)	• Eliminates gravitational effect on pharyngeal residue
Head tilt to stronger side	• Directs the bolus down stronger side

Motor with Swallow

Behavioral techniques that fall within the classification of "motor with swallow" (Robbins et al., 2008) include those swallowing maneuvers performed while swallowing food or drink (Table 1–9). The purpose of these maneuvers is to exert voluntary control over specific aspects of swallowing, thereby altering swallow physiology. Direct visual feedback during VFSE or ESE can be useful to help patients to learn these techniques and the benefits of consistently implementing these procedures.

Motor without Swallow

The motor without swallow (Robbins et al., 2008) group of behavioral techniques contains the range of movement, strength, and endurance exercises that are designed to improve swallowing physiology in the absence of actual swallow activity, as shown in Table 1–10.

CONCLUSION

Successful management of dysphagia post-trauma requires the following: detailed assessment of the swallowing impairment; minimization of aspiration risk; and implementation of physiologically-based rehabilitation techniques to optimize the swallow. To achieve these outcomes the clinician must have a working knowledge of normal swallow physiology, rehabilitation strategies, and treatment principles. It is acknowledged throughout this initial chapter that more detailed explanations of dysphagia, its assessment, and rehabilitation have been provided elsewhere (see list of textbooks in Further Reading list). The current content, however, provides

Table 1–9. Motor with Swallow Behavioral Techniques

Therapy strategy	*Intended physiological effect*	*References/further reading*
Supraglottic swallow	• Facilitates closure of the true vocal folds both before and during the swallow to prevent penetration	Logemann (1983, 1991, 1993); Martin, Logemann, Shaker, & Dodds (1993); Ohmae, Logemann, Kaiser, Hanson, & Kahrilas (1996)
Supraglottic swallow	• Tilts arytenoid cartilage anteriorly to base of epiglottis to close airway before and during the swallow to prevent penetration • Produces earlier cricopharyngeal opening • Alters extent of vertical laryngeal position before swallow	Martin et al. (1993); Logemann (1991, 1993); Ohmae et al. (1996)
Mendelsohn maneuver	• Extends and prolongs laryngeal elevation during the swallow • Indirectly results in prolonged cricopharyngeal opening • Technique also assists in normalizing timing of pharyngeal events during the swallow	Cook et al. (1989); Huckabee & Cannito (1999); Jacob, Kahrilas, Logemann, Shah, & Ha (1989); Kahrilas, Logemann, Krugler, & Flanagan (1991); Lazarus, Logemann, & Gibbons (1993); Logemann (1991, 1993); Logemann & Kahrilas (1990)
Effortful swallow	• Improves base of tongue retraction; this action generates: increased tongue propulsive force; increased oral pressure; increased duration of pharyngeal pressure and UES relaxation; increased extent of hyoid movement and laryngeal vestibule closure	Hind et al. (2001); Hiss & Huckabee (2005); Huckabee & Cannito (1999); Kahrilas, Lin, Logemann, Ergun, & Facchini (1993); Logemann (1991, 1993); Pouderoux & Kahrilas (1995)
Tongue-holding maneuver (Masako)	• Increases anterior bulging of posterior pharyngeal wall at the level of the tongue base • Improves posterior pharyngeal wall adduction to tongue base	Fujiu & Logemann (1996)

the basis for the following four chapters, which will discuss in detail how dysphagia assessment and management vary for patients who experience traumatic brain injury, spinal cord injury, burn injury, multitrauma, and/or iatrogenic trauma.

Table 1–10. Motor without Swallow Behavioral Tasks

Targeted component	*Therapy techniques*
Labial function	Range of motion exercises; labial compression around tongue depressors or IOPI bulb
Buccal compression	Buccal compression against a tongue depressor or IOPI bulb (placed laterally in cheek)
Lingual function	Compression against a tongue depressor or IOPI bulb (repositioning tongue depressor or IOPI bulb to specific targets; e.g., tongue tip, middle, and back)
Jaw	Passive stretching (use of tongue blades or Therabite system; see Chapters 4 and 5); range of motion and resistance exercises
Velar elevation and closure	Velar elevation in nasal and nonnasal speech drills; velar elevation exercises against resistance during CPAP therapy
Pharyngeal contraction	Pharyngeal gargle
Upper esophageal sphincter opening	Head-lifting maneuver (Shaker et al., 1997)
Laryngeal elevation and closure	Vocal fold adduction exercises to assist vocal fold adduction; laryngeal elevation exercises (pitch glides)
Respiratory capacity and timing	Enhancing respiratory capacity: improving respiratory capacity and forced expiratory volumes (training devices such as an incentive spirometer (see Chapter 3); requires liaison with physiotherapy and/or respiratory clinicians

Note: IOPI = Iowa Oral Pressure Instrument, CPAP therapy = continuous positive airway pressure therapy.

FURTHER READING

Chicero, J. A. Y., & Murdoch, B. E. (2006). *Dysphagia: Foundation, theory and practice*. Chichester, UK: WileyBlackwell.

Crary, M. A., & Groher, M. E. (2003). *Introduction to adult swallowing disorders*. Boston: Butterworth-Heinemann.

Groher, M. E. (1997). *Dysphagia: Diagnosis and management* (3rd ed.). Boston: Butterworth-Heinemann.

Huckabee, M.-L., & Pelletier, C. A. (1999). *Management of adult neurogenic dysphagia.* San Diego, CA: Singular.

Logemann, J. A. (1998). *Evaluation and treatment of swallowing disorders* (2nd ed.). Austin, TX: Pro-Ed.

Miller, A. J. (1999). *The neuroscientific principles of swallowing and dysphagia.* San Diego, CA, and London: Singular.

Murry, T., & Carrau, R. (2006). *Clinical management of swallowing disorders.* San Diego, CA: Plural.

Perlman, A. L., & Schulze-Delrieu, K. S. (1997). *Deglutition and its disorders: Anatomy, physiology, clinical diagnosis and management.* San Diego, CA, and London: Singular.

REFERENCES

Akkersdijk, W. L., Roukema, J. A., & van der Werken, C. (1998). Percutaneous endoscopic gastrostomy for patients with severe cerebral injury. *Injury*, *29*(1), 11-14.

Akkersdijk, W. L., van Bergeijk, J. D., van Egmond, T., Mulder, C. J. J., Henegouwen, G. P. V., Vanderwerken, C., et al. (1995). Percutaneous endoscopic gastrostomy (PEG): Comparison of push and pull methods and evaluation of antibiotic prophylaxis. *Endoscopy*, *27*, 313-316.

Annoni, J. M., Hubert, V., Frischknecht, R., & Uebelhart, D. (1998). Percutaneous endoscopic gastrostomy in neurological rehabilitation: A report of six cases. *Disability and Rehabilitation*, *20*(8), 308-314.

Aviv, J. E., & Murry, T. (2005). *FEEST: Flexible endoscopic evaluation of swallowing with sensory testing*. San Diego, CA: Plural.

Bakke, M., Møller, E., Thomsen, C. E., Dalager, T., & Werdelin, L. M. (2007). Chewing in patients with severe neurological impairment. *Archives of Oral Biology*, *52*, 399-403.

Bastian, R. W. (1998). Contemporary diagnosis of the dysphagia patient. *Otolaryngologic Clinics of North America*, *31*(3), 489-506.

Bussone, M., Lalo, M., Piette, F., Hirsch, J. F., & Senecal, P. (1992). Percutaneous endoscopic gastrostostomy: Its value in assisted alimentation in malnutrition in elderly patients: Apropos of 101 consecutive cases in patients over 70 years of age. *Annales de Chirurgie*, *46*(1), 59-66.

Ciocon, J. O., Silverstone, F. A., Graver, L. M., & Foley, C. J. (1988). Tube feedings in elderly patients: Indications, benefits and complications. *Archives of Internal Medicine*, *148*(2), 429-433.

Cook, I. J., Dodds, W. J., Dantas, R. O., Massey, B., Kern, M. K., Lang, I. M., et al. (1989). Opening mechanism of the human upper esophageal sphincter. *American Journal of Physiology*, *257*, G748-G759.

DePippo, K. L., Holas, M. A., & Reding, M. J. (1992). Validation of the 3-oz water swallow test for aspiration following stroke. *Archives of Neurology*, *49*, 1259-1261.

Dodds, W. J., Stewart, E. T., & Logemann, J. A. (1990). Physiology and radiology of the normal oral and pharyngeal phases of swallowing. *American Journal of Radiology*, *154*, 953-963.

Figueiredo, F. A., da Costa, M. C., Pelosi, A. D., Martins, R. N., Machado, L., & Francioni, E. (2007). Predicting outcomes and complications of percutaneous endoscopic gastrostomy. *Endoscopy*, *39*(4), 333-338.

Fujiu, M., & Logemann, J. A. (1996). Effect of a tongue holding maneuver on posterior pharyngeal wall movement during deglutition. *American Journal of Speech-Language Pathology*, *5*(1), 23-30.

Gonzalez Rothi, L. J., Musson, N., Rosenbek, J., & Sapienza, C. M. (2008). Neuroplasticity and rehabilitation research for speech, language and swallowing disorders. *Journal of Speech, Language and Hearing Research*, *51*(1), S222-S224.

Groher, M. E. (1997). *Dysphagia: Diagnosis and management* (3rd ed.). Boston: Butterworth-Heinemann.

Har-El, F., & Balwally, A. N. (1995). Transcutaneous cervical minioesophagostomy. *Otolaryngology-Head and Neck Surgery*, *113*, 387-392.

Hind, J. A., Nicosia, M., Roecker, E., Carnes, M., Doyle, J., Dengal, G. A., et al. (2001). Comparison of effortful and noneffortful swallows in healthy middle aged and older adults. *Archives of Physical Medicine and Rehabilitation*, *82*, 1661-1665.

Hiss, S. G., & Huckabee, M. L. (2005). Timing of pharyngeal and upper esophageal sphincter pressures as a function of normal and effortful swallowing in young healthy adults. *Dysphagia*, *20*, 149-156.

Huckabee, M. L., & Cannito, M. P. (1999). Outcomes of swallowing rehabilitation in chronic brainstem dysphagia: A retrospective evaluation. *Dysphagia*, *14*, 93-109.

Humbert, I. A., & Robbins, J. (2007). Normal swallowing and functional magnetic resonance imaging: A systematic review. *Dysphagia*, *22*, 266-275.

Ibuki, T., Ando, N., & Tanaka, Y. (1994). Vocal fold paralysis associated with difficult gastric tube insertion. *Canadian Journal of Anaesthesiology*, *41*, 431-434.

Ichord, R. N. (1994). Neurology of deglutition. In D. Tuchman & R. S. Walter (Eds.), *Disorders of feeding and swallowing in infants and children: Pathophysiology, diagnosis, and treatment* (pp. 37-52). San Diego, CA: Singular.

Jacob, P., Kahrilas, P. J., Logemann, J. A., Shah, V., & Ha, T. (1989). Upper esophageal sphincter opening and modulation during swallowing. *Gastroenterology*, *97*, 1469-1478.

Jean, A., & Dallaporta, M. (2006). *Electrophysiologic characterization of the swallowing pattern generator in the brainstem*. GI Motility Online, doi:10.1038/gimo9. Retrieved February 27, 2007, from http://www.nature.com/gimo/contents/pt1/full/gimo9.html

Jones, B., & Donner, M. W. (1988). Examination of the patient with dysphagia. *Radiology*, *167*, 319-326.

Kahrilas, P. J., Lin, S., Logemann, J. A., Ergun, G. A., & Facchini, F. (1993). Deglutitive tongue action: Volume accommodation and bolus propulsion. *Gastroenterology*, *104*, 152-162.

Kahrilas, P. J., Logemann, J. A., Krugler, C., & Flanagan, E. (1991). Volitional augmentation of upper esophageal sphincter opening during swallowing. *American Journal of Physiology*, *260* (Gastrointestinal and Liver Physiology, 23), G450-G456.

Kennedy, J. G., & Kent, R. D. (1988). Physiologic substrates of normal deglutition. *Dysphagia*, *3*, 24-27.

Kidder, T. M., Langmore, S. E., & Martin, B. J. W. (1994). Indications and techniques of endoscopy in evaluation of cervical dysphagia: Comparison with radiographic techniques. *Dysphagia*, *9*(4), 256-261.

Kleim, J. A., & Jones, T. A. (2008). Principles of experience-dependent neural plasticity: Implications for rehabilitation after brain damage. *Journal of Speech, Language and Hearing Research*, *51*(1), S225-S239.

Langmore, S. E., Schatz, K., & Olson, N. (1991). Endoscopic and videofluoroscopic evaluations of swallowing and aspiration. *Annals of Otolaryngology, Rhinolology and Laryngology*, *100*, 678-681.

Larson, D. E., Burton, D. D., Schroeder, K. W., & DiMagno, E. P. (1987). Percutaneous endoscopic gastrostomy: Indications, success, complications and mortality in 314 consecutive patients. *Gastroenterology*, *93*, 48-52.

Lazarus, C. L., Logemann, J. A., & Gibbons, P. (1993). Effects of maneuvers on swallowing function in a dysphagic oral cancer patient. *Head and Neck Surgery*, *15*, 419-424.

Leopold, N. A., & Kagel, M. C. (1983). Swallowing, ingestion, and dysphagia: A reappraisal. *Archives of Physical Medicine and Rehabilitation*, *64*, 371-373.

Leopold, N. A., & Kagel., M. C. (1997). Dysphagia—Ingestion or deglutition? A proposed paradigm. *Dysphagia*, *12*, 202-206.

Logemann, J. A. (1983). Anatomy and physiology of normal deglutition. In J. A. Logemann (Ed.), *Evaluation and treatment of swallowing disorders* (pp. 11-36). San Diego, CA: College-Hill Press.

Logemann, J. A. (1991). Approaches to management of disordered swallowing. *Bailliere's Clinical Gastroenterology*, *5*(2), 269-280.

Logemann, J. A. (1993). *Manual for the videofluorographic study of swallowing* (2nd ed.). Austin, TX: Pro-Ed.

Logemann, J. A. (1994). Multidisciplinary management of dysphagia. *Acta Oto-Rhino-Laryngologica-Belgica*, *48*(2), 235-238.

Logemann, J. A. (1997). Therapy for oropharyngeal swallowing disorders. In A. L. Perlman & K. Schulze-Delrieu (Eds.), *Deglutition and its disorders, anatomy, physiology, clinical diagnosis and management* (pp. 449-462). San Diego, CA: Singular.

Logemann, J. A. (2007). Swallowing disorders. *Best Practice & Research in Clinical Gastroenterology*, *21*(4), 563-573.

Logemann, J. A., Gensler, G., Robbins, J., Lindblad, A. S., Brandt, D., Hind, J. A., et al. (2008). A randomized study of three interventions for aspiration of thin liquids in patients with dementia or Parkinson's disease. *Journal of Speech, Language and Hearing Research*, *51*, 173-183.

Logemann, J. A., & Kahrilas, P. J. (1990). Relearning to swallow post CVA: Application of manoeuvres and indirect biofeedback: A case study. *Neurology*, *40*, 1136-1138.

Logemann, J. A., Pauloski, B. R., Colangelo, L., Lazarus, C., Fujiu, M., & Kahrilas, P. J. (1995). Effects of sour bolus on oropharyngeal swallowing measures in patients with neurogenic dysphagia. *Journal of Speech and Hearing Research*, *38*, 556-563.

Logemann, J. A., Pepe, J., & Mackay, L. E. (1994). Disorders of nutrition and swallowing: Intervention strategies in the trauma center. *Journal of Head Trauma Rehabilitation*, *9*(1), 43-56.

Ludlow, C. L., Hoit, J., Kent, R., Ramig, L., Shrivastav, R., Strand, E., et al. (2008). Translating principles of neural plasticity into research on speech motor control recovery and rehabilitation. *Journal of Speech, Language and Hearing Research*, *51*(1), S240-S239.

Martin, B. J. W., Logemann, J. A., Shaker, R., & Dodds, W. J. (1993). Normal laryngeal valving patterns during three breath hold manoeuvres: A pilot investigation. *Dysphagia*, *8*, 11-20.

McGowan, S. L., Hirsch, N., Shuldman, C. M., Gleeson, M., & Smith, M. (2007). A pilot study of fiberoptic endoscopic evaluation of swallowing in patients with cuffed tracheostomies in neurological intensive care. *Neurocritical Care*, *6*(2), 90-93.

Miller, A. J. (1986). Neurophysiological basis of swallowing. *Dysphagia*, *1*, 91-100.

Miller, R. E., Castlemain, B., Lacqua, F. J., & Kotler, D. P. (1989). Percutaneous endoscopic gastrostomy. Results in 316 patients and review of literature. *Surgical Endoscopy*, *3*(4), 186-190.

Norton, J. A., Ott, L. G., McClain, C., Adams, L., Dempsey, R. J., Hauck, D., et al. (1988). Intolerance to enteral feeding in the brain injured patient. *Journal of Neurosurgery*, *68*, 62-66.

Ohmae, Y., Logemann, J. A., Kaiser, P., Hanson, D. G., & Kahrilas, P. J. (1996). Effects of two breath holding manoeuvres on oropharyngeal swallow. *Annals of Otology, Rhinology and Laryngology*, *105*(2), 123-131.

Plant, R. L. (1998). Anatomy and physiology of swallowing in adults and geriatrics. *Otolaryngologic Clinics of North America*, *31*(3), 477-488.

Pouderoux, P., & Kahrilas, P. J. (1995). Deglutitive tongue force modulation by volition, volume and viscosity in humans. *Gastroenterology*, *108*, 1418-1426.

Robbins, J., Butler, S. G., Daniels, S. K., Gross, R. D., Langmore, S., Lazarus, C. L., et al. (2008). Swallowing and dysphagia rehabilitation: Translating principles of neural plasticity into clinically oriented evidence. *Journal of Speech, Language and Hearing Research*, *51*(1), S276-S300.

Shaker, R., Kern, M., Bardan, E., Taylor, A., Stewart, E., Hoffmann, R., et al. (1997). Augmentation of deglutitive upper esophageal sphincter opening in the elderly by exercise. *American Journal of Physiology*, *272*, G1518-G1522.

Shinghai, T., & Shimada, K. (1976). Reflex swallowing elicited by water and chemical substances applied in the oral cavity, pharynx, and larynx of the rabbit. *Japanese Journal of Physiology*, *26*, 455-469.

Smith-Hammond, C. (2008). Cough and aspiration of food and liquids due to oral pharyngeal dysphagia. *Lung*, *186*, S35-S40.

Sonies, B. C. (1991). Instrumental procedures for dysphagia diagnosis. *Seminars in Speech and Language*, *12*(3), 185-197.

Sorin, R., Somers, S., Austin, W., & Bester, S. (1988). The influence of videofluoroscopy on the management of the dysphagic patient. *Dysphagia*, *2*(3), 127-135.

Steffes, C., Weaver, D. W., & Bouwman, D. L. (1989). Percutaneous endoscopic gastrostomy. New technique—Old complications. *American Surgery*, *55*, 273-277.

Stiegman, G. V., Goff, J. S., Silas, D., Pearlman, N., Sun, J., & Norton, L. (1990). Endoscopic versus operative gastrostomy: Final results of a prospective randomized trial. *Gastrointestinal Endoscopy*, *36*, 1-5.

Storey, A. T. (1968). A functional analysis of sensory units innervating epiglottis and larynx. *Experimental Neurology*, *20*, 366-383.

Suiter, D. M., & Leder, S. B. (2008). Clinical utility of the 3-ounce water swallow test. *Dysphagia*, *23*, 244–250.

Takahashi, K., Groher, M. E., & Michi, K.-I. (1994). Symmetry and reproducibility of swallowing sounds. *Dysphagia*, *9*(3), 168–173.

Teismann, I, K., Steinstraeter, O., Stoeckigt, K., Suntrup, S., Wollbrink, A., Pantev, C., Dziewas, R. (2007). Functional oropharyngeal sensory disruption interferes with the cortical control of swallowing. BMC Neuroscience, 2(8), 62

Tsuboi, A., Kolta, A., Chen, C. C., & Lund, J. P. (2003). Neurons of the trigeminal main sensory nucleus participate in the generation of rhythmic motor patterns. *European Journal of Neuroscience*, *17*(2), 229–238.

Warms, T., & Richards, J. (2000). "Wet voice" as a predictor of penetration and aspiration in oropharyngeal dysphagia. *Dysphagia*, *15*(2), 84–88.

2 Traumatic Brain Injury

ANGELA T. MORGAN AND ELIZABETH C. WARD

INTRODUCTION

Traumatic brain injury (TBI) is one of the most prevalent causes of death or lifelong disability (Thurman, Alverson, Dunn, Guerrero, & Sniezek, 1999). TBI is often associated with a broad spectrum of comorbid injury and prolonged hospitalization (Scott-Jupp, Marlow, Seddon, & Rosenbloom, 1992). Patterns of recovery are equally diverse and may take place over a long period of time. In light of the complex, multifactorial nature of TBI, optimal dysphagia management depends on the speech language pathologists (SLP) having a thorough understanding of the interplay of factors that will influence the nature, severity, and rate of recovery of swallowing for this population.

INCIDENCE AND EPIDEMIOLOGY OF TBI

The incidence of TBI is significantly high, having been reported at approximately 300 to 400 per 100,000 individuals in the population (Tennant, 2005; Yates, Williams, Harris, Round, & Jenkins, 2006). Mortality is reported in approximately 24 to 27% (Morris, Ridley, Lecky, Munro, & Christensen, 2008; Myburgh et al., 2008) of admitted cases. Of those who survive, the majority of cases experience mild TBI. Only 8 to 10% of survivors are reported to experience moderate to severe brain injury (von Wild & Wenzlaff, 2005; Yates et al., 2006). Although moderate to severe brain injury is more commonly associated with poorer long-term outcomes, there is increasing evidence that individuals with mild TBI will also show long-term deficits in everyday functioning across a wide range of domains.

Brain injury is most common in three demographic groups: (a) adults younger than 45 years of age (Jennett, 1996), (b) children and adolescents (Kraus, Rock, & Hemyari, 1990), and (c) adults over 70 (who largely sustain a TBI due to falls; Koskinen & Alaranta, 2008). Males are typically at an increased risk of acquiring TBI (Koskinen & Alaranta, 2008).

PATHOPHYSIOLOGY OF TRAUMATIC BRAIN INJURY

Brain injury refers to a structural and/or physiological change in the nerve tissue of the brain to a pathological degree. TBI is typically associated with diffuse axonal injury, but may also be accompanied by focal or multifocal brainstem or cortical injuries. These neural lesions occur as a result of the mechanisms by which the injury is caused.

The type of brain injury sustained may be classified in a number of ways. Two important distinctions that relate to the biomechanics of brain injury include open versus closed and direct versus indirect injury. For the purposes of medical management, further classification can be made on the basis of the neuropathophysiology of TBI, by differentiating between primary and secondary brain injury. The following sections define each of these possible methods for describing brain injury post-trauma.

Open vs. Closed Head Injury

Open head injury is defined as exposure of the meninges following scalp and/or skull penetration. The neural damage associated with open head injury is typically focal, that is, localized around the point of penetration. Historically associated with wartime injuries, the incidence of open head trauma is now relatively low. In contrast, closed head trauma is prevalent, and it may result from a broad range of activities of daily living (e.g., falls when walking on unsteady surfaces or motor vehicle accidents associated with driving). A closed head injury is distinct from an open head injury in that the meninges remain intact. Brain damage associated with closed head injury can result from either compression or acceleration forces. Generalized or diffuse cerebral involvement is common following closed head injury, but is often accompanied by some degree of focal lesion. A further important division in relation to closed head injury includes the distinction between direct and indirect injury as described in the following section. Please note that the term TBI will refer to closed head injury throughout the remainder of this chapter, unless otherwise specified.

Direct vs. Indirect Brain Injury

Direct injury results from three possible mechanisms: (a) the head being hit by an object, (b) the motion of the head being arrested by another object, or (c) compression of the head. Direct injuries are more commonly associated with focal lesions, such as scalp bleeding, skull fractures, epidural hematoma, or brain contusion. Direct injury in isolation is rare, as the acceleration of the direct impact will typically set the head in motion, resulting in simultaneous indirect injury on the opposite side of the skull. The point of original direct impact is referred to as the coup; the indirect injury to the cerebral area opposite the blow is the contrecoup (also contracoup). The force of the blow may cause the brain to rebound from the skull, causing contusions (or bruising) to the brain tissue where it strikes the skull. Both coup and contrecoup lesions may result in the specific behavioral and physiological impairments associated with TBI.

Indirect injury occurs as a result of acceleration of the brain when there is no direct contact of the skull with another object. More specifically, indirect injury is where the brain undergoes violent motion inside the skull, for example, as in a motor vehicle accident (MVA) or in cases of nonaccidental or inflicted injury. Typical manifestations of indirect injury include concussion, subdural hematoma, or diffuse axonal injury (DAI). The acceleration-deceleration forces and rotation of the brain inside the skull place strain on the nerve fibers and blood vessels, resulting in axonal sheering as seen in DAI or concussion, as described further later in this chapter.

Primary Neuropathophysiological Effects of TBI

Primary injuries occur almost instantaneously at the time of the initial injury, including skull fracture, cranial nerve damage, contusion, cerebral concussion, and diffuse axonal injury (Finfer & Cohen, 2001; Moppett, 2007). Secondary injuries are classed as physiological events that are consequential to the original injury. Primary injuries were once thought to be irreversible, whereas secondary injuries could be offset to some degree through medical intervention. More recently, however, studies have reported that "primary injury" may also be altered through medical management, and that some aspects of TBI previously referred to as "secondary injury" may actually occur at the time of original trauma (Moppett, 2007). Despite the fact that debate is continuing regarding the definitions and mechanisms of injury, the primary versus secondary framework is still useful for conceptualizing brain injury, and key features of these categories are detailed below.

Skull Fracture

Skull fractures are frequently associated with brain injury. A variety of fractures may result from neurologic trauma, including linear (where the impact causes the direct area of damage to the skull to bend inwards and the area surrounding this focal region to bend outwards), depressed (comminuted fractures where the bone may be displaced inward), and comminuted fractures (where a bone is broken into many pieces that may penetrate the cerebrum). As regards the specific region of the skull fractured, a basilar or base of skull fracture is more commonly associated with worse outcome post-TBI than fractures to other skull regions (Fabbri, Servadei, Marchesini, Stein, & Vandelli, 2008). This poor outcome is likely due to cranial nerve damage given their intracranial course throughout the base of the skull. Base of skull fractures commonly result from a large impact to the back of the head, such as a fall or a horse kick to the base of skull. Fracture in this region may consist of a break in the basal sections of the frontal, ethmoid, sphenoid, temporal, or occipital bones.

Depressed skull fractures may also be associated with poorer neurological outcome as a result of causing cortical bruising. Brain dysfunction resulting from skull fracture can impact upon the swallowing mechanism as a result of damage to: (a) the cortex, affecting the more voluntary phases of the swallowing process, and/or (b) the brainstem, resulting in impairment at any level of oropharyngeal swallowing function, dependent upon the cranial nerves involved (see Chapter 1, Table 1-2).

Cranial Nerve Damage

TBI may cause cranial nerve dysfunction either by damaging the cranial nerve nuclei in the brainstem or by disrupting the nerves themselves in their intra- or extracranial course. Extracranial trauma to the face may result in damage to branches of the facial (VII) and trigeminal (V) nerves. With the exception of cranial nerve palsies resulting from contusions of the extracranial branches of the nerves, many traumatic cranial nerve palsies are permanent. Despite how the injury was incurred, and whether it is permanent or temporary, damage to the cranial nerves at any point in their course may result in dysfunction at numerous levels in both the swallowing and speech mechanisms. The reader is referred to Chapter 5 for further discussion of the impact of physical cranial nerve damage on swallowing function.

Brain Contusion

A brain contusion (bruise) consists of diffuse areas of hemorrhage and edema within the brain tissue following TBI. As discussed, the initial direct impact may also produce contrecoup areas of hemorrhage on the opposite side of the direct injury. In the past, contusions were considered to occur in cortical regions only; however, improved neuroimaging methods have since identified contusions within deep areas of the brain. The presence of contusions may signify secondary injury because they are commonly associated with intracellular swelling of adjacent structures. Symptoms resulting from a brain contusion are dependent upon the size and location of the contusion, and potential symptoms may include hemiparesis, speech, language, and swallowing dysfunction, and visual deficits (Murdoch, 1990).

Cerebral Concussion

A cerebral concussion refers to a transient loss of awareness or responsiveness immediately after brain injury. Loss of consciousness may last from minutes to hours, and occurs due to shearing and stretching forces on the brainstem. The term *concussion* is generally used to refer to patients who show full neurological recovery within 1 to 2 hours. Loss of consciousness was once considered a relatively benign feature of trauma. If it occurred in the absence of any obvious signs of neurological impairment (e.g., facial palsy, dysarthria, and visual deficits), loss of consciousness was historically associated with few negative long-term impacts. It is now well recognized, however, that loss of consciousness may be associated with both acute neurological damage (i.e., damage occurring due to intracranial injury; Clement et al., 2006; Da Dalt et al., 2006) and longer term psychosocial issues (e.g., Hessen, Nestvold, & Sundet, 2006; Lee, 2007).

Diffuse Axonal Injury

(DAI occurs due to the rapid acceleration and subsequent deceleration (rotational forces) that accompany high-velocity impact. Specifically, stretching and straining of the axons results in torn axonal fibers, damaged glial cells, and degeneration of neuronal fibers that are distal to the main focal area of shearing. Secondary brain injuries resulting from DAI include the degeneration of viable brain tissue by prolonged ischemia, cerebral edema, hypoxia, hypotension, seizures, or increased intracranial pressure. DAI commonly affects the brainstem (Mannion et al., 2007), hippocampus, corpus callosum, and subcortical white matter (Guthrie, Mast, Richards, McQuaid, & Pavlakis, 1999).

Traditionally, DAI has been considered a primary injury, given that some axonal death occurs in the most severely damaged regions at the time of impact. More recently, however, this concept has been challenged, as current findings show that most axotomy occurs within 12 to 24 hours post-injury (e.g., Reilly, 2001). More specifically, many of the axons that will eventually die do not experience axotomy until around 6 hours or greater post-injury (Maxwell, Bullock, Landhold, & Fujisawa, 1994; Reilly, 2001; Teasdale & Graham, 1998). This model implies that the deterioration in patients following the immediate injury may be due to this progressive axonal loss (Letarte, 1999). Consequently, there are some authors who argue that, although some traumatic axotomy occurs immediately, the majority of the damage occurs later (Letarte, 1999); hence, DAI could be classified as both a primary and secondary effect.

Secondary Neuropathophysiological Effects of TBI

Secondary injuries are central nervous system insults that occur hours or days following the initial primary damage and that may worsen neurological outcome (Finfer & Cohen, 2001; Moppett, 2007). Secondary complications are primarily the result of (a) raised intracranial pressure (ICP) leading to reduced cerebral perfusion and potential cell damage through lack of oxygen; (b) infarction, or death of tissue due to regional blood deprivation; (c) hypoxia, or oxygen deprivation; (d) hematomas, or bleeding/clotting within the skull; (e) edema, or brain swelling due to an increase in fluid content; (f) hemorrhage, or rupture of cortical veins; and/or (g) infection. A range of pharmacological approaches has been investigated to try to reduce the impact of secondary effects; however, the evidence for the benefit of these interventions in improving human patient outcomes has been limited to date (see Moppett, 2007, for brief review).

Raised Intracranial Pressure

Raised ICP is known to worsen over the days following the injury, although it may also occur early post-TBI (Stocchetti et al., 2007). A recent study found that 77.11% (155/201) of cases developed raised ICP, despite active preventative treatment being used in almost all cases (200/201; Stocchetti et al., 2007). The authors reported that cases with raised ICP experienced their highest average ICP reading during the first 3 days post-injury. Twenty-five percent of cases, however, had delayed ICP increases, reaching their highest average ICP reading greater than 5 days post-injury. Patients who developed ICP earlier required more aggressive therapy (Stocchetti et al., 2007). When levels of intracranial pressure cannot be controlled or reversed with medical management, neurosurgical intervention is warranted (neurosurgical management is discussed further in Chapter 5).

Hemorrhage and Hematoma

Traumatic brain injury may be associated with intra- or extra-axial hemorrhage or hematoma (straining or tearing of blood vessels). Intra-axial hemorrhage is associated with blood vessel damage within the skull and brain tissue (also known as cerebral hemorrhage), whereas extracranial hemorrhage is damage to the blood vessels within the skull but external to the brain. Intra- and extra-cranial hemorrhages can be further divided into a number of specific subtypes of blood vessel damage, dependent upon where the bleed is situated.

Intra-axial hemorrhage can include two subtypes of damage: intraparenchymal (bleeding within the brain tissue) or intraventricular (bleeding within the brain's ventricles). Extra-axial hemorrhages may be divided into three main subtypes: epidural (blood buildup between the dura mater and the skull), subdural (between the dura mater and the arachnoid or middle meninges), and subarachnoid hemorrhage (bleeding into the arachnoid space, i.e., the area between the arachnoid membrane and pia mater).

Immediate symptoms of hemorrhage include an intense headache ("thunderclap headache"), stiff neck, nausea, vomiting, and dysarthria. The presence of hemorrhage or hematoma can lead to increased intracranial pressure, subsequently leading to brain tissue damage. The regions of the frontal and temporal lobes are particularly susceptible to damage from subdural hematoma lesions. Hemorrhage is reported to impact upon behavior, memory, and attention. These problems may in turn impact upon feeding and swallowing in patients with TBI.

Seizures and Epilepsy

There is an increased risk of epilepsy or seizures following TBI, with the risk varying dependent upon injury severity and time post-injury (Annegers, Rocca, Hauser, & Coan, 1998). In a population-based study of seizure development post-TBI, overall incidence was reported at 3.1% (Annegers et al., 1998). However, seizure incidence has been reported to range from 4 to 25% in smaller cohort studies (Formisano et al., 2007; Moppett, 2007). The incidence of seizures categorized by injury severity has been reported as 1.5% after mild injuries, 2.9% after moderate injuries, and 17% after severe injuries (Annegers et al., 1998). Key risk factors for seizure development reportedly include: Glasgow Coma Score (GCS) <10, brain contusion, subdural, or intracranial hematoma, depressed skull fracture, penetrating head wound, loss of consciousness or amnesia for more than 1 day, an age of 65 years or older, or presence of a seizure within the first 24 hours of injury (Annegers et al., 1998; Temkin et al., 1990). Patients considered to be at high risk for developing seizures may be treated with antiepileptics as a preventative measure (Brain Trauma Foundation, 2000).

CLASSIFICATION AND DIAGNOSTIC TOOLS

It is well documented that patients with TBI may be predisposed to dysphagia (Morgan, Ward, Murdoch, Kennedy, & Murison, 2003; Ward, Green, & Morton, 2007). With severe brain injury in particular, there is a possibility of focal, multifocal, and/or diffuse cortical and brainstem damage, which may affect the neurological control of swallowing. Information obtained from diagnostic assessments such as computed tomography (CT) and magnetic resonance imaging (MRI) investigations can provide insight into the severity and extent of neural injury. Subsequently, this information may indicate the likely impact of this damage on swallowing function.

Computed Axial Tomography

The structural neurological damage resulting from TBI is most commonly evaluated through the use of CT (or CAT) scan. In particular, CT is used for the detection of acute hematoma and of contusions of the cortex. CT is reported to have poor ability to detect brainstem and posterior fossa lesions and DAI compared to MRI (Mannion et al., 2007).

A number of classification systems have been developed to try to encourage standard reporting of CT lesions across centers internationally. Informal systems involve documentation of key injury types, that is, brainstem injury, midline shift, basal cisterns status, subarachnoid hemorrhage, and intracranial lesions. The most widely used scale is the Marshall CT classification of TBI (Marshall, Marshall, Klauber, & Clark, 1992; Table 2–1). There are, however, a large number of limitations of the Marshall CT classification, including: poor inter-rater reliability (Havill et al., 2001); the lack of a classification category for a normal scan (Moppett, 2007); its retrospective nature (i.e., knowledge of clinical course is required to define a mass lesion as evacuated or not), and the difficulty of measuring mass volumes (Stocchetti et al., 2007). Prognostic sensitivity of the Marshall CT system may be improved by recording the presence of additional structural lesions to those typically reported (e.g., intraventricular hemorrhage, subdural hematoma, status of basal cisterns, presence of different types of mass lesions; Maas, Hukkelhoven, Marshall, & Steyerberg, 2005; Maas et al., 2007).

Magnetic Resonance Imaging

If an individual has a normal CT scan, but an abnormal Glasgow Coma Scale score (i.e., less than 15, as detailed further

Table 2–1. Marshall CT Classification of TBI

Category	*Definition*
Diffuse Injury I (no visible pathology)	No visible intracranial pathology
Diffuse Injury II	Cisterns present with midline shift <5 mm and/or lesion densities present No high-or-mixed-density lesion >25 ml; may include bone fragments and foreign bodies
Diffuse Injury III	Cisterns compressed or absent with midline shift of 0–5 mm No high-or-mixed-density lesion >25 ml
Diffuse Injury IV	Midline shift >5 mm No high-or-mixed-density lesion >25 ml
Evacuated Mass Lesion	Any lesion surgically evacuated
Nonevacuated Mass Lesion	High-or-mixed-density lesion >25 ml; not surgically evacuated

Note. From "A New Classification of Head Injury Based on Computerized Tomography," by L. F. Marshall, S. B. Marshall, M. R. Klauber, and M. V. Clark, 1992, *Journal of Neurosurgery*, *75*, pp. 5S, S14–S20. Reprinted with permission.

below) after 24 hours of admission, a repeat CT or an MRI is warranted. MRI is known to be more sensitive than CT for documenting lesions such as brainstem injury and posterior fossa lesions and for detecting DAI (Mannion et al., 2007). A recent study comparing the clinical application of MRI and CT scans in 55 patients with closed TBI revealed that MRI was more sensitive at detecting DAI, subarachnoid hemorrhage, cortical contusions, and acute subdural hematoma, but was less sensitive at detecting skull fracture (Morais, Spotti, Tognola, Gaia, & Andrade, 2008). In addition, it has been proposed that MRI is more sensitive for detecting soft tissue damage such as spinal cord injury in the absence of any vertebrae fracture. Consequently, MRI is typically used where there are suspected neural lesions not detectable using CT.

Diffusion Weighted Image Acquisition and Analysis

Further developments in MRI and analysis have enabled more sensitive and specific detection and quantification of white matter damage, specifically, a data acquisition technique known as diffusion weighted imaging (DWI) and analysis techniques of fractional anisotropy (FA) and fiber tractography.

DWI is based on principles of water diffusivity, that is, the random movement of water molecules. The random movement of water molecules is more restricted in white matter tracts than in the remaining cortex of the brain, and as a result, the anisotropy (restricted directionality of diffusion) in white matter is higher than in grey matter. FA measures can therefore be calculated for different areas of brain tissue, and FA maps or white matter fiber maps can be generated. FA values range from 0 to 1, where 0 represents complete lack of directional restriction (isotropic diffusion) and 1 represents very organized tissues such as in white matter tracts (anisotropic diffusion; see Le Bihan et al., 2001, for review). From the generation of FA maps, white matter fiber tracts can be determined through a process known as tractography. Once the white matter pathways are identified, the volume or integrity of the tracts can be measured. These developments in MR data acquisition and analysis have potential application for examining the extent of injury following TBI, where white matter damage is common as a result of DAI. For example, DWI is useful for objectively documenting the subtle neural damage often present in mild TBI (Kraus et al., 2007), and can also be used to document white matter damage associated with a wide range of behavioral impairments associated with TBI (e.g., Salmond et al., 2006).

Classifying Severity of Injury

Coma results from severe DAI of the brainstem reticular formation. Consequently, degree of coma or altered cognitive functioning post-injury is a common method of establishing the severity of TBI. The Glasgow Coma Scale (GCS) remains the most commonly used scale to measure the depth of coma and severity of brain injury. Eye, motor, and verbal responses are assessed within the first 24 hours after trauma. The GCS rates these three responses according to set criteria (Table 2–2) on a scale from 3 to 15. The greater the GCS score, the more conscious the patient. The total score is then equated to a particular severity level. A score of 8 or less indicates that the

Table 2–2. Glasgow Coma Scale (GCS)

Category	*Criteria*	*Score*
Eye opening (E)	Spontaneous	4
	To speech	3
	To pain	2
	No response	1
Best motor response (M)	Follows commands	6
	Localization of pain	5
	Withdrawal of pain	4
	Flexion to pain	3
	Extension to pain	2
	No response	1
Verbal response (V)	Oriented	5
	Confused conversation	4
	Inappropriate words	3
	Incomprehensible sounds	2
	No response	1

Note. Coma score = E + M + V.

patient is in a coma, and denotes a severe brain injury. A score of 9 to 12 indicates a moderate brain injury, and a score of 13 to 15 represents a mild brain injury. The GCS is also used to measure change in a patient's acute condition.

Post-traumatic amnesia (PTA) is another method used for ongoing monitoring of brain injury severity. PTA includes the period of unconsciousness following brain injury, and extends until the patient's memory for ongoing events becomes reliable and accurate. Russell (1932) attempted to classify diffuse brain damage due to acceleration/deceleration injuries according to the duration of PTA. Russell's classification of injury severity by length of PTA is listed in Table 2-3.

Table 2–3. Post-Traumatic Amnesia (PTA) Classification System

PTA Duration	*Severity Rating*
<1 hour	Mild
1–24 hours	Moderate
1–7 days	Severe
>7 days	Very severe

Both GCS and duration of PTA are clinically used to classify injury severity, and there is little consensus between health professionals regarding the best index for defining injury severity. Research into the best method for determining injury severity is ongoing. For example, the Mayo Classification System for Traumatic Brain Injury has recently been proposed. The classification system uses a range of existing measures (e.g., GCS, PTA, trauma-related neuroimaging abnormalities) to classify the type and severity of TBI (Malec et al., 2007). Until a consensus on the optimal classification system is reached, it is likely that depth of coma (as measured via GCS) and duration of PTA will remain the most commonly used clinical tools.

Monitoring Cognitive and Medical Recovery

As outlined above, duration of PTA is defined as the period in which a patient is unconscious, to the point when a patient's memory for ongoing events becomes reliable and accurate. By definition, PTA consists of anterograde amnesia, in which the patient is unable to store or recall ongoing events post-injury. Historically, it was believed that a patient was severely limited or unable to learn new material while in PTA. Recently, however, it has been reported that new learning can occur in relation to functional situations (e.g., tasks of daily living likely using procedural memory; Weir, Doig, Fleming, Wiemers, & Zemljic, 2006).

PTA is monitored as an indicator of change in patient status during recovery. Although seminal work was first conducted in this field by Russell and colleagues (e.g., Russell, 1932; Russell & Smith, 1961), two of the most commonly used tools to measure PTA in recent times include the Modified Oxford Post-Traumatic Amnesia Scale (MOPTAS) and the Westmead Post-Traumatic Amnesia Scale (WPTAS). The WPTAS was developed based on the MOPTAS.

- The MOPTAS is adapted from the original Oxford PTA scale by Fortuny, Briggs, Newcombe, Ratcliff, and Thomas (1980), in which three target pictures are presented to the patient, and recall is tested on the following day. If the patient is not able to attain 100% recall, recognition testing is used where the target pictures are interspersed among five foils. Twenty-one sets of foils were used in the original procedure by Fortuny et al. (1980), allowing new foils to be presented each day for 3 weeks, with repetition of the foils after this time if the patient is still in PTA.
- The WPTAS is reported to differ from the MOPTAS on two key aspects, first, that the foils consist of one single set of six pictures, and second, that the three target pictures are altered after the first day on which the maximum score is obtained, and a new set of target pictures is chosen from the foils. The old targets are then used as foils (Tate et al., 2006). The WPTAS has been reported as a more challenging task for the patient than the MOPTAS, because the foils and targets are not independent. Consequently, the recognition task in the WPTAS is more demanding. Recently a randomized trial compared the WPTAS and MOPTAS to test whether there were differences between the scales (Tate et al., 2006). The study demonstrated no statistically significant difference in the duration of PTA between the two measures, with the exception that there was a slightly protracted period of resolution in the end stage of PTA with the WPTAS (Tate et al., 2006). Further information on the WPTAS PTA protocol is available from Marosszeky, Ryan, Shores,

Batchelor and Marosszeky (1997) and http://www.psy.mq.edu.au/pta/

In addition to ongoing measurements of coma, consciousness, or alertness, many centers use their own informal systems for documenting cognitive improvement during the acute phase when more formalized and higher level neuropsychological assessments are precluded. One scale that has been used in the early phase of acute cognitive management in the patient with TBI is the Rancho Los Amigos (RLA) cognitive scale (Hagen, Malkmus, & Durham, 1979). Although the RLA is less commonly used in clinical settings to date, it is important to highlight this scale here given its use in much of the research literature in relation to predictive and prognostic factors for dysphagia (e.g., Mackay, Morgan, & Bernstein, 1999a, 1999b; Winstein, 1983), discussed later in this chapter. The RLA consists of eight levels ranging from level 1: No Response (e.g., unresponsive to any stimulus), to level 8: Purposeful-Appropriate (alert, oriented, defects in stress tolerance, judgment, abstract reasoning persist; Table 2-4). Ratings are conducted following observations of the patients' performance during interactions with the assessing clinicians and supplemented by input from other professionals involved with the patient.

MEDICAL MANAGEMENT

A number of guidelines for medical management of TBI are available, as developed by various brain injury consortia (see Brain Trauma Foundation, 2000; Maas et al., 2007; Vos et al., 2002). Despite the existence of many different guidelines, there is a degree of consensus regarding the primary objectives of acute care, specifically: maintaining stable and adequate cerebral perfusion (including neurosurgical intervention to ensure this), ensuring adequate patient ventilation, and avoiding development of any secondary injury effects.

Neurosurgery

In instances where brain edema and raised ICP cannot be treated effectively with medical management, neurosurgery may be required. Craniectomy, or *decompressive craniectomy*, is a common surgical procedure used to help relieve ICP and improve cerebral perfusion pressure and cerebral blood flow. The procedure involves removal of part the skull, thereby providing the brain tissues with room to expand and subsequently lowering pressure within the skull.

Following intracranial hemorrhage, blood can enter the cerebral ventricles and prevent drainage of the cerebrospinal fluid (CSF), resulting in a buildup of CSF. When the ventricles in the brain become enlarged with fluid, a ventriculoperitoneal (VP) shunt may be used to manage the increased ICP. The VP procedure involves insertion of a catheter into a ventricle (usually in the anterior horn of the lateral ventricle, close to the foramen of Monro) in order to drain CSF from the ventricular system into the peritoneal space in the abdominal cavity.

Intubation and Ventilation

The majority of patients who experience TBI will require a period of ventilatory support via endotracheal intubation.

Table 2–4. Rancho Los Amigos Scale	
Level	***Description of Behavior***
1: No response	Appears to be in a deep sleep and is unresponsive to stimuli.
2: Generalized Response	Reacts inconsistently and nonpurposefully to stimuli in a nonspecific manner. Responses are limited and often the same regardless of stimuli presented.
3: Localized Response	Responses are specific, (i.e. are directly related to the type of stimulus presented, such as turning head toward a sound or focusing on a presented object) but are inconsistent. May follow simple commands in an inconsistent or delayed manner.
4: Confused-Agitated	The individual is in a heightened state of activity and severely confused, disoriented, and unaware of present events. Behavior is frequently bizarre and inappropriate to immediate environment. Patient is unable to perform self-care. If not physically disabled, she may perform automatic motor activities such as sitting, reaching, and walking as part of the agitated state, but not necessarily as a purposeful act.
5: Confused-Inappropriate, Non-agitated	Appears alert and responds to simple commands. More complex commands, however, produce responses that are nonpurposeful and random. The individual may show some agitated behavior in response to external stimuli rather than internal confusion. She is highly distractible and generally has difficulty learning new information. Can manage self-care activities with assistance. Memory is impaired and verbalization is often inappropriate.
6: Confused-Appropriate	Shows goal-directed behavior but relies on cueing for direction. Can relearn old skills such as activities of daily living, but memory problems interfere with new learning. Has beginning of awareness of self and others.
7: Automatic-Appropriate	Goes through familiar daily activities automatically with appropriate behavior and minimal confusion, but is highly dependent on predictable/repetitive routine. Has shallow recall of activities and superficial awareness of, but lack of insight into, present condition. Requires supervision because judgment, problem-solving, and planning skills are impaired.
8: Purposeful-Appropriate	Is alert, orientated and able to recall and integrate past and recent events. Can learn new activities. Deficits in attention, stress tolerance, judgment, abstract reasoning, and social, emotional, and intellectual capacities may persist. Apparently mild residual deficits may have significant detrimental impact on participation in social and work activities and roles.

Note. From *Rehabilitation of the Head Injured Adult: Comprehensive Physical Management,* by C. Hagen, D. Malkmus, & P. Durham, 1979, Downey, CA: Professional Staff Association of the Rancho Los Amigos Hospital, Inc. Adapted with permission.

Specifically, patients who present with rapidly deteriorating levels of consciousness or coma (GCS <8), loss of protective reflexes, ventilatory insufficiency, hyperventilation, or respiratory arrhythmia will require immediate intubation and ventilation. This is critical to prevent additional injury due to hypoxia and hypotension.

In a recent study of 117 patients referred to speech-language pathology (SLP) for dysphagia management, all patients had received a period of mechanical ventilation, with the average duration received by the group being around 1 week (range 1–28 days; Ward et al., 2007). Duration of ventilation, however, was found to be dependent upon injury severity. Patients with severe injury (GCS <8) were ventilated for almost twice as long (approximately 9 days) as those with less severe GCS scores.

Patients with persistent coma or complicated medical conditions that necessitate long-term ventilation will require conversion from an endotracheal tube (ETT) to a tracheostomy. Ward et al. (2007) reported that the average duration of endotracheal intubation for their total group was around 5 days, with half the group requiring ongoing intubation via a tracheotomy. Optimal timing for conversion from ETT to tracheostomy, however, is still under consideration in the literature. A recent study reported that patients with severe TBI who had "early" tracheostomy (< or = 7 days, n = 27) experienced a statistically significantly shorter stay in the critical care unit than patients in the "late" group (>7 days, n = 28; Ahmed & Kuo, 2007). For patients who require a tracheostomy, intubation may continue for a number of weeks. Once converted from ETT to a tracheostomy tube, Ward et al. (2007) noted that the average duration of intubation via tracheostomy tube for their patients was approximately 2 weeks.

As for all populations, the need for ventilation and often protracted periods of intubation (both ETT and tracheostomy) may be an additional factor contributing to impaired swallow function post-TBI. Complications following translaryngeal intubation (i.e., ETT; such as reduced mobility or paralysis of the vocal folds, formation of ulceration, vocal nodules, granulomas, polyps, and/or posterior and subglottic stenosis) may affect glottic anatomy and function and precipitate swallowing dysfunction (Morgan & Mackay, 1999). In addition, for patients who require ongoing intubation, the presence of a tracheostomy tube may also have a negative impact on the movement of key structures during the swallow, such as laryngeal elevation. Similarly, the absence of airflow through the glottis and upper airways can further disrupt swallow function due to reduced/impaired efficacy and timing of vocal fold closure during the swallow; increased secretion production; and an inability to cough and clear secretions or penetrated/aspirated content. For further reading regarding the potential impact of ventilation and intubation on swallow function, the reader is directed to the work by Dikeman and Kazandjian (2003).

DYSPHAGIA POST-TRAUMATIC BRAIN INJURY

Dysphagia has long been recognized as a negative sequela of TBI, yet the exact nature of the swallowing features associated with the disorder has not been well defined. This is likely due in part to the wide variety of swallowing impairments resulting from the diverse neurological damage associated with the condition. Furthermore, even individuals with similar underlying brain pathology have been noted to present with markedly different behavioral swallowing deficits. As a result, it has been challenging to determine those factors predictive of the nature and presentation of dysphagia associated with TBI.

Prevalence and Predictive Factors

Early studies reporting on the frequency of dysphagia in the adult population with brain injury were inconsistent in their findings, with prevalence figures ranging from 26 to 82% (Cherney & Halper, 1989; Field & Weiss, 1989; Lazarus & Logemann, 1987; Winstein, 1983; Yorkston, Honsinger, Mitsuda, & Hammen, 1989; Table 2-5). Possible reasons for the dis-

Table 2–5. Dysphagia Incidence Figures Reported for the Adult Population with Traumatic Brain Injury

Dysphagia Incidence	*Subject Population*	*Setting*	*Author*
4.5%	9 of 199 consecutive TBI admissions	A	Field & Weiss (1989)
77.5%	31of 40 consecutive TBI admissions	A	Yorkston, Honsinger, Mitsuda, & Hammen (1989)
61%	33 of 54 severe TBI admissions	A	Mackay, Morgan, & Bernstein (1999b)
65%	96 of 148 consecutive TBI admissions (73% severe TBI)	AR	Halper, Cherney, Cichowski, & Zhang (1999)
27%	55 of 201 TBI admissions to a rehabilitation program only	R	Winstein (1983)
26%	49 of 189 consecutive TBI admissions	R	Cherney & Halper (1989)
30%	9 of 30 patients admitted to TBI program of original 199 consecutive admissions	R	Field & Weiss (1989)
41.6%	218 of 524 consecutive TBI admissions	R	Cherney & Halper (1989)
13%	8 of 62 consecutive TBI admissions	OR	Yorkston et al. (1989)
40%	406 of 1016 TBI rehabilitation admissions (n = 2447 missing data)	R	Brown, Malec, Diehl, N. N., Englander, J., & Cifu (2007)

Note: A = acute; R = rehabilitation; AR = acute rehabilitation; OR = outpatient rehabilitation.

crepancies in prevalence figures between studies may include different assessment methods or definitions of dysphagia used by different health professionals, and the different settings in which prevalence studies were performed (e.g., acute vs. rehabilitation). During the past 10 years, however, more consistent dysphagia prevalence figures have been reported in clinical samples with TBI, ranging from 40 to 65.1% (Brown, Malec, Diehl, Englander, & Cifu, 2007; Cherney & Halper, 1996; Halper, Cherney, Cichowski, & Zhang, 1999; Mackay et al., 1999b; Schurr et al., 1999). It has been suggested that the higher prevalence figures reported in more recent literature may reflect the trend for earlier admission of TBI patients to acute rehabilitation settings (Halper et al., 1999).

Research is continuing to define factors that may help: (a) predict the likelihood of dysphagia occurring in the acute phase post-TBI (predictive factors) and (b) determine longer term dysphagia outcomes (prognostic factors). Primary variables of interest in research exploring predictive or prognostic factors include: the extent of injury (duration of coma, GCS, CT findings), the presence of tracheostomy and duration of ventilation, physical damage to the swallowing structures, the presence of cognitive impairment, and the duration to first swallow assessment (Mackay et al., 1999; Morgan, Ward, Murdoch, Kennedy, et al., 2003; Ward et al., 2007). Research in each of these three areas is outlined below.

Extent of Injury

One could assume that the greater the extent of brain injury, the greater the impairment to the swallowing mechanism. For this reason researchers have explored a number of measures of the extent of brain injury in an attempt to elucidate the relationship between injury severity and dysphagia outcome, including the duration of coma, GCS score, and the extent of neurological damage (as determined via radiological measures).

- Duration of coma. An association has been documented between a prolonged duration of coma and a greater severity of dysphagia (Lazarus & Logemann, 1987). Lazarus and Logemann (1987) documented swallowing impairment and coma duration in 53 adult patients with TBI. Patients who had been in a coma for longer than 24 hours exhibited more severe swallowing problems than patients whose coma lasted less than 24 hours. The authors were cautious to point out, however, that this was not a direct association, and that some patients with no coma history, or only short durations of coma, were also found to present with severe swallowing problems. Furthermore, some patients who were not comatose also presented with dysphagia, and others who were comatose for an extended duration demonstrated only mild swallowing difficulties (Lazarus & Logemann, 1987).
- Glasgow Coma Scale (GCS). A lower GCS score on admission is indicative of greater neurological impairment. Lower GCS scores, in particular those denoting severe injury (≤8), have been found to place patients at greater risk for swallowing impairment and aspiration (Mackay et al., 1999b; Morgan, Ward, Murdoch, Kennedy, et al., 2003). Mackay et al. (1999b) reported that adult patients with TBI and a GCS score from 3 to 5 on admission have significantly

longer durations until the initiation of oral feeding, longer durations until achieving total oral intake, and almost three times the duration between initial oral trials and achieving total oral feeding. In addition, these patients have almost twice as many swallowing abnormalities identified via a videofluoroscopic swallowing examination (VFSE) than patients with GCS scores of 6 to 8 (Mackay et al., 1999a). Morgan, Ward, Murdoch, Kennedy, et al. (2003) found similar results for the pediatric population with a GCS of ≤8 being the strongest variable for predicting the presence of dysphagia in children post-TBI.

- CT and MRI findings. CT or MRI data can also indicate the extent or severity of brain injury. Patients with CT scans indicating more severe TBI (e.g., midline shift, brainstem injury, or intracranial bleeds requiring emergent operative intervention) have been reported to have more than twice as many swallowing abnormalities (as determined on instrumental assessment) than patients with CT scans indicating less severe TBI (Mackay et al., 1999a). In terms of prognosis, adult patients with CT scans indicative of more severe TBI also presented with significantly longer durations before achieving oral feeding, and had longer intervals from initiation to total oral feeding than patients with less severe TBI (Mackay et al., 1999a). Ward et al. (2007) also reported preliminary evidence to suggest that a prolonged time until the first swallowing assessment and a CT finding indicative of severe TBI were predictive of a longer duration before returning to a normal oral diet.

Intubation and Ventilation

Increased duration of ventilation, endotracheal intubation, and the presence of a tracheostomy may also be associated with greater severity of dysphagia. Duration of ventilation in patients with TBI is reported to be related to the number of abnormal swallowing characteristics (rated on VFSE) and the prevalence of aspiration (Mackay et al., 1999a). Specifically, Mackay et al. (1999a) reported that a ventilation duration of 15 days was associated with statistically higher percentages (90%) of abnormal swallowing in adults with TBI, compared to the 8 to 14 day ventilated group (75%) and the 7 day ventilated group (42.9%). A ventilation duration of more than 15 days also was found to be associated with statistically higher prevalence rates of aspiration (60%), compared to the group ventilated for 8 to 14 days (56%), and the group ventilated for 7 days (25%) (Mackay et al., 1999a). In contrast, however, in children a key risk factor for dysphagia occurring post-TBI has been reported to be a ventilation duration exceeding just 1.5 days (Morgan, Ward, Murdoch, Kennedy, et al., 2003), being markedly less than the duration of ventilation that places adults in a higher risk category for dysphagia onset.

Cognitive Impairment

Studies have also examined the association between cognitive impairment and resolution of dysphagia. Mackay et al. (1999b) found that three key factors were more commonly associated with aspiration: increased injury severity (i.e., GCS scores of 3 to 5), CT scan results indicating midline shift, brainstem pathology, or operative procedures, and a lower RLA; Hagen, 1981) level (RLA II versus

RLA III to IV). These factors were also associated with twice as many swallowing deficits in TBI patients. Evaluation of the various admitting factors documented for each patient (e.g., CT data, GCS, and RLA) revealed that the RLA level was the most important independent predictor of the duration to normal oral diet. A similar pattern of resolution of cognition in parallel with the return to oral intake has also been reported for the pediatric population post-TBI (for further reading on the resolution of dysphagia in children post-TBI, see Morgan, Ward, & Murdoch, 2004).

Duration to Initial Swallow Assessment

Recent research has suggested that global measures, such as the duration to the initial swallowing assessment, may serve as useful predictors for determining when a patient will commence oral intake and resume a normal oral diet. Ward et al. (2007) examined the predictive power of parameters available at the time of the initial swallowing assessment (including injury severity, ventilation, and presence of a tracheostomy), and found that the duration to the first swallowing assessment (DFSA) was the most significant variable predictive of the duration to achieving an oral diet (without supplementation). Although a high level of variance was observed in the group data, an overall pattern was revealed. Specifically, patients' assessed within the first 4 days of admission had a rapid return to oral intake (without supplementation). If a patient was medically and cognitively unable to be assessed until 1 week post-TBI, however, the number of days until the patient could manage sufficient oral intake (and not require supplementation) doubled. Both DFSA and CT were found to be predictive of a return to full oral diet by patient discharge.

As no prior studies had explored the DFSA as a parameter in their prediction models, these findings require further verification. It is not unexpected, however, that such a parameter would be sensitive for predicting return to oral intake and recovery, considering that the timing of initial swallow assessment is influenced by all of the other individual parameters discussed previously (extent of injury, duration of ventilation, and cognitive level). Indeed, Mackay et al. (1999b) noted that as more information becomes available from acute care management, the ability to predict oral intake improves. In their studies, ventilation duration, the CT scan results, and whether or not aspiration was noted on a VFSE were all factors independently associated with prognosis or longer term dysphagia outcome, that is, the number of days to achieving oral feeding and the duration of the delay between initial swallowing trials and total oral intake.

Assessment of Dysphagia Following Traumatic Brain Injury

The prevalence of swallowing disorders following severe TBI is relatively high, with the presenting dysphagia typically characterized by a combination of oral and pharyngeal stage deficits. TBI may manifest in a wide array of physical and cognitive-behavioral deficits, typically as a result of the diffuse nature of the brain damage sustained during trauma. It is therefore anticipated that dysphagia will present differently between patients. Consequently, the need for thorough and sensitive individual evaluation of swallow function incorporating both clinical and instrumental assessment procedures is crucial in the TBI population.

It is also important to highlight that dysphagia assessment is an ongoing process for patients with TBI. Multiple reassessments are required over the course of the acute care and rehabilitative period. Even for patients requiring long-term rehabilitation, best practice management would involve regular repeat assessment to continually reevaluate current physiological status and rehabilitation outcomes. The need for multiple reassessment of patient status is highlighted in the single case study reports of dysphagia management post-TBI in the literature, with the majority of cases undergoing at least two and sometimes three or four instrumental studies of swallowing behavior during the rehabilitation period (Drake, O'Donoghue, Bartram, Lindsay, & Greenwood, 1997; Hoppers & Holm, 1999; Rowe, 1999; Tippett, Palmer, & Linden, 1987; Yuen & Hartwick, 1992).

Clinical Swallowing Examination

Although a clinical swallowing examination (CSE) is known to provide limited data on the functioning of the pharyngeal phase of the swallow, it does provide clinicians with a wealth of information. Clinical assessment assists the clinician to gain a quick indication of the nature and severity of dysphagia, to gauge the patient's cognitive-behavioral status, to establish a baseline of orofacial functioning, to noninvasively explore feeding options such as diet choice or compensatory feeding strategies, and to help determine the optimal positioning for feeding. Early diet or postural adjustments determined from the CSE can help reduce aspiration risk in the population with traumatic brain injury (Logemann, Pepe, & Mackay, 1994). It is also an important assessment tool for monitoring progress. In addition to the key components of a standard CSE (see Chapter 1), the following section discusses specific issues for consideration when conducting a CSE for a patient following TBI.

Positioning and Control for Self-Feeding. Dysphagia may occur through inadequate airway protection, oral and pharyngeal dysfunction, or difficulties with self-feeding, all of which may occur with improper positioning and body alignment (Avery-Smith & Dellarosa, 1994). Following brain injury, abnormal muscle tone, reflexes, and sensory deficits may result in postural problems that may affect the ability to assume and maintain a seated upright position. It is important to determine the presence and extent of any postural or positioning issues and the potential impact these may have on oral intake. Close liaison with physiotherapy and occupational therapy services can help maximize posture and control for feeding.

Cognitive-Behavioral Considerations. A greater emphasis is now placed on the importance of cognition in the return to oral intake. A number of investigations have highlighted that severe cognitive and communication disorders co-occur with severe oral intake problems in the TBI population (Cherney & Halper, 1989; Mackay et al., 1999a,b; Morgan et al., 2004; Ward et al., 2007; Winstein, 1983). Consequently, it can be beneficial for the clinician to monitor cognitive-behavioral characteristics as part of the CSE.

Winstein (1983) was the first to investigate the impact of cognition on swallowing impairment in an adult population with TBI using the Rancho Los Amigos Hospital cognitive scale (Hagen et al., 1979; see Table 2-4). Impaired cognition was the most frequently identified problem interfering with swallowing. Findings from this study suggested that although oral feeding may be indicated earlier, progression to a functional eating level is usually not seen until the patient reaches at least level V (confused and inappropriate). As discussed previously, Mackay et al. (1999a,b) also found an association between level of cognitive function and oral intake. Regardless of the presence of a swallowing disorder, they noted that patients were functioning at least at RLA level IV (confused and agitated) when commencing oral feeding, and RLA level VI (confused but displaying more appropriate behavior) when managing a full oral intake.

A range of cognitive-behavioral features that should be considered during the CSE are outlined in Table 2-6. Reduced patient awareness of dysphagia is of special concern, as these patients are less likely to comply with suggested treatment or management strategies. For example, patients with reduced awareness in other populations (i.e., post-stroke) have been found to have poorer outcomes at 3 months post-injury compared to those with appropriate dysphagia awareness (Parker et al., 2004). Further, patients with good awareness of the clinical indicators of dysphagia are reported to comply with taking smaller volumes of drink and drinking more slowly than those with poor awareness (Parker et al., 2004). Patient awareness in the study by Parker et al. (2004) was defined via a list of simple questions including: Did you have difficulty keeping drink in your mouth? Did you cough when you were drinking? Did it take a long time to drink?

Boczko (2006) recently examined the association between patient awareness of dysphagia and clinician-identified dysphagia using a screening tool of nine closed yes/no questions including: difficulty keeping liquids in the mouth; coughing after drinking; shortness of breath while drinking; voice change after drinking; coughing after eating; shortness of breath after eating; food getting stuck in the mouth/throat when eating; voice change after eating; and difficulty with saliva. This screening tool was reported to be a consistent and reliable generalized indicator of the potential for dysphagia (Boczko, 2006). There was good agreement between patient and clinician identification of a swallowing problem. The type of problem identified, however, and its intensity and manifestation were not always consistent between patient and clinician.

Oral-Structural Deficits. As discussed in Chapter 1, a thorough assessment of the oromotor, pharyngeal, and laryngeal structures is an important component of the CSE. Although this aspect of assessment provides information regarding the potential underlying neurological injury (e.g., facial palsy suggesting cranial nerve VII injury), it also involves determining the extent of physical/structural damage. Due to the often traumatic nature of TBI (e.g., high-speed MVA), there is a high probability of comorbid structural deficits including damage to the oral, pharyngeal, laryngeal, and esophageal structures. Examples may include: soft tissue damage such as tearing of the buccal tissue, torn labial tissue, or palatal punctures that can impact on the oral stage of the swallow; fractures of the jaw affecting jaw opening and movement; laryngeal trauma (from either injury or intubation),

Table 2–6. Characteristics of Oropharyngeal Dysphagia Following Traumatic Brain Injury

Phase	***Deficit***
Oral	Altered muscle tone and oral reflexes affecting mouth opening and movement
	Reduced lip closure leading to drooling and loss of saliva control
	Pooling of food in the lateral sulcus due to unilateral buccal weakness
	Reduced lingual control
	Reduced velopharyngeal closure resulting in nasal regurgitation
	Prolonged oral transit
Pharyngeal	Absence/delay in trigger of swallow reflex
	Reduced pharyngeal peristalsis
	Pharyngeal residue/pooling in valleculae and pyriform sinus (possibly due to reduced movement of the base of tongue or reduced laryngeal elevation)
	Premature entry of bolus into hypopharynx
	Laryngeal dysfunction (reduced closure, elevation, spasm)
	Silent aspiration
	Aspiration with reflexive cough
	Cricopharyngeal disorder

Note: Compiled from "Dysphagia with Head Injury," by L. H. Field and C. J. Weiss, 1989, *Brain Injury, 3*(1), pp. 19–26; "The Role of Fiberoptic Endoscopy in Dysphagia Rehabilitation," by P. Hoppers and S. E. Holm, 1999, *Journal of Head Trauma Rehabilitation, 14*(5), pp. 475–485; "Swallowing Disorders in Closed Head Trauma Patients," by C. Lazarus and J. A. Logemann, 1987, *Archives of Physical Medicine and Rehabilitation, 68*(2), pp. 79–84 ; "Disorders of Nutrition and Swallowing: Intervention Strategies in the Trauma Center," by J. A. Logemann, J. Pepe, and L. E. Mackay, 1994, *Journal of Head Trauma Rehabilitation, 9*(1), pp. 43–56; "Swallowing Disorders in Severe Brain Injury: Risk Factors Affecting Return to Oral Intake," by L. E. Mackay, A. S. Morgan, and B. A. Bernstein, 1999, *Archives of Physical Medicine and Rehabilitation, 80*, pp. 365–371; "Acute Characteristics of Pediatric Dysphagia Subsequent to Traumatic Brain Injury: Videofluoroscopic Assessment," by A. T. Morgan, E. C. Ward, B. E. Murdoch, and K. Bilbie, 2002, *Journal of Head Trauma Rehabilitation, 17*(3), pp. 220–241; Morgan et al. (2003); "Clinical Progression and Outcome of Pediatric Dysphagia Following Traumatic Brain Injury," by A. T. Morgan, E. C. Ward, and B. E. Murdoch, 2004, *Brain Injury, 18*(4), pp. 359–376; "Resolution of Paediatric Dysphagia Following Traumatic Brain Injury: Radiological Assessment," by A. T. Morgan, E. C. Ward, and B. E. Murdoch, 2005, *Medical Journal of Speech-Language Pathology, 13*(2), pp. 109–125; "Prospective Evaluation of Oro-Pharyngeal Dysphagia after Severe Traumatic Brain Injury," by R. Terre and F. Mearin, 2007, *Brain Injury, 21*(13–14), 1411–1417; "Evolución de la Aspiración Laringo-Traqueal en la Disfagia Orofaríngea Secundaria a Lesión Cerebral Traumática: Cuantificación Videofluoroscópica," by R. Terre and F. Mearin, 2007, *Revista Espanola de Enfermedades Digestivas, 88*(1), pp. 7–12; "Patterns and Predictors of Swallowing Resolution Following Adult Traumatic Brain Injury," by E. C. Ward, K. Green, and A. L. Morton, 2007, *Journal of Head Trauma Rehabilitation, 22*(3), pp. 184–191.

which may lead to reduced laryngeal elevation or closure; scar tissue formation on the tissues of the pharynx leading to possible pooling or reduced pharyngeal wall movement; and wounds to the chest, which may cause esophageal perforation or fistula formation. Particularly in the initial stages of acute hospital management, the coexistence of such physical damage can significantly affect swallowing function and impede, or even delay, the initial stages of swallowing rehabilitation. The reader is referred to Chapter 5 for more detailed discussion of physical and structural trauma.

Oral Trials. Oral trials to determine aspiration risk proceed largely as outlined in Chapter 1. However, considering the potential for cognitive-behavioral factors to influence oral intake safely, it is especially important to assess swallow safety under both (a) clinician/carer controlled intake and (b) patient self-feeding conditions. Impulsivity can lead to inappropriate amounts of food and fluid being placed in the oral cavity, and a lack of dysphagia awareness may lead to unsafe food choices and intake of unsafe consistencies (e.g., food acquired from other patients, the cafeteria, or other visitors). When the person with TBI cannot adequately self-monitor or learn techniques for enhancing swallow safety, the benefits of compensatory techniques such as consistency, temperature, taste modification, as well as postural adjustments should be explored. External factors such as the impact of noise or other distractions on swallowing safety should be considered. For some individuals, oral intake may be optimized when they are in a quiet room with minimal distractions, rather than in a general multiple-bed ward. Joint assessment with occupational therapy can help the SLP to explore ways for enhancing safe independent feeding so that swallowing safety can be maintained.

Instrumental Assessment

Objective measurement of the oral, pharyngeal, and esophageal phases for swallowing requires utilization of instrumental diagnostic imaging techniques. Instrumental methods are of particular importance for the evaluation of the pharyngeal phase of swallowing, and for determining the presence of aspiration. As the risk for aspiration is high following TBI, and may have no observable clinical indications (i.e., silent aspiration), instrumental or objective assessment to support the clinical assessment findings is warranted.

Of the instrumental techniques available to assess swallow function, the endoscopic swallowing examination (ESE) is most useful during the early acute state of admission. Leder (1999) reported the use of ESE with a group of 47 TBI patients in an acute care setting. The author reported that ESE provided objective information upon which feeding recommendations could be based, and concluded that ESE was a valuable technique for assessing dysphagia and aspiration status in acute TBI patients. Advantages of the ESE procedure highlighted by Leder (1999) included: the ability to use the tool at the bedside, the use of real foods (i.e., not barium impregnated), and the noninvasive repeatability of the procedure (no radiation exposure). Hoppers and Holm (1999) also noted that twice as many ESE studies were conducted compared with VFSE procedures in their clinical rehabilitation center. The authors reported that ESE is "an effective tool to evaluate all of the common physiologic dysphagia symptoms in the population with brain injury" (p. 481).

Although ESE may be considered "uniquely suited for assessing patients with acute TBI" (Leder, 1999, p. 449), as discussed further in Chapter 1, this procedure does not allow visualization of tongue control or oral phase deficits (Bastian, 1998; Hoppers & Holm, 1999;

Willging & Thompson, 1995). This ESE limitation is of relevance to the TBI population who commonly present with oral physiological deficits that contribute to their dysphagia (Field & Weiss, 1989; Lazarus & Logemann, 1987; Morgan, Ward, & Murdoch, 2003, Morgan et al., 2004; Ward, 2007). Consequently, once the patient is mobile and able to be transported to the radiology suite, additional assessment using a VFSE (see procedure in Chapter 1) is warranted to enable a full and comprehensive analysis of swallowing physiology.

Characteristics of Dysphagia Post-TBI

Patients may present with a range of feeding and swallowing issues after TBI. Neurological damage resulting from the primary and secondary effects of TBI can cause both motor and sensory deficits that impact on swallow physiology. Adding to this, the presence of postural and tonal deficits and cognitive-behavioral dysfunction can further limit swallowing safety and the resumption of independent oral intake. The anticipated presenting characteristics of dysphagia, its natural history, and prognosis will be described in detail below.

Oropharyngeal Deficits

Details of specific oral and pharyngeal stage deficits that have been reported for the TBI population have been summarized in Table 2-7. One of the most commonly reported deficits across studies is a delay or absence of a swallow trigger (Field & Weiss, 1989 Lazarus & Logemann, 1987). The high prevalence of disorders involving the swallowing reflex may reflect the importance of cortical as well as brainstem input into triggering a swallow reflex. Although the brainstem controls the swallowing center, voluntary tongue initiation of the swallow also plays a role in triggering the reflexive swallow.

Aspiration rates in the adult TBI population are consistently high, with figures of up to 71% reported in some studies (Schurr et al., 1999). The reported physiological cause of the aspiration, however, has varied between studies. Lazarus and Logemann (1987) found an aspiration rate of 38% in their group of 53 dysphagic patients, and reported that the majority of aspiration events occurred before the swallow (13 patients) due to either an absent or delayed swallowing reflex, or a combination of reduced lingual control with a delayed reflex. Two of the 53 patients were found to aspirate during the swallow, as a result of reduced laryngeal closure. Aspiration after the swallow was observed in four cases, reportedly due to reduced pharyngeal peristalsis in three cases, and due to cricopharyngeal dysfunction in the remaining case (Lazarus & Logemann, 1987). A slightly higher aspiration rate of 41% (22 of 54) was documented by Mackay et al. (1999b). In contrast to Lazarus and Logemann's (1987) findings, Mackay et al. (1999b) noted that the majority of the aspiration occurred during the swallow (77%), before the swallow (41%), and in a few cases after the swallow (18%).

"Silent" aspiration is a significant issue in the TBI population, with a number of authors identifying evidence of frank aspiration on VFSE investigations with no coughing or distress observed (Horner & Massey, 1991; Lazarus & Logemann, 1987). Leder (1999) examined the swallowing function of TBI patients in an acute care setting using fiberoptic endoscopic evaluation of swallowing (FEES). Within the group of 47 patients studied, 17 (36%)

Table 2–7. Cognitive-Behavioral Features for Consideration during CBE

Cognitive-Behavioral Feature	***Criterion Indicating Presence of Deficit***
Alertness	Reduced level of alertness/lethargic: patient requires verbal/tactile stimulation to remain alert, or may fall asleep
Cooperation	Agitated/uncooperative: patient verbally/physically refuses to complete task/accept food, patient is agitated
Attention	Distractible: patient requires constant verbal or tactile prompts to remain on task
Interaction	Patient is pragmatically incorrect: e.g., poor eye contact, talking incessantly while ignoring task at hand
Dysphagia awareness	Lack of awareness: patient seems unaware/will not admit to difficulty with eating/swallowing affecting ability to self-regulate feedings

Note: Adapted from "Clinical Progression and Outcome of Pediatric Dysphagia Following Traumatic Brain Injury," by A. T. Morgan, E. C. Ward, and B. E. Murdoch, 2004, *Brain Injury, 18*(4), pp. 359–376; and "Frequency, Progression and Outcome in Adults Following Head Injury," by C. J. Winstein, 1989, *Physical Therapy, 63*, pp. 1922–1997.

were found to be aspirating, with 9 patients (53%) reported to silently aspirate.

Following TBI, patients may also display disorders of oral or pharyngeal sensation, that is, hyper- or hyposensitive responses to touch. Disordered sensory function has been reported to occur as frequently as in 73% of TBI cases (Winstein, 1983). Both pediatric and adult patients with brain injury presenting with hyposensitivity display characteristics such as loss of food from the mouth, pooling of food in the buccal cavities, loss of food particles in the mouth, and premature entry of the bolus into the pharynx (e.g., Morgan, Ward, & Murdoch, 2003). For case study discussion of the impact of these deficits, the reader is referred to Gilmore et al. (2003).

Absent or limited sensation is thought to be responsible for a poor motor response to bolus presentation, or leftover bolus in the mouth, although inattention to motor deficits may also be implicated (Lazarus & Logemann, 1987; Veis & Logemann, 1985). Neglect of food in the mouth can create potential for aspiration. Different foods possess a wide array of sensory qualities with respect to temperature, texture, and taste. These sensory qualities in combination may stimulate oral movements and result in triggering of the swallowing reflex. Changing the volume and viscosity of boluses, which can be achieved through the use of different foods, has been shown to change oral movement responses (Dantas et al., 1990). In the presence of reduced oral sensitivity, the swallow reflex may often be absent or delayed. Alternatively, hypersensitivity may be associated with abnormal reflexive responses to oral stimulation including tonic or clonic bite reflex, hyperactive gag reflex, rooting reflex, or tongue thrusting.

Reduced pharyngeal sensation can also cause severely impaired swallowing

(Morgan & Mackay, 1999). Pharyngeal peristalsis may be weak or uncoordinated and this may result in pharyngeal residue and possible aspiration after swallowing. The patient may have reduced airway protection due to an absent or delayed cough reflex. Lazarus and Logemann (1987) reported decreased pharyngeal sensation and an absent reflexive cough during or after aspiration of material into the airway. Patients with this array of deficits will need to be instructed to cough to optimize airway protection.

Impact of Cognitive Impairment and Behavioral Dysregulation

Cognitive and behavioral impairments may compound the physical causes of dysphagia. Potential cognitive-behavioral deficits may include: poor memory, limited insight, reduced alertness and attention, poor organization and sequencing skills, impulsivity, poor judgement and reasoning, and communication deficits (Cherney & Halper, 1989; Morgan et al., 2004; Ward et al., 2007). Lazarus and Logemann (1987) expressed concern in regard to the potential additional risk of impulsivity for some patients with dysphagia post-TBI. Impulsivity may result in the rapid intake of large amounts of food without the existing physiological control to handle food at such a rapid rate of ingestion. Authors have stressed that cognitive deficits can interfere with the eating process to the extent that they may cause aspiration, even in the absence of a physiological cause for dysphagia (Cherney & Halper, 1989).

Natural History and Prognosis

Although dysphagia associated with TBI is highly heterogeneous, data from group studies can provide some useful indication of the natural history and prognosis of dysphagia post-injury. In a recent study of 117 patients referred to SLP for dysphagia management (of whom 78% were severe TBI), the first swallowing assessment occurred on average between 8 to 10 days post-admission to an acute care setting (Ward et al., 2007). At the time of initial assessment, one patient was fully ventilated, 11 were in the process of being weaned, and 105 of the patients had been weaned. Half of the group had a tracheostomy in situ. Initial assessment determined that 50% of patients were safe for some oral intake, and these patients were able to immediately commence supervised oral trials. Between 2 and 3 weeks following admission, the majority of the group were managing oral intake without need for additional supplementation (Ward et al., 2007). At an average of 22 days following admission, 47% had returned to a normal oral diet (i.e., able to manage a diet of food and fluids of similar consistency as eaten pre-injury). By discharge, only two patients failed to achieve any safe oral intake. For the other 115 patients, approximately half had returned to a full normal (food + fluid) diet, 82% were safely managing thin fluids, and the remainder safely achieved some modified oral intake by discharge.

Terre and Mearin (2007b) also reported positive long-term outcomes following TBI. They found that 45% of their 48 patients with dysphagia post-TBI referred for neurorehabilitation were managing a normal oral diet at discharge (at an average of 6 months post-injury), 27% were on a modified oral diet, 14% were on combined oral intake and gastrostomy feeding, and 14% were fed exclusively by gastrostomy. Early research by Winstein (1983) reported an average time from non-oral intake at admission to successful oral intake to be approximately 3 months, with a range of between 5 and 21 weeks. Of the total group of 55 dysphagic patients studied, Winstein (1983) found that 94% of patients with dysphagia on admission achieved functional oral intake, the majority within 5 months post-injury.

Management of Dysphagia Post-TBI

The importance of early assessment and intervention for dysphagia cannot be underestimated in the neurological recovery of patients with severe TBI (Mackay et al., 1999b; Logemann et al., 1994). Detailed information regarding the nature and type of deficit contributing to swallowing dysfunction is essential for enhancing sensitive and accurate diagnosis of swallowing impairment, and for maximizing the efficacy of intervention strategies.

Non-Oral Supplementation

Maintaining adequate nutrition is critical for achieving optimal recovery from TBI. The rehabilitation team must determine which patients are at risk for aspiration, reduce the impact or burden of the dysphagia, and ensure that the patients' hydration and nutritional needs are being met (Groher, 1992). The duration of supplemental nutrition is often prolonged in the TBI population. An average period of approximately 2 to 3 weeks of non-oral supplemental feeding has been reported for individuals *without dysphagia* post-TBI (Mackay et al., 1999a; Ward et al., 2007). In comparison, patients *with dysphagia* have been reported to be on supplementary feeding for periods of between 2 and 4 weeks (Ward et al., 2007), and for as long as up to 8 weeks (Mackay et al., 1999a).

Patients who have acquired TBI require vigilant monitoring of their nutritional support due to increased metabolic needs (Pepe, Morgan, & Mackay, 1997), gastric difficulties complicating nutritional intake, and swallowing impairments affecting oral intake. A study of nutritional status of 53 closed head injury patients, 56% of whom had dysphagia, found that from the time of injury until admission to a rehabilitation facility, patients lost an average of 29 pounds (Brooke & Barbour, 1989). In addition, 31% of the group was identified to have protein malnutrition. The difficulty of obtaining early nutritional stability post-TBI is acknowledged, however, considering the number of potential coexisting problems that may limit the attainment of this goal, including hypermetabolism, aspiration, gastric dysfunction, cognitive-behavioral problems, and swallowing disorders (Logemann et al., 1994). When determining the optimal method of nutritional support, early evaluation of swallowing ability and aspiration risk is of paramount importance. A multidisciplinary approach must also be applied, involving the physician, dietitian, respiratory therapist, and SLP (Logemann, 1994; Logemann et al., 1994). The degree of swallowing impairment in particular will help to guide the medical team in their determination of how nutritional support can safely be provided, and whether or not non-oral nutritional support or supplementary feeds are required in the short or long term

Although oral feeding is the optimal method of enteral nutrition, both non-oral enteral (via the gastrointestinal system) and parenteral (via the bloodstream) feeding can provide adequate nutrition for critically injured patients (detailed further in Chapter 1). Following TBI, however, the majority of patients receive nutritional supplementation via enteral feeding, typically via nasogastric feeding. For patients who present with concomitant base of skull or midfacial fractures, enteral feeding is provided via orogastric tube (see Chapter 5). Patients with protracted swallowing dysfunction will be managed via percutaneous gastrostomy (PEG).

Swallow Rehabilitation

It is recognized that there is a lack of efficacy data regarding the rehabilitation of the patient with dysphagia (Logemann, 2007). This holds true for patients with TBI where limited efficacy data exist for specific therapeutic strategies and treatment programs. Consequently, there is an absence of an established, formalized, or standardized rehabilitation program for dysphagia post-TBI.

Given the diverse nature of TBI, however, no one specific rehabilitation program will likely account for an individual patient's complete needs. Therefore, based on detailed clinical and instrumental assessment, the clinician must determine the potential benefit of postural modifications, dietary modification, swallowing maneuvers, sensory stimulation techniques, rehabilitation exercises, or combination of these approaches (for more detail see Chapter 1). A recent examination of neurorehabilitation programs experienced by 48 patients with clinically suspected oropharyngeal dysphagia revealed that multiple techniques and approaches may be utilized to optimize outcome. The range of techniques applied in the study included: dietetic changes (increase in bolus viscosity, 63%); postural maneuvers (cervical flexion, 31%), motor control exercises (to improve orolingual mobility, 29%), and active maneuvers (supraglottal swallowing and the Mendelsohn maneuver, 21%; Terre & Mearin, 2007b).

Rehabilitation programs implementing a range of techniques and strategies have been found to improve swallowing outcomes for individual patients post-TBI. Schurr et al. (1999) detailed the therapeutic modifications introduced with a subgroup of patients with TBI previously identified as aspirating via a VFSE. Authors reported the use of various compensatory strategies including diet modification, postural adjustment, and head flexion in order to prevent aspiration in each of the cases. Each patient was also reported to undergo active treatment for dysphagia; however, the exact details of the therapeutic interventions were not stated. The authors reported that dysphagia intervention (involving a combination of dietary, postural, and behavioral modifications) had facilitated 20 of 24 patients (83%) in the group to return to oral dietary intake.

Early research by Winstein (1983) commented on the use of three different types of rehabilitation programs for patients with dysphagia following head injury, dependent upon the status of swallowing function on admission to therapy. The programs included:

1. A nonfeeding program: designed as a stimulation program for very low level patients, in preparation for later feeding. This program was described as encompassing desensitization techniques such as stroking and applying pressure or stretching to facilitate normal swallowing, sucking, and interoral responses.
2. A facilitation and feeding program: used to facilitate normal feeding pat-

terns using a small amount of puree consistency.

3. A progressive feeding program: where specialized techniques (not detailed by the author) were used to help the patient build swallowing endurance by systematically increasing the amount of oral intake.

This progressive feeding program was continued until the patient could manage a whole meal within half an hour without any difficulties (Winstein, 1983). This article highlighted the issue that dysphagia intervention programs for the TBI patient can be undertaken at all stages of the rehabilitation process regardless of the functional swallowing status of the patient. Although it is recognized that there is no benefit in introducing oral feedings when this may place the patient at risk, many authors (Winstein, 1983; Ylvisaker & Logemann, 1985) strongly support the aggressive early introduction of indirect treatment strategies designed to improve neuromotor function for swallowing.

In addition to considering the specific nature of the dysphagia treatment program, conducting dysphagia rehabilitation as part of a coordinated holistic multidisciplinary program is critical. Research has revealed that patients managed in facilities with formalized TBI programs have significantly improved outcomes compared to patients managed in nonformalized programs, specifically, reduced coma duration (formalized programs = 18.9 days, nonformalized programs = 53.8 days), shorter rehabilitation stays (formalized = 106.5, nonformalized = 239.5 days), and higher cognitive levels on discharge (Mackay, Bernstein, Chapman, Morgan, & Milazzo, 1992). It has also been found that an increased proportion of patients managed under a formalized TBI service are discharged to home rather than to extended care facilities (Mackay et al., 1992). Such evidence reflects the value of dedicated rehabilitation services for patients post-TBI, in which intervention programs include early and aggressive trauma rehabilitation, family education and involvement in patient care, and coordination between medical and rehabilitation professionals.

Managing Cognitive-Behavioral Deficits

In addition to the physiological basis of the swallowing impairment, cognitive deficits that affect safe swallowing need to be addressed in the TBI population. It is recognized that coexisting cognitive and communicative deficits may, in some cases, influence the type of management program and its functional outcomes more than the extent of physiological impairment in the swallowing mechanism (Cherney & Halper, 1989; Halper et al., 1999; Mackay et al., 1999a). The existence of cognitive deficits may limit the application of various techniques in the process of rehabilitation. Training a patient to employ compensatory strategies and incorporate them into mealtime routines requires a level of cognitive function in areas such as attention, concentration, and memory, all of which are frequently compromised after TBI (Tippett et al., 1987). In addition, the ability for new learning may also be reduced following brain injury, further complicating the introduction and training of rehabilitation techniques (Ylvisaker & Logemann, 1985). Ylvisaker and Logemann (1985) highlighted the need to consider the environment, the patient's behavior and judgment, and the ability for new learning when managing the patient with cognitive impairments.

A range of subskills that influence swallowing ability in the TBI population has been reported, including alertness and orientation; cognitive behavior and behavioral dysregulation; positioning and proximal control; self-feeding; oral and pharyngeal sensory disorders; and the physiological impairments (oral and pharyngeal movement disorders) (Avery-Smith & Dellarosa, 1994). Based on the literature containing methods purported to improve deficits in these areas, Avery-Smith and Dellarosa (1994) specified a number of techniques that may have application for the brain-injured patient. At present, though, there is little evidence for the effect of these techniques on swallowing outcome in the TBI population. Case studies discussing cognitive-behavioral aspects of dysphagia rehabilitation post-TBI that have been described in the literature will be described in further detail below:

- Halper et al. (1999) discussed two case studies of TBI patients in which details on the process of swallowing rehabilitation were noted. The first case presented with severe dysphagia and moderately severe cognitive-communicative deficits. The rehabilitative process for this patient involved an oral feeding program with compensatory strategies (modified consistencies, quiet environment, encouraging the patient to take multiple swallows) and simultaneous therapy targeting improving memory, attention, and reasoning. Concomitant improvement in chewing and swallowing were noted in parallel with improvements in cognitive state. The second case presented with a similar pattern of severe dysphagia and moderately severe cognitive-communicative function, as reported in case one. Some improvement was noted in swallowing function for the second case; however, this patient had more persistent moderately severe cognitive deficits. Due to his continued cognitive impairments, the patient required individual supervision for all oral intake to ensure safe swallowing. The authors concluded that the patient's potential for functional feeding was limited by his cognitive impairments.
- Tippett et al. (1987) reported on dysphagia management of a single patient with TBI with cognitive and language impairments that further complicated dysphagia management. Specifically, the patient presented with deficient attention skills, impaired short-term memory, impulsivity, faulty verbal reasoning, and poor abstract thinking, all of which were contraindications for safe oral feeding. A combination of techniques was used to address the cognitive issues impacting upon dysphagia including reduced bolus size, the use of multiple swallows and throat clearing, and verbal cues to reinforce behaviors such as encouraging a reduced rate of oral intake. Furthermore, a structured environment was introduced by maintaining staff consistency, reducing distractions in the room and on the food tray, enforcing patient supervision while feeding to encourage monitoring and feedback of behaviors, the use of clear explanations, and family education and involvement to facilitate their understanding and reinforce

adherence to dietary recommendations. The patient was also supported in keeping a diary where appropriate dietary consistencies were documented. The diary could be reviewed by the patient to assist safe food choices in environments outside of the hospital room, such as the hospital cafeteria. This process was introduced to help the generalization of dietary modifications to other external situations (Tippett et al., 1987).

Caregiver/Family Involvement

With the introduction of any form of swallowing intervention program, the importance of involving family members along with the patient in the process of goal setting and daily therapy cannot be overemphasized. Where cognitive and behavioral issues compound the difficulties of ensuring safe oral intake, educating family members about the nature of the patient's swallowing difficulties and teaching strategies to counteract these difficulties during mealtimes can facilitate the rehabilitative process. Where possible, education of the family/carer can be enhanced with clear explanations using instrumental swallow assessment footage (VFSE/ESE recordings; Ylvisaker & Logemann, 1985).

ASSOCIATED SPEECH AND LANGUAGE COMORBIDITY

Patients with TBI may experience widespread injuries including associated spinal cord injury (see Chapter 3), burns (see Chapter 4), or physical/structural damage to the swallowing mechanism (i.e., maxillofacial, tracheal, or pharyngeal damage; see Chapter 5). Given the close proximity or shared neural and physiological substrates and the shared use of many of the same oropharyngeal structures for the production of speech and swallowing, it is not surprising that dysphagia is commonly associated with comorbidly presenting communication disorder. In particular, patients with TBI may present with comorbid language and motor speech deficits.

Language Disorders

The linguistic deficits arising from TBI during the acute period may be debilitating, especially for individuals with moderate or severe TBI. For many weeks post-injury, patients may be able to understand and/or express only a few words and limited phrases. Although there is good prognosis for the recovery of functional communication abilities, patients with TBI will often experience long-term difficulties with cognitive-communicative impairments, including those arising due to difficulties with attention, memory, and reasoning. To this end, it is difficult to dissociate specific communication deficits from cognitive impairment in individuals with linguistic deficits post-TBI. For further reading in this area, the reader is referred to: (for adults) Coelho (2007); Cummings (2007); Leblanc, De Guise, Feyz, & Lamoureux (2006); (for pediatric) Ewing-Cobbs and Barnes (2002).

Motor Speech Disorders

Dysarthria is the most commonly occurring motor speech disorder to arise post-TBI, with apraxia of speech and stuttering occurring much less frequently. Apraxia of speech is more frequently associated with focal lesions to Broca's area or the inferior frontal gyrus (e.g., Hillis et al., 2004), as seen most commonly following stroke. Dysarthria, however, may arise subsequent to direct or indirect damage to a variety of neurological areas (such as cerebellum, cortex, brainstem, basal ganglia). Given the often widespread nature of neurological damage associated with DAI post-TBI, it is not surprising that dysarthria is the most commonly presenting motor speech disorder seen in this population. The dysarthria may resolve relatively quickly within a matter of weeks or months during the acute phase post-TBI. In a number of cases, however, dysarthria may persist for years, especially when associated with moderate or severe injury. Typically, dysarthria will manifest as a mixed speech disorder (e.g., mixed spastic-flaccid or spastic-ataxic dysarthria) when associated with TBI, again likely due to the widespread neurological damage associated with DAI. For further reading see: (for adults) Kuruvilla, Murdoch, and Goozèe (2007); Sellars, Hughes, and Langhorne (2005); Wang, Kent, Duffy, and Thomas (2005); (for pediatric) Cahill, Murdoch, and Theodoros (2005); Morgan, Liegeois, and Occomore (2007).

CONCLUSION

Traumatic brain injury typically results in diffuse neurological injury, resulting from a wide range of possible external factors, each associated with different mechanisms of damage. As a result, patients with TBI experience multiple deficits across a range of physical and cognitive domains. Careful consideration must be applied to the patient's nutritional status, existing physiological deficits, cognitive-behavioral impairments, and quality of life. These features must be carefully monitored, with sensitive application of assessments applied at multiple time points in order to reassess current level of functioning and guide each stage of the rehabilitative process to produce the optimal outcomes for each individual.

REFERENCES

Ahmed, N., & Kuo, Y. H. (2007). Early versus late tracheostomy in patients with severe traumatic head injury. *Surgical Infection*, *8*(3), 343–347.

Annegers, J. F., Rocca, W. A., Hauser, W. A., & Coan, S. P. (1998). Prognostic value of computerized tomography scan characteristics in traumatic brain injury: Results from the IMPACT Study. *New England Journal of Medicine*, *338*(1), 20–24.

Avery-Smith, W., & Dellarosa, D. M. (1994). Approaches to treating dysphagia in patients with brain injury. *The American Journal of Occupational Therapy*, *48*(3), 235–239.

Bastian, R. W. (1998). Contemporary diagnosis of the dysphagia patient. *Otolaryngologic Clinics of North America*, *31*(3), 489–506.

Boczko, F. (2006). Patients' awareness of symptoms of dysphagia. *Journal of the American Medical Directors Association*, *7*(9), 587–590.

Brain Trauma Foundation. (2000). *Management and prognosis of severe traumatic brain injury*. New York: Author.

Brooke, M. M., Barbour, P. G., Cording, L. G., Tolan, C., Bhoomkar, S., McCall, G. W., et al. (1989). Nutritional status during rehabilitation after head injury. *Neurorehabilitatino and Neural Repair*, *3*(1), 27–33.

Brown, A. W., Malec, J. F., Diehl, N. N., Englander, J., & Cifu, D. X. (2007). Impairment at rehabilitation admission and 1 year after moderate-to-severe traumatic brain injury: A prospective multi-centre analysis. *Brain Injury, 21*(7), 673-680.

Cahill, L. M., Murdoch, B. E., & Theodoros, D. G. (2005). Articulatory function following traumatic brain injury in childhood: A perceptual and instrumental analysis. *Brain Injury, 19*(1), 41-58.

Cherney, L. R., & Halper, A. S. (1989). Recovery of oral nutrition after head injury in adults. *Journal of Head Trauma Rehabilitation, 4*, 42-50.

Cherney, L. R., & Halper, A. S. (1996). Swallowing problems in adults with traumatic brain injury. *Seminars in Neurology, 16*(4), 349-353.

Clement, C. M., Stiell, I. G., Schull, M. J., Rowe, B. H., Brison, R., Lee, J. S., et al. CCC Study Group. (2006). Clinical features of head injury patients presenting with a Glasgow Coma Scale score of 15 and who require neurosurgical intervention. *Annals of Emergency Medicine, 48*(3), 245-251.

Coelho, C. A. (2007). Management of discourse deficits following traumatic brain injury: Progress, caveats, and needs. *Seminars in Speech & Language, 28*(2), 122-135.

Cummings, L. (2007). Pragmatics and adult language disorders: Past achievements and future directions. *Seminars in Speech & Language, 28*(2), 96-110.

Da Dalt, L., Marchi, A. G., Laudizi, L., Crichiutti, G., Messi, G., Pavanello, L., et al. (2006). Predictors of intracranial injuries in children after blunt head trauma. *European Journal of Pediatrics, 165*(3), 142-148.

Dantas, R. O., Kern, M. K., Massey, B. T., Dodds, W. J., Kahrilas, P. J., Brasseur, J. G., et al. (1990). Effect of swallowed bolus variables on oral and pharyngeal phases of swallowing. *American Journal of Physiology, 258*, G675-G681.

Dikeman, K. J., & Kazandjian, M. S. (2003). *Communication and swallowing management of tracheostomized and ventilator dependent adults* (2nd ed.). Clifton Park, New York: Thompson Delmar Learning.

Drake, W., O'Donoghue, S., Bartram, C., Lindsay, J., & Greenwood, R. (1997). Eating in side-lying facilities rehabilitation in neurogenic dysphagia. *Brain Injury, 11*(2), 137-142.

Ewing-Cobbs, L., & Barnes, M. (2002). Linguistic outcomes following traumatic brain injury in children. *Seminars in Pediatric Neurology, 9*(3), 209-217.

Fabbri, A., Servadei, F., Marchesini, G., Stein, S. C., & Vandelli, A. (2008). Early predictors of unfavourable outcome in subjects with moderate head injury in the emergency department. *Journal of Neurology, Neurosurgery & Psychiatry, 79*(5), 567-573.

Field, L. H., & Weiss, C. J. (1989). Dysphagia with head injury. *Brain Injury, 3*(1), 19-26.

Finfer, S. R., & Cohen, J. (2001). Severe traumatic brain injury. *Resuscitation, 48*(1), 77-90.

Formisano, R., Barba, C., Buzzi, M. G., Newcomb-Fernandez, J., Menniti-Ippolito, F., & Zafonte, R. (2007). The impact of prophylactic treatment on post-traumatic epilepsy after severe traumatic brain injury. *Brain Injury, 21*(5), 499-504.

Fortuny, L. A., Briggs, M., Newcombe, F., Ratcliff, G., & Thomas, C. (1980). Measuring the duration of post traumatic amnesia. *Journal of Neurology, Neurosurgery & Psychiatry, 43*, 377-379.

Gilmore, R., Aram, J., Powell, J., & Greenwood, R. (2003). Treatment of oro-facial hypersensitivity following brain injury. *Brain Injury, 17*(4), 347-354.

Groher, M.E. (1992). *Dysphagia: Diagnosis & Management* (2nd ed.). Boston: Butterworth-Heinemann.

Guthrie, E., Mast, J., Richards, P., McQuaid, M., & Pavlakis, S. (1999). Traumatic brain injury in children and adolescents. *Child and Adolescent Psychiatric Clinics of North America, 8*(4), 807-826.

Hagen, C. (1981). Language disorders secondary to closed head injury: Diagnosis and management. *Topics in Language Disorders, 1*, 73-87.

Hagen, C., Malkmus, D., & Durham, P. (1979). *Rehabilitation of the head injured adult: Comprehensive physical management.* Downey, CA: Professional Staff Association of the Rancho Los Amigos Hospital, Inc.

Halper, A. S., Cherney, L. R., Cichowski, K., & Zhang, M. (1999). Dysphagia after head trauma: The effect of cognitive-communicative impairments on functional outcomes. *Journal of Head Trauma Rehabilitation, 14*(5), 486-496.

Havill, J. H., Sleigh, J. W., Davis, G. M., Chatterton, B. J., Gilbert, K. W., Marsh, N. V., et al. (2001). Observer error and prediction of outcome—Grading of head injury based on computerized tomography. *Critical Care Resuscitation, 3*, 15-18.

Hessen, E., Nestvold, K., & Sundet, K. (2006). Neuropsychological function in a group of patients 25 years after sustaining minor head injuries as children and adolescents. *Scandinavian Journal of Psychology*, 47(4), 245-251

Hillis, A. E., Work, M., Barker, P. B., Jacobs, M. A., Breese, E. L., & Maurer, K. (2004). Re-examining the brain regions crucial for orchestrating speech articulation. *Brain, 127*(7), 1479-1487.

Hoppers, P., & Holm, S. E. (1999). The role of fiberoptic endoscopy in dysphagia rehabilitation. *Journal of Head Trauma Rehabilitation, 14*(5), 475-485.

Horner, J., & Massey, E. W. (1991). Managing dysphagia: Special problems in patients with neurologic disease. *Postgraduate Medicine, 89*(5), 203-213.

Jennett, B. (1996). Epidemiology of head injury. *Journal of Neurology, Neurosurgery & Psychiatry, 60*, 362-369.

Koskinen, S., & Alaranta, H. (2008). Traumatic brain injury in Finland 1991-2005: A nationwide register study of hospitalized and fatal TBI. *Brain Injury, 22*(3), 205-214.

Kraus, J. F., Rock, A., & Hemyari, P. (1990). Brain injuries among infants, children, adolescents, and young adults. *American Journal of Disability in Childhood, 144*(6), 684-691.

Kraus, M., Susmaras, T., Caughlin, B. P., Walker, C. J., Sweeney, J. A., & Little, D. M. (2007). White matter integrity and cognition in chronic traumatic brain injury: A diffusion tensor imaging study. *Brain, 130*, 2508-2519.

Kuruvilla, M., Murdoch B., & Goozèe, J. (2007). Electromagnetic articulography assessment of articulatory function in adults with dysarthria following traumatic brain injury. *Brain Injury, 21*(6), 601-613.

Lazarus, C., & Logemann, J. A. (1987). Swallowing disorders in closed head trauma patients. *Archives of Physical Medicine and Rehabilitation, 68*(2), 79-84.

LeBihan, D., Mangin, J., Poupon, C., Clark, C., Pappata, S., Molko, N., et al. (2001). Diffusion tensor imaging: Concepts and applications. *Journal of Magnetic Resonance Imaging, Neuroradiology, 13*, 534-546.

Leblanc, J., De Guise, E., Feyz, M., & Lamoureux, J. (2006). Early prediction of language impairment following traumatic brain injury. *Brain Injury, 20*(13-14), 1391-1401.

Leder, S. B. (1999). Fiberoptic endoscopic evaluation of swallowing in patients with acute traumatic brain injury. *Journal of Head Trauma Rehabilitation, 14*(5), 448-453.

Lee, L. K. (2007). Controversies in the sequelae of pediatric mild traumatic brain injury. *Pediatric Emergency Care, 23*(8), 580-583.

Letarte, P. B. (1999). Neurotrauma care in the new millennium. *Surgical Clinics of North America, 79*(6), 1449-1470.

Logemann, J. A. (1994). Non-imaging techniques for the study of swallowing. *Acta Oto-Rhino-Laryngologica Belgica, 48*(2), 139-142.

Logemann, J. A. (2007). Oropharyngeal dysphagia and nutritional management. *Current Opinion in Clinical Nutrition and Metabolic Care, 10*(5), 611-614.

Logemann, J. A., Pepe, J., & Mackay, L. E. (1994). Disorders of nutrition and swallowing: Intervention strategies in the trauma center. *Journal of Head Trauma Rehabilitation, 9*(1), 43-56.

Maas, A. I. R., Hukkelhoven, C. W. P. M., Marshall, L. F., & Steyerberg, E. W. (2005). Prediction of outcome in traumatic brain injury with computed tomographic characteristics: A comparison between the computed tomographic classification and combinations of computed tomographic predictors. *Neurosurgery*, *57*, 1173–1182.

Maas, A. I., Steyerberg, E. W., Butcher, I., Dammers, R., Lu, J., Marmarou, A., et al. (2007). Prognostic value of computerized tomography scan characteristics in traumatic brain injury: Results from the IMPACT Study. *Journal of Neurotrauma*, *24*(2), 303–314.

Mackay, L. E., Bernstein, B. A., Chapman, P. E., Morgan, A. S., & Milazzo, L. S. (1992). Early intervention in severe head injury: Long-term benefits of a formalized program. *Archives of Physical Medicine and Rehabilitation*, *73*(7), 635–641.

Mackay, L. E., Morgan, A. S., & Bernstein, B. A. (1999). Factors affecting oral feeding with severe TBI. *Journal of Head Trauma Rehabilitation*, *14*(5), 435–447.

Mackay, L. E., Morgan, A. S., & Bernstein, B. A. (1999). Swallowing disorders in severe brain injury: Risk factors affecting return to oral intake. *Archives of Physical Medicine and Rehabilitation*, *80*, 365–371.

Malec, J. F., Flaada, J. T., Perkins, P. K., Leibson, C. L., Mandrekar, J. N., Brown, A. W., et al. (2007). The Mayo Classification System for traumatic brain injury severity. *Journal of Neurotrauma*, *24*(9), 1417–1424.

Mannion, R. J., Cross, J., Bradley, P., Coles, J. P., Chatfield, D., Carpenter, A., et al. (2007). Mechanism-based MRI classification of traumatic brainstem injury and its relationship to outcome. *Journal of Neurotrauma*, *24*(1), 128–135.

Marshall, L. F., Marshall, S. B., Klauber, M. R., & Clark, M. V. (1992, November). A new classification of head injury based on computerised tomography. *Journal of Neurosurgery*, *75*, 5S, S14–S20.

Maxwell, W. L., Bullock, R., Landhold, H., & Fujisawa, H. (1994). Massive astrocytic swelling in response to extracellular glutamate —A possible mechanism for post-traumatic brain swelling? *Acta Neurochirurgica Supplementum* (Wien), *60*, 465–467.

Marosszeky, N.E.V., Ryan, L., Shores, E.A., Batchelor, J. & Marosszeky, J.E. (1997). *The PTA Protocol: Guidelines for using the Westmead Post-Traumatic Amnesia (PTA) Scale.* Sydney, Australia: Wild & Wooley. http://www.psy.mq.edu.au/pta/page2.html

Moppett, L. K. (2007). Traumatic brain injury: Assessment, resuscitation and early management. *British Journal of Anaesthesia*, *99*(1), 18–31.

Morais, D. F., Spotti, A. R., Tognola, W. A., Gaia, F. F., & Andrade, A. F. (2008). Clinical application of magnetic resonance in acute traumatic brain injury. *Arquivos de Neuropsiquiatria*, *66*(1), 53–58.

Morgan, A. S., & Mackay, L.E. (1999). Causes and complications associated with swallowing disorders in traumatic brain injury. *Journal of Head Trauma Rehabilitation*, *14*(5), 454–461.

Morgan, A. T., Liegeois, F., & Occomore, L. (2007). Electropalatography treatment for articulation impairment in children with dysarthria post-traumatic brain injury. *Brain Injury*, *21*(11), 1183–1193.

Morgan, A. T., Ward, E. C., & Murdoch, B. E. (2003). Acute clinical characteristics of paediatric dysphagia following traumatic brain injury. *Journal of Head Trauma Rehabilitation*, *19*(3), 226–240.

Morgan, A. T., Ward, E. C., & Murdoch, B. E. (2004). Clinical progression and outcome of pediatric dysphagia following traumatic brain injury. *Brain Injury*, *18*(4), 359–376.

Morgan, A. T., Ward, E. C., & Murdoch, B. E. (2005). Resolution of paediatric dysphagia following traumatic brain injury: Radiological assessment. *Medical Journal of Speech-Language Pathology*, *13*(2), 109–125.

Morgan, A. T., Ward, E. C., Murdoch, B. E., & Bilbie, K. (2002). Acute characteristics of pediatric dysphagia subsequent to traumatic brain injury: Videofluoroscopic assessment. *Journal of Head Trauma Rehabilitation, 17*(3), 220-241.

Morgan, A. T., Ward, E., Murdoch, B., Kennedy, B., & Murison, R. (2003). Incidence, characteristics and predictive factors for dysphagia following paediatric traumatic brain injury. *Journal of Head Trauma Rehabilitation, 18*(3), 239-251.

Morris, S., Ridley, S., Lecky, F. E., Munro, V., & Christensen, M. C. (2008). Determinants of hospital costs associated with traumatic brain injury in England and Wales. *Anaesthesia, 63*(5), 499-508.

Murdoch, B. E. (1990). *Acquired speech and language disorders: A neuroanatomical and functional neurological approach*. London: Chapman & Hall.

Myburgh, J. A., Cooper, D. J., Finfer, S. R., Venkatesh, B., Jones, D., Higgins, A., et al. (2008). Australasian Traumatic Brain Injury Study (ATBIS): Investigators for the Australian and New Zealand Intensive Care Society Clinical Trials Group. Epidemiology and 12-month outcomes from traumatic brain injury in Australia and New Zealand. *Journal of Trauma, 64*(4), 854-862.

Parker, C., Power, M., Hamdy, S., Bowen, A., Tyrrell, P., & Thompson, D. G. (2004). Awareness of dysphagia by patients following stroke predicts swallowing performance. *Dysphagia, 19*(1), 28-35.

Pepe, J., Morgan, A. S., & Mackay, L. E. (1997). The metabolic response to acute traumatic brain injury and associated complications. In L. E. Mackay, P. E. Chapman, & A. S. Morgan (Eds.), *Maximising brain injury recovery:Iintegrating critical care and early rehabilitation* (pp. 396-443). Gaithersburg, MD: Aspen.

Reilly, P. L. (2001). Brain injury: The pathophysiology of the first hours. Talk and die revisited. *Journal of Clinical Neuroscience, 8*, 398-403.

Rowe, L. A. (1999). Case studies in dysphagia after pediatric brain injury. *Journal of Head Trauma Rehabilitation, 14*(5), 497-504.

Russell, W. R. (1932). Cerebral involvement in head injury. *Brain, 55*, 549-603.

Russell, W. R., & Smith, A. (1961). Post-traumatic amnesia in closed head injury. *Archives of Neurology, 5*, 4-17.

Salmond, C. H., Menon, D. K., Chatfield, D. A., Williams, G. B., Pena, A., Sahakian, B. J., et al. (2006). Diffusion tensor imaging in chronic head injury survivors: Correlations with learning and memory indices. *Neuroimage, 29*(1), 117-124.

Schurr, M. J., Ebner, K. A., Maser, A. L., Sperling, K. B., Helgeson, R. B., & Harms, B. (1999). Formal swallowing evaluation and therapy after traumatic brain injury improves dysphagia outcomes. *The Journal of Trauma: Injury, Infection and Critical Care, 46*(5), 817-821.

Scott-Jupp, R., Marlow, N., Seddon, N., & Rosenbloom, L. (1992). Rehabilitation and outcome after severe head injury. *Archives of Disability in Childhood, 67*(2), 222-226.

Sellars, C., Hughes, T., & Langhorne, P. (2005). Speech and language therapy for dysarthria due to non-progressive brain damage (a review). *Cochrane Database Systematic Reviews 20*(3). DOI: 10.1002/14651858.CD002088.pub2.

Stocchetti, N., Colombo, A., Ortolano, F., Videtta, W., Marchesi, R., Longhi, L., et al. (2007). Time course of intracranial hypertension after traumatic brain injury. *Journal of Neurotrauma, 24*(8), 1339-1346.

Tate, R. L., Pfaff, A., Baguley, I. J., Marosszeky, J. E., Gurka, J. A., Hodgkinson, A. E., et al. (2006). A multicentre, randomised trial examining the effect of test procedures measuring emergence from post-traumatic amnesia. *Journal of Neurology, Neurosurgery & Psychiatry, 77*, 841-849.

Teasdale, G. M., & Graham, D. I. (1998). Craniocerebral trauma: Protection and retrieval of the neuronal population after injury. *Neurosurgery, 43*(4), 723-737.

Temkin, N. R., Dikmen, S. S., Wilensky, A. J., Keihm, J., Chabal, S., & Winn, H. R. (1990). A randomized, double-blind study of phenytoin for the prevention of post-traumatic seizures. *New England Journal of Medicine, 323*(8), 497-502.

Tennant, A. (2005). Admission to hospital following head injury in England: Incidence and socio-economic associations. *BMC Public Health, 5*, 21.

Terre, R., & Mearin, F. (2007). Evolución de la aspiración laringo-traqueal en la disfagia orofaríngea secundaria a lesión cerebral traumática: Cuantificación videofluoroscópica. *Revista Espanola de Enfermedades Digestivas, 88*(1), 7-12.

Terre, R., & Mearin, F. (2007). Prospective evaluation of oro-pharyngeal dysphagia after severe traumatic brain injury. *Brain Injury, 21*(13-14), 1411-1417.

Thurman, D. J., Alverson, C., Dunn, K. A., Guerrero, J., & Sniezek, J. E. (1999). Traumatic brain injury in the United States: A public health perspective. *Journal of Head Trauma Rehabilitation, 14*(6), 602-615.

Tippett, D. C., Palmer, J., & Linden, P. (1987). Management of dysphagia in a patient with closed head injury. *Dysphagia, 1*, 221-226.

Veis, S. L., & Logemann, J. A. (1985). Swallowing disorders in persons with cerebrovascular accident. *Archives of Physical Medicine and Rehabilitation, 66*(6), 372-375.

von Wild, K. R., & Wenzlaff, P. (2005). Quality management in traumatic brain injury (TBI): Lessons from the prospective study in 6.800 patients after acute TBI in respect of neurorehabilitation. *Acta Neurochirurgica Supplementum, 93*, 15-25.

Vos, P. E., Battistin, L., Birbamer, G., Gerstenbrand, F., Potapov, A., Prevec, T., et al. (2002). European Federation of Neurological Societies. EFNS guideline on mild traumatic brain injury: Report of an EFNS task force. *European Journal of Neurology, 9*(3), 207-219.

Wang, Y. T., Kent, R. D., Duffy, J. R., & Thomas, J. E. (2005). Dysarthria associated with traumatic brain injury: Speaking rate and emphatic stress. *Journal of Communication Disorder, 38*(3), 231-260.

Ward, E. C., Green, K., & Morton, A. L. (2007). Patterns and predictors of swallowing resolution following adult traumatic brain injury. *Journal of Head Trauma Rehabilitation, 22*(3), 184-191.

Weir, N., Doig, E., Fleming, J. M., Wiemers, A., & Zemljic, C. (2006). Objective and behavioral assessment of the emergence from post-traumatic amnesia. *Brain Injury, 20*(9), 927-935.

Willging, J. P., & Thompson, D. M. (2005). Pediatric FEESST: Fiberoptic endoscopic evaluation of swallowing with sensory testing. *Current Gastroenterology Report, 7*(3), 240-243.

Winstein, C. J. (1983). Neurogenic dysphagia: Frequency, progression, and outcome in adults following head injury. *Physical Therapy, 63*(12), 1992-1997.

Yates, P. J., Williams, W. H., Harris, A., Round, A., & Jenkins, R. (2006). An epidemiological study of head injuries in a UK population attending an emergency department. *Journal of Neurology, Neurosurgery & Psychiatry, 77*, 699-701.

Ylvisaker, M., & Logemann, J. A. (1985). Therapy for feeding and swallowing disorders following head injury. In M. Ylvisaker (Ed.), *Head injury rehabilitation: Children and adolescents* (pp. 195-215). Boston: College Hill Press.

Yorkston, K. M., Honsinger, M. J., Mitsuda, P. M., & Hammen, V. (1989). The relationship between speech and swallowing disorders in head-injured patients, *Journal of Head Trauma Rehabilitation, 4*(4), 1-16.

Yuen, H. K., & Hartwick, J. A. (1992). Diet manipulation to resume regular food consumption for an adult with traumatic brain injury. *The American Journal of Occupational Therapy, 46*(10), 943-945.

3 Traumatic Spinal Cord Injury

MAURA M. SOLLEY AND ELIZABETH C. WARD

INTRODUCTION

Formal rehabilitation programs for adults with spinal cord injury (SCI) were not widely available until world events in the 1940s required a response to the large numbers of wounded veterans returning from military conflicts. Since that time there have been numerous advancements in SCI care, resulting in the current model of coordinated rehabilitation services for this group of patients (for a comprehensive summary of current thinking underpinning SCI service, the reader is referred to Scott, 2001). Within this current model of care, there is increased recognition of the impact and implications of dysphagia for patients with SCI.

However, although dysphagia management is now an integral part of the rehabilitation process post-SCI, limited research evidence continues to hamper the development of comprehensive, evidence-based clinical services for this population. Existing data suggest that early swallowing complications post-SCI largely resolve during the acute and subacute phases of care. Patients then typically return to a regular diet and thin fluids during the rehabilitation phase. It is recognized, however, that some patients present with mild (where modified textures with or without swallowing techniques enable safe oral intake) to severe dysphagia (where non-oral supplementation is needed) for a protracted period of time. These individuals require specialized dysphagia assessment and intensive long-term swallowing rehabilitation.

Determining the nature and extent of dysphagia services provided for this population necessitates an understanding of the wide impact of SCI. Specifically, important areas of knowledge include awareness of: the mechanisms of SCI; the impact of SCI on other body systems (e.g., impaired respiration); the impact of medical and surgical SCI management; the influence of cooccurring medical conditions; and the effect of injury on the psychological state of the individual. Provision of dysphagia services to this specialized trauma population includes close consultation between the speech-language pathologist (SLP) and the multidisciplinary team in order to ensure that interventions are safely applied to each patient. Equally important is the clinician's need to hold clinical competency in dysphagia practice, including at least minimum levels of competency, clinical privileges or credentialing required for tracheostomy management, a working knowledge of assisted ventilation, and familiarity with caring for the patient within the critical care setting. In recognition of the breadth of information and skills required to work with this population, the current chapter will provide the reader with a basic orientation to SCI and its management in addition to detailed information regarding dysphagia characteristics and population-specific dysphagia management issues. Further readings and resources are also referred to throughout the chapter to assist the clinician in preparation for their role in the management of dysphagia post-SCI.

THE SPINE AND SPINAL CORD

Optimal clinical management of the SCI population requires an understanding of the anatomy of the spinal cord and its functions. Readers are advised to participate in multidisciplinary education in the field of spinal cord injury, avail themselves of a detailed anatomy and physiology text, and seek further information from on-line services such as the American Spinal Injury Association (http://www.asia-spinalinjury.org) and http://www.spinalcord.org to support their clinical practice. The following information is provided to facilitate basic orientation to the vertebral column, the spinal cord, and the spinal nerves.

The spinal cord receives sensory information from the skin, muscles and joints of the upper and lower limbs and torso as well as the viscera. The motor neurons of the spinal cord regulate both voluntary and reflex movements. The processing of spinal reflexes may occur entirely within the spinal cord system. Higher brain function can mediate responses to some spinal reflexes as sensory information about local neural activity is relayed through ascending neural pathways. The spinal cord is protected by the vertebral column. The vertebral column serves many functions, including distribution of the weight of the head, neck, chest, and upper extremities down through the column to the large sacral vertebrae and pelvic cradle; provision of a stable place of attachment for muscles, ligaments, ribs, and visceral structures; flexibility of movement through the torso; protection to the spinal cord; and production of red blood cells. The vertebral column consists of 32 or 33 individual vertebrae (7 cervical, 12 thoracic, 5 lumbar, 5 sacral, and 3 [or 4] fused coccygeal vertebrae) bound to one another by interlocking bony processes, muscles, and ligaments, and separated by fibrocartilagenous disks (Figure 3-1 and Table 3-1). The design of the vertebral column allows limited movement between adjacent vertebrae while permitting extensive movement in the vertebral column as a whole. The muscles and ligaments of the spine support vertebral stability and flexibility. As such, the vertebral muscles can be broadly classified according to function: forward flexors, lateral flexors, rotators, and extensors.

Along the length of the vertebral column, the shape and size of the vertebrae vary, with the atlas (C1) being the smallest and the lumbar vertebrae being the largest. The column is divided into regions including the cervical, thoracic, lumbar, sacral, and coccygeal. Of these, the *cervical* region is of particular importance to the SLP because it provides the skeletal support to the oropharyngeal, laryngeal, and upper esophageal anatomy.

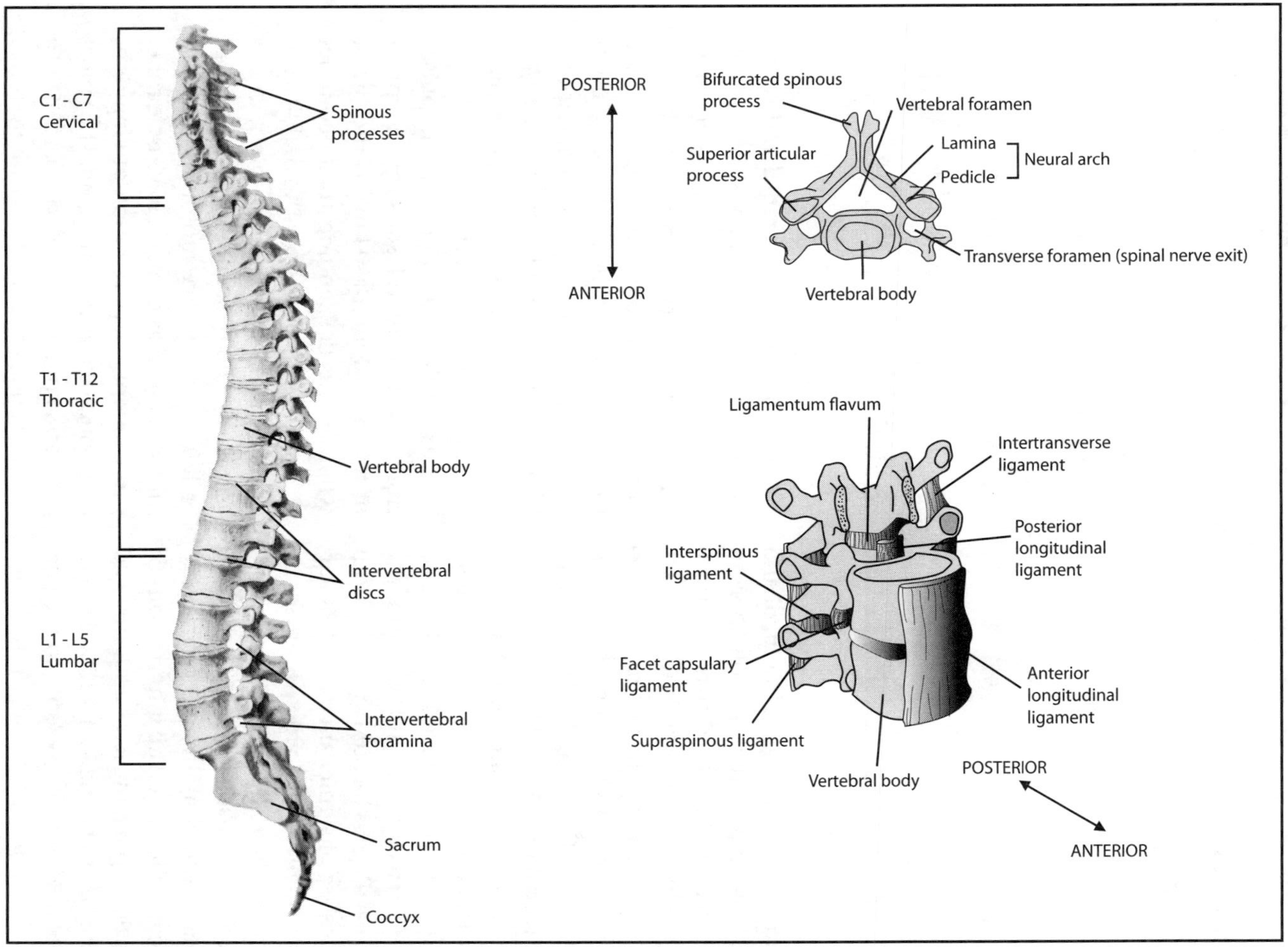

Figure 3–1. Anatomy of the human vertebral column with close-up detail of a cervical vertebra (*upper right-hand detail*) and the ligaments of the vertebral column (*lower right-hand detail*).

Table 3–1. Summary of the Anatomical Divisions of the Human Vertebral Column

Anatomical Division	*Number of Vertebrae*	*Body Region*	*Vertebrae Abbreviation*
Cervical	7	Neck	C1–C7
High cervical region	(2)	Upper neck/base of skull	C1–C2
Low cervical region	(5)	Mid-lower neck	C3–C7
Thoracic	12	Chest	T1–T12
Lumbar	5	Low back	L1–L5
Sacral	5 (fused)	Pelvis	S1–S5
Coccygeal	3 (or 4)	Tailbone	None

In addition, it is the atlanto-occipital and atlanto-axial joints that largely permit skull movement (up and down) and turning of the neck. The atlas and axis (C1 and C2) are referred to as the *high cervical region* and the remaining cervical vertebrae (C3–C7) form the *low cervical region* (see Table 3–1). There are other dysphagia-relevant anatomical landmarks that correspond with cervical vertebrae; for instance, the thyroid cartilage is located between C4 and C5 and the cricoid cartilage is located at C6-C7. Both cartilages are of significance for SLPs during both clinical and videofluoroscopy evaluations where these structures may be palpated and visually tracked to monitor laryngeal excursion in the pharyngeal phase of swallowing. The innervations of the cervical spinal muscles and the head movements that these facilitate have been detailed in Table 3–2 due to the particular relevance of these muscles for dysphagia interventions.

Contained within the vertebral column is the spinal cord. The brain, brainstem, and spinal cord constitute the *central nervous system*. The *peripheral nervous system* consists of the cranial and spinal nerves. The spinal cord consists of a core of grey matter surrounded by white matter where the grey matter largely contains nerve cell bodies and glial cells, and the white matter is made of bundles (tracts) of myelinated sensory and motor neuron fibers. These tracts of white matter conduct impulses towards (ascending) and away from (descending) the brain. The ascending tracts conduct impulses from the peripheral sensory receptors of the body (such as skin) to the brain, whereas the descending tracts conduct the motor impulses from the brain to the muscles and glands of the body. These ascending and descending tracts assist in reflex and voluntary motor and sensory functions such as changes in muscle tone, proprioception, perception of vibration, light touch, balance, and so on. The spinal cord and spinal nerves form parts of the somatic and autonomic nervous systems. The somatic nervous system governs voluntary actions including musculoskeletal functions and skin responses to external stimuli (like heat and cold). The autonomic nervous system aids in maintaining

Table 3–2. Cervical Spine Muscles, Their Actions, and Innervations

Action	*Innervation*	*Muscles*
Head extension	Suboccipital	Rectus capitus posterior minor
Head extension and rotation	Middle/lower cervical	Spinalis capitus and spinalis cervicus
	Suboccipital	Rectus capitus posterior major
Head extension and rotation and vertebral flexion	C2–C3	Sternocleidomastoid
Head extension and lateral head movement	Suboccipital	Obliquus capitus superior
Head rotation and backwards movement	Middle/lower cervical	Longissimus capitus
	C1–C5	Semispinalis capitus
Atlas rotation	Suboccipital	Obliquus capitus inferior
Lateral head movement	C2–C3	Rectus capitus lateralis
Head flexion	C1, C2, C3	Longus capitus and rectus capitus anterior
Neck flexion and rotation	Lower cervical	Scalenus
Cervical flexion	C2–C7	Longus colli cervicis
Cervical extension	Middle/lower cervical	Iliocostalis cervicis, splenius cervicis, and longissimus cervicis
Cervical rotation	Middle/lower cervical	Semispinalis cervicis

Note. Adapted from *Muscles of the Spine*, by K. Bridwell, (2007). *Spine Universe*. Retrieved July 27, 2008, from http://www.spineuniverse.com/displayarticle.php/article1272.html .

homeostasis (normal function) throughout the body through involuntary responses in glands and cardiac and other smooth muscles to regulate functions including blood pressure, sexual responses and sweating. The autonomic nervous system is further specialized into the sympathetic (e.g., "fight or flight" responses) and parasympathetic (conserving body resources, slowing digestion, regulating heartbeat) nervous systems.

The spinal cord begins at the terminus of the brainstem and extends from the foramen magnum of the occipital bone to end at the first lumbar vertebra, where it becomes the conus medullaris (Figure 3–2). Spinal nerves are clumped together at the conus medullaris; these are known as the cauda equina (because they bear resemblance to a horse's tail). At the cauda equina, the spinal nerves radiate out through the vertebral column inferiorly (Bridwell, 2008). The posterior of each vertebra accommodates the spinal cord within an arch that surrounds the space known as the vertebral foramen

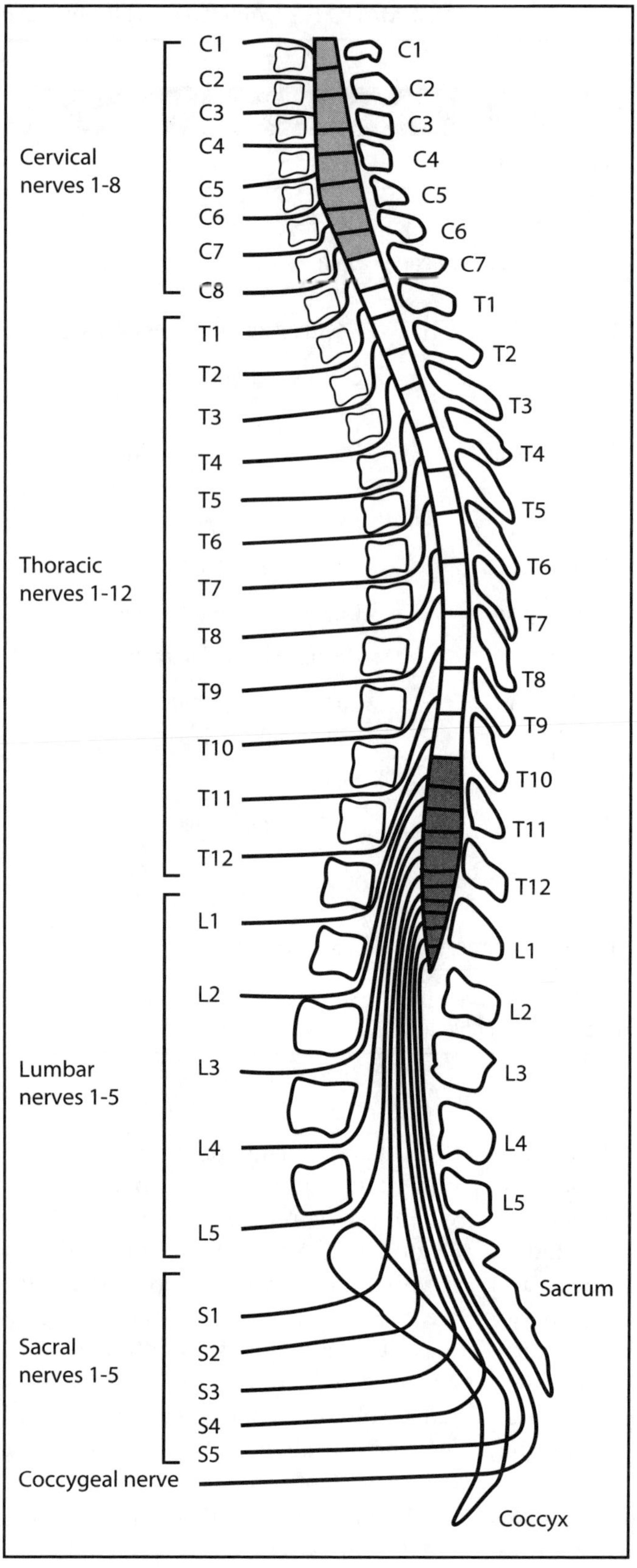

Figure 3–2. Schematic of spinal cord and spinal nerves within the vertebral canal (vertebral body and arch illustrated with the transverse processes omitted to demonstrate the position of the spinal cord and spinal nerves in relationship to each vertebra).

(see Figure 3-1). This bony canal provides a degree of protection from physical injury. In addition, the spinal cord is protected, and in part maintained, by cerebrospinal fluid and three layers of meninges, the outer layer of dura, then the arachnoid, and the innermost pia mater. The spinal cord is nourished by blood vessels, which travel through the intervertebral foramina (openings on each side of the vertebra).

In correspondence with the surrounding vertebral body, the length of the spinal cord is referred to in four anatomical regions: the cervical, thoracic, lumbar, and sacral regions. Thirty-one pairs of spinal nerves (8 cervical, 12 thoracic, 5 lumbar, 5 sacral, and 1 coccygeal pair) progressively enter and exit the vertebral canal via intervertebral foramina. Nerves are named in reference to the foramina through which they enter or exit the spinal cord. This is with the exception of the first cervical nerve, which emerges between the occipital bone and the atlas. The cervical spinal nerves, C2-C7, exit *above* the correspondingly numbered vertebrae, while C8 exits between C7 and T1. The remaining pairs of spinal nerves emerge *below* the vertebrae for which they are named (see Figure 3-2).

TRAUMATIC SPINAL CORD INJURY

To ensure consistent national and international reporting, Australia has adopted The United States Centers for Disease Control and Prevention definition of SCI. This defines SCI as the occurrence of an acute, traumatic lesion of neural elements in the spinal canal (spinal cord and cauda equina) that results in temporary or permanent sensory deficit, motor deficit, or bowel/bladder dysfunction (Thurman, Sniezek, Johnson, Greenspan, & Smith, 1995).

Mechanisms of Traumatic Spinal Cord Injury

Injury to the spinal cord may result from a combination of: direct tissue damage caused by the trauma; compression damage resulting from displaced bony fragments, pooled fluids, and swelling; or ischemic injury due to damage to or impingement of spinal arteries. Spinal cord transection, where the cord is completely severed, is rare. Rather, most SCIs result from violent motions of the head, neck, and trunk, causing neural, bone, vascular, and ligament damage. The spinal column has most mobility at C4 to C7 and T11 to L2. Mobility is associated with vulnerability to damage in the case of trauma, and these two spinal column regions are where most SCI occurs. Indeed, research has reported that 58% of SCI in Australia involved the cervical spine, with damage to C4, C5, and C6 found to be three of the top four injury locations (O'Connor, 2005). A number of mechanisms can force movements of the head, neck, and trunk in relation to each other causing vertebral column damage in isolation, or in combination with SCI. These mechanisms include hyperflexion (a decrease in the angle between vertebral joints as the chin moves towards the chest beyond the usual range of motion), hyperextension (straightening or extension beyond the normal range of the joint), axial loading (vertical compression), rotation, and penetrating injuries. A range of recognized presentations of vertebral damage is summarized in Table 3-3.

Table 3–3. Types of Vertebral Fractures

Mechanism of Injury	***Type of Fracture***	***Physiological Effect***
Complex	Odontoid fracture	Type 1 odontoid fracture is associated with life-threatening atlanto-occipital dislocation. The odontoid bone provides an axis for the rotation movement of the atlanto-occipital unit.
Vertical compression (axial loading)	Jefferson fracture	Burst fracture of all aspects of the C1 ring.
	Burst fracture of vertebral body	Vertebral body shatters outward. Associated with anterior cord syndrome.
Flexion	Wedge fracture	Anterior body of vertebra bears most of the force. Ligament swelling. Associated with osteoporosis and low falls.
	Flexion teardrop fracture	Anterior bony fragment displacement through a combination of flexion and compression forces. Associated with motor vehicle accidents.
	Atlantoaxial subluxation and dislocation	Rupture of atlantoaxial ligaments without bony injury (strong ligaments normally provide the stability to this joint). Associated with motor vehicle accidents. Facial and skull fractures often cooccur.
	Bilateral facet dislocation	Displacement of more than half of the diameter of the vertebral body following extreme spinal flexion.
Flexion-rotation	Unilateral facet dislocation	Some bony projection into the neural foramina.
	Hangman fracture	Occurs at C2. Most common cervical fracture. Associated with hangings and motor vehicle accidents.
Extension	Extension teardrop fracture	Usually low cervical level. Associated with central cord syndrome.

Note. Adapted from *Fracture, Cervical Spine*, by M. Davenport, 2008, *eMedicine*. Retrieved May 23, 2008, from http://www.emedicine.com/emerg/TOPIC189.HTM .

Spinal cord injury may arise from multiple mechanisms, which can include the "primary" injury, and the "secondary" injury caused from pathological processes. Primary injury occurs following compression of the bony vertebral canal, direct trauma from fragments of vertebral fractures or foreign bodies, and/or misalignment of one or more vertebrae or discs. Secondary processes of injury include hemorrhage, other vascular disruptions, edema, inflammation, demyelination, scarring, and necrosis. The presenting range of physiological responses is dependent upon the type of injury. These physiological changes begin at the time of injury and continue over many years, spanning the acute, secondary, and chronic injury phases. At each of these phases, there are cellular, vascular, neurological, and muscular responses to the injury that contribute to the medical state and functional ability of the patient. Outlined in Table 3–4 are some of the known physiological responses that may occur at each stage.

Classification of Traumatic Spinal Cord Injury

The nature of SCI may be considered in a number of ways. The first feature of the cord injury relates to whether the spinal cord surface is *breached*. Injuries caused by laceration (tearing and severing) or maceration (i.e., a softening of spinal cord due to exposure to fluids) create a breach to the surface of the spinal cord. In comparison, contusion (where the spinal cord is bruised and blood from the capillaries seeps into surrounding tissues) and solid cord injuries do not breach the cord surface (Hulsebosch, 2002).

The injury is then classified according to the *neurological level of injury*. The neurological level of injury refers to the lowest segment of the spinal cord that has retained motor and sensory function on both sides of the body. To provide a consistent way of reporting the severity level and types of SCI, the American Spinal Injury Association developed a simple impairment rating scale (Marino, 2002), (Figure 3–3). The ASIA scale identifies the sensory, motor, neurological, and vertebral levels at which spinal cord functioning remains intact. This five-step process (see "Steps in Classification" in Figure 3–3) begins with performing sensory testing to light touch and a pin prick at each of the dermatomes.

Table 3–4. Phases of Physiological Change in Response to Spinal Cord Injury

Time Post-Onset	*Phases of Evolving Spinal Cord Injury*
Acute: From the moment of injury to the first few days following SCI	During the acute phase the following processes begin: • Mechanical damage to neural and other soft tissue. • Electrolytic changes leading to *spinal shock*—a term that describes a transient neuronal disruption in distal spinal function. • Hemorrhage within the vertebral canal causing localized edema, thrombosis (blood clot), vasospasm (spasm and constriction of blood vessels), and loss of vascular auto regulation. The acute phase evolves differently depending on the way that the spinal cord was injured.

continues

Table 3–4. *continued*

Time Post-Onset	*Phases of Evolving Spinal Cord Injury*
Acute: From the moment of injury to the first few days following SCI *continued*	The following are specific features of the acute phase arising in two different types of cord damage, contusion and compression: • Contusion—a necrotic core develops in the grey matter with ongoing cell loss in all directions from the site of injury. • Cord compression (following vertebral displacement)—edema is followed by excessive production of connective tissue as a reparative response (fibrosis), worsening the neural injury with tissue scarring.
Secondary: During the first few minutes through to the first weeks of cord injury	The spinal cord lesion grows in size. Within the first 15 minutes after injury, biochemical injury to the spinal cord begins, incorporating the following: • Muscle cell breakdown causes release of amino acids and other cell substrates to a level that is toxic to spinal cord tissue. • Electrolytic shifts and edema within the vertebral canal continue to interrupt adequate blood supply. An inadequate blood supply for the provision of oxygen to the damaged spinal cord (ischemia) contributes to cellular death. • Lipid peroxidation is also thought to be triggered at this time, where lipid molecules lose electrons and the lipid cell membrane is damaged. Lipid peroxidation is associated with the formation of carcinogenic and mutagenic agents. • A process of apoptosis (preprogrammed cell death or "cell suicide") begins and other barriers to cord regeneration (such as inflammation) are expressed in the area around the SCI.
Chronic: Days to years following the spinal cord injury	Again, the physiological changes in the spinal cord following SCI are influenced by the mechanism of injury. For example, in penetrating injuries there will be ongoing development of scarring and tethering of the cord. • In approximately 20% of individuals with SCI, syringomyelia, a condition where cerebrospinal fluid collects within the spinal cord and forms a fluid-filled cavity (syrinx) or cyst, eventually develops. The syrinx can expand over time and cause further destruction of the spinal cord. • Apoptosis continues above and below the spinal cord injury site, in some cases including brain regions. • Cut axons regenerate and sprout but can extend no farther than 1 mm from their origin, limiting functional recovery of movement and sensation. • Demyelination occurs during the chronic phase of injury, resulting in neuronal conduction deficits. • In many sensory reception cell types, permanent hyperexcitability develops, leading to chronic pain syndromes in a majority of patients with spinal cord injury.

Note. Adapted from "Recent Advances in Pathophysiology and Treatment of Spinal Cord Injury," by C. E. Hulsebosch, 2002, *Advances in Physiology Education*, *26*(4), pp. 238–255.

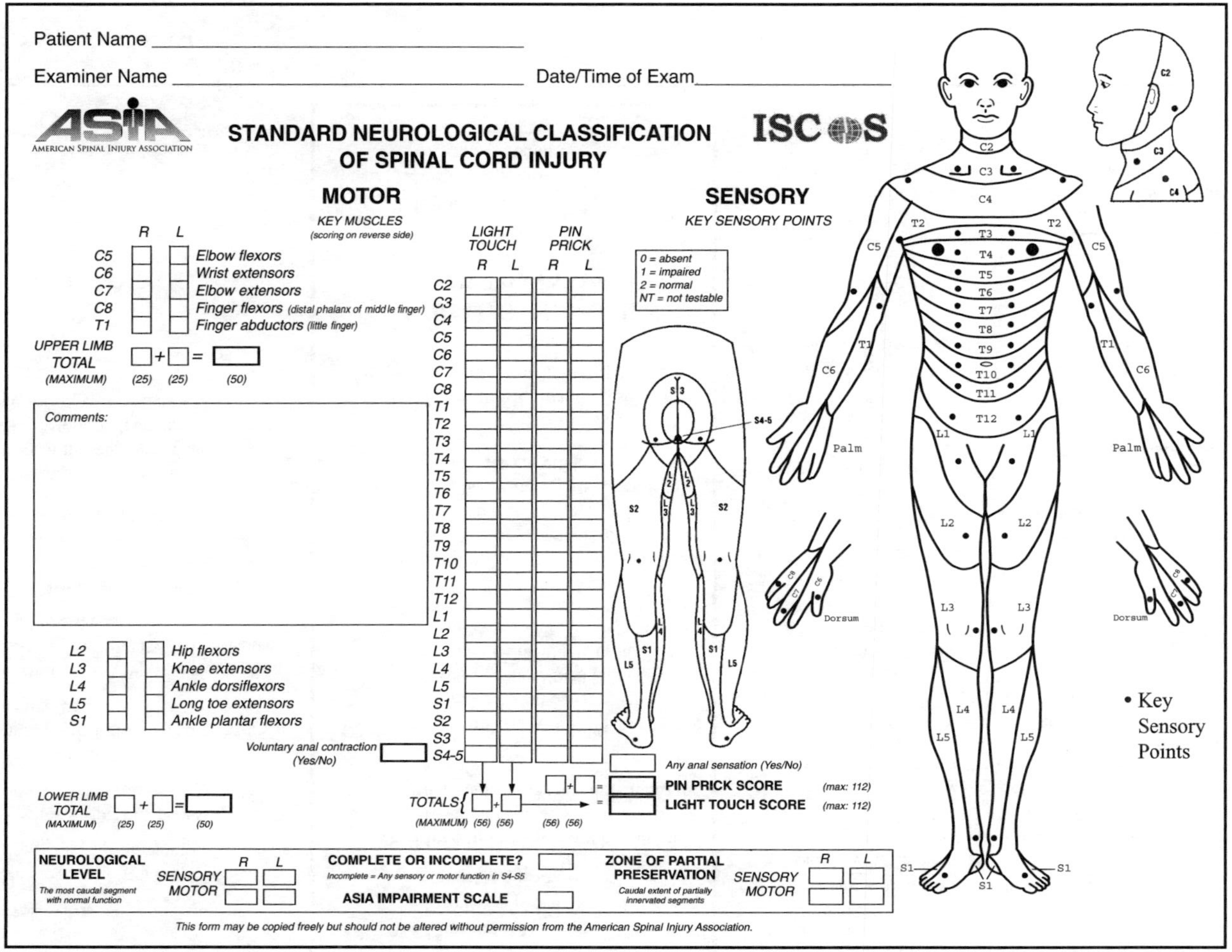

Figure 3–3. ASIA Impairment Scale. From American Spinal Injury Association Web site. Available at http://www.asia-spinalinjury.org/publications/2006_Classif_worksheet.pdf *continues*

MUSCLE GRADING

0 total paralysis

1 palpable or visible contraction

2 active movement, full range of motion, gravity eliminated

3 active movement, full range of motion, against gravity

4 active movement, full range of motion, against gravity and provides some resistance

5 active movement, full range of motion, against gravity and provides normal resistance

5* muscle able to exert, in examiner's judgement, sufficient resistance to be considered normal if identifiable inhibiting factors were not present

NT not testable. Patient unable to reliably exert effort or muscle unavailable for testing due to factors such as immobilization, pain on effort or contracture.

ASIA IMPAIRMENT SCALE

☐ **A = Complete**: No motor or sensory function is preserved in the sacral segments S4-S5.

☐ **B = Incomplete:** Sensory but not motor function is preserved below the neurological level and includes the sacral segments S4-S5.

☐ **C = Incomplete:** Motor function is preserved below the neurological level, and more than half of key muscles below the neurological level have a muscle grade less than 3.

☐ **D = Incomplete:** Motor function is preserved below the neurological level, and at least half of key muscles below the neurological level have a muscle grade of 3 or more.

☐ **E = Normal:** Motor and sensory function are normal.

CLINICAL SYNDROMES (OPTIONAL)

☐ Central Cord
☐ Brown-Sequard
☐ Anterior Cord
☐ Conus Medullaris
☐ Cauda Equina

STEPS IN CLASSIFICATION

The following order is recommended in determining the classification of individuals with SCI.

1. Determine sensory levels for right and left sides.
2. Determine motor levels for right and left sides.
   Note: in regions where there is no myotome to test, the motor level is presumed to be the same as the sensory level.
3. Determine the single neurological level.
   This is the lowest segment where motor and sensory function is normal on both sides, and is the most cephalad of the sensory and motor levels determined in steps 1 and 2.
4. Determine whether the injury is Complete or Incomplete (sacral sparing).
   If voluntary anal contraction = **No** *AND all S4-5 sensory scores =* **0** *AND any anal sensation =* **No**, *then injury is COMPLETE. Otherwise injury is incomplete.*
5. Determine ASIA Impairment Scale (AIS) Grade:

Is injury Complete? — If **YES**, AIS=A Record ZPP (For ZPP record lowest dermatome or myotome on each side with some (non-zero score) preservation)

NO ↓

Is injury motor incomplete? — If **NO**, AIS=B (Yes=voluntary anal contraction OR motor function more than three levels below the motor level on a given side.)

YES ↓

Are at least half of the key muscles below the (single) neurological level graded 3 or better?

NO ↓ AIS=C

YES ↓ AIS=D

If sensation and motor function is normal in all segments, AIS=E
Note: AIS E is used in follow up testing when an individual with a documented SCI has recovered normal function. If at initial testing no deficits are found, the individual is neurologically intact; the ASIA Impairment Scale does not apply.

Figure 3–3. *continued*

Dermatomes are the regions of the skin that have sensory innervations from a given spinal cord level. For example, C3 receives the sensory input from the region of the lower part of the neck to the clavicle. Motor function is then determined by testing the myotomes, the groups of muscles served by a single nerve. The result of the combined motor and sensory testing informs the neurological level of injury.

The ASIA impairment scale then classifies the *completeness* of injury (signified by ratings along a scale of A: complete to E: incomplete). *Complete injuries* imply loss of all motor, sensory, and reflex functioning below the level of SCI with both sides of the body equally impaired. *Incomplete injuries* imply some sparing of any of these domains. When the injury is complete, the zone of partial preservation is also noted. The term *zone of partial preservation* identifies all spinal segments below the neurological level of injury with preservation of motor or sensory findings. A rating of A–E is made based on the results of neurological level and completeness, where A refers to complete injuries and B–D incomplete (see Figure 3–3).

The ASIA scale also allows for the identification of spinal cord injury clinical *syndromes*. These include:

- Central cord syndrome: when there is greater motor function preserved in the lower limbs than in the upper limbs, in combination with bladder dysfunction and variable sensory loss below the level of the spinal cord injury. This is more likely to occur in a hyperextension injury in those with long-standing cervical spondylosis (degeneration and deformity in the joints of two or more adjoining vertebrae; Alpert, 2007).
- Brown-Sequard syndrome: when there is contralateral loss of pain and temperature sensation and ipsilateral loss of motor function and proprioception. This syndrome may follow unilateral hemisection of the spinal cord (e.g., gunshot wound).
- Anterior cord syndrome: describes paraplegia, loss of pain, and decrease in body temperature below the level of the injury. This is caused by disc herniation into the canal space that leads to damage in the anterior and lateral portions of the spinal cord with sparing of the posterior portion of the cord.
- Conus medullaris syndrome: relates to the presence of symptoms of hypertonicity of some reflexes (anal sphincter) and spasticity in muscles below the injury. Damage to the conus medullaris will produce both upper motor neuron and lower motor neuron responses because it forms the junction between the spinal cord and the spinal nerves. The syndrome may arise from lumbar trauma, vertebral deformity, and medical conditions (such as infections, cancer).
- Cauda equina syndrome: describes symptoms of bilateral leg pain, saddle anesthesia, urinary continence and retention disorders, and loss of anal tone in addition to other signs that indicate compromise of the nerve roots from L1–L5 to S1–S5. A lesion to the cauda equina is a lower motor neuron injury because this is part of the peripheral nervous system. This syndrome may follow lumbar disc herniation into the vertebral canal or

disease processes like epidural abscess (Dawodu, 2007).

Other terminology exists relating to the *level and pattern* of impairment. *Tetraplegia* (previously *quadriplegia*) is the term for neurological impairment following injury to the cervical segments. Because damage to the cervical segments is most frequently associated with swallowing impairments, patients with tetraplegia constitute the majority of the SLP's clinical caseload. In tetraplegia, neurological function to the neck, upper and lower limbs, trunk, and pelvic organs is impaired. The term *paraplegia* describes neurological injury to the thoracic, and/or lumbar, and/or sacral spinal cord segments, while all cervical segments remain intact. Paraplegia presents with intact upper limb functioning and variable levels of functional impairment to the trunk, lower limbs, and pelvic organs.

Patterns of impairment are largely predicted by the level and completeness of SCI. Table 3-5 provides the reader with an outline of functional capacity following different levels of SCI.

Incidence and Epidemiology of Traumatic Spinal Cord Injury

Information regarding trends in SCI is collected in different ways in different countries, limiting the direct comparability of epidemiological data. For example, the National Spinal Cord Injury Statistical Center in the United States captures data from federally sponsored SCI care systems across the United States and excludes data from other types of care. The Australian Institute of Health and Welfare reports on data drawn from the Australian Spinal Cord Injury Register that represents the total national adult population and includes Australian residents who incurred a SCI while overseas. Comparison of data from these two primary sources (Cripps, 2007; National Spinal Cord Injury Statistical Center, 2008) as well as other referenced studies reveals the following patterns in the population of adults with SCI:

- Incidence: In the population aged 15 years and over, new cases of SCI average 15.7 cases per million

Table 3–5. Levels of Spinal Cord Injury and Corresponding Functional Abilities

Spinal Nerves	***Spinal Level***	***Extent of Compromised Function***
Cervical 1–8[1]	C1–C3	Limited head/neck movements—flexion, extension, and rotation. Requires assisted ventilation (usually via tracheostomy tube). Vital capacity is only 5–10% of normal. Cough is absent. Unable to clear pharyngeal and chest secretions. Communication may be achieved with tracheostomy speech or may require augmentative communication and assistive technology. Independent mobilization is possible in a power chair via head, chin, or breath control systems (e.g., "sip and puff" switch).

Table 3–5. *continued*		
Spinal Nerves	***Spinal Level***	***Extent of Compromised Function***
Cervical 1–8[1] *continued*	C3–C4	Assisted ventilation required initially, but many individuals will be weaned from long-term ventilatory assistance. Reduced vital capacity due to paralysis of intercostals. Cough is weak. Typically has some head and neck control and, if C4 preserved, may be able to shrug shoulders.
	C5	Spontaneous breathing with reduced respiratory endurance and vital capacity. May require assistance to clear secretions completely but can self-assist cough. Has head and neck control and can bend elbows and turn palm. No wrist or hand control. Able to feed independently once full assistance has been provided to set up adapted utensils, etc.
	C6	Spontaneous breathing with reduced respiratory endurance, vital capacity, and cough effectiveness. Has movement in head, neck, shoulders, arms, and wrists. Capacity for self-feeding with adapted utensils. May propel manual wheelchair for short distances and use hand controls for power chair.
	C7	Spontaneous breathing with reduced respiratory endurance and vital capacity. Has similar movement as C6 injury. Driving may be possible with modifications to vehicle.
	C8	Spontaneous breathing with reduced respiratory endurance and vital capacity. Has near normal hand function. Able to transfer to manual wheelchair independently. Can live independently with home modifications.
Thoracic 1–12	T1–T9	T2–T4 vital capacity is 30–50% of normal, and cough remains weaker than non–spinal cord injured individuals. Uses manual wheelchair independently.
	T10–T12	Respiratory dysfunction is minimal. Vital capacity is essentially normal, and cough is strong. Independent in car (including loading wheelchair). Some independent walking.
Lumbar 1–5	L1–L5	Return of additional movement in hips and knees. Improvement in walking with supportive devices.
Sacral 1–5	S1–S5	Some return of voluntary bowel, bladder, and sexual functions.

[1]Cervical spinal vertebrae = 1–7 only.

Note. Adapted from *Spinal Cord Injury Information Network—Functional Goals Following SCI*, 2008. Retrieved July 30, 2008, from http://www.spinalcord.uab.edu/ and *The consortium for spinal cord medicine.* (1999). *Outcomes following traumatic spinal cord injury: clinical practice guidelines for health-care professionals.* Paralyzed Veterans of America. Retrieved June 27, 2008, from http://www,pva.org/site/News2?page=NewsArticle&id=7655 .

annually in Australia compared to the much higher 32 to 40 cases per million reported in the United States.

- Prevalence: Approximately 9000 patients in Australia and 255,702 in the United States present with persisting neurological deficits (at 90 days post-SCI or at discharge from rehabilitation). The discrepancy between these figures reflects in part the larger U.S. general population.
- Etiology: Both Australian and U.S. data suggest that physical trauma is the cause for the majority of new cases of SCI each year (e.g., in Australia over 70% of new cases of SCI are due to motor vehicle accidents, low and high falls, water sports, and other causes including industrial accidents and acts of violence). There is a higher representation of acts of violence (gunshot, stabbing, being struck with fists or an object) as a cause of SCI in the United States, where this was the third most likely cause of SCI. This is in contrast with Australia, where such cases were rare (less than 10 cases in 2005–2006). In Australia in 2005 to 2006, 22% of traumatic SCIs were work-related accidents. Non-traumatic SCI in both the United States and Australia is associated with conditions such as ischemia, cancer, abscesses, spinal canal stenosis, disc disease, myelitis, and medical interventions.
- Nature of injury: Data from the United States and Australia indicate that incomplete tetraplegia is most common post-SCI (Table 3–6).
- Age: Younger adults are most likely to have a SCI, with over 50% of new cases occurring in people aged 30 years and less. A quarter of all new traumatic SCIs occurred in

Table 3–6. Comparison of Incidence of Persisting Traumatic Spinal Cord Injury between Australia (2005–2006 data)[1] and United States (2000 data)[2]

Spinal Cord Injury by Neurological Level	*Australian Incidence*	*U.S. Incidence*
Incomplete tetraplegia	37%	34.1%
Complete tetraplegia	16%	18.3%
Incomplete paraplegia	28%	18.5%
Complete paraplegia	19%	23%
Complete recovery	Nil reported	Less than 1%

[1]From *2005–6 Spinal Cord Injury, Australia*, by R. A. Cripps, 2007, Research and Statistic Series Number 36. Adelaide. Australian Institute of Health and Welfare. (AIHW cat.no. INJCAT 102). Retrieved July 30, 2008, from http://www.nisu.flinders.edu.au/pubs/reports/2007/injcat102.php .

[2]From National Spinal Cord Injury Statistical Center (2008 dated reports). Retrieved August 1, 2008, from http://www.spinalcord.uab.edu/show.asp?durki=19775&site=1021&return=19679 .

individuals aged 15 to 24 years in Australia. An increasing representation of aged persons in the general population of industrialized countries suggests potential for a similar rise in the proportion of aged persons in the SCI population. In Australia, people 75 years and older accounted for 6% of all new cases in 2004 to 2005.

- Gender: The data collected in the United States and Australian populations demonstrate that approximately 80% of new cases of SCI occur in males. This gender imbalance is greatest in the young and least in those over 65 years in both countries.
- Occupational status: A majority of U.S. and Australian residents with SCI were employed at the time of injury. In 2005 to 2006, 65% of Australians were employed at the time of their SCI, with a degree of overrepresentation in both highly skilled occupations (e.g., managers, supervisors, and professionals) and less skilled occupations (e.g., laborers, clerical) when compared to the general population.
- Concurrent injuries: Injuries likely to cooccur with SCI include traumatic brain injury (Glasgow Coma Score of 12 or below at discharge); non-vertebral fractures requiring surgery; severe facial injuries affecting sense organs; major chest injury requiring chest-tube or assisted ventilation; traumatic amputations of a limb; and severe hemorrhaging or damage to any internal organ requiring surgery (Biering-Sorensen et al., 2006).
- Neurological recovery: Current data describe a low rate of full neurological recovery (1%) in patients admitted to acute care following SCI. However, international research is investigating a range of approaches including biological therapies to improve spinal cord regeneration and bionics to restore lost motor function.
- Length of stay: SCI has been described as the most expensive condition among all causes for hospitalization (McCrory, Samsa, Hamilton, Govert, Matcha, & Goslin, 2001). The median duration of initial care (i.e., from accident retrieval to discharge from rehabilitation) for persisting SCI in Australian hospitals in 2005 to 2006 was approximately 4.3 months (130 days). Individuals with complete tetraplegia exceeded the median duration of inpatient care for those with paraplegia with a stay of 7.5 months (226 days). Many factors influence these figures, including national and local government policies for health funding (e.g., socialized medicine or privately funded health care); the availability of suitable accommodation and trained carers; and whether the patient completes rehabilitation as an inpatient or is discharged earlier from inpatient care to transitional programs that provide community-based rehabilitation. This information was not available from the U.S. data.
- Life expectancy: Between 1.4 and 4% of individuals with SCI die during acute hospitalization, and mortality rates are higher in older patients. Longevity for survivors approaches normal life expectancy in the industrialized world (Table 3-7). In adults of all ages, life expectancy following SCI is best when there is some sparing of motor function at any level. As may be expected, the

Table 3–7. Comparison of Life Expectancy between Individuals with and without Spinal Cord Injury (who have survived for 1 year post-injury)

Age at Injury	*Level of Spinal Cord Injury*	*Remaining Life Expectancy*
20 years	**No spinal cord injury**	**58.4 years**
	Ventilator assisted	23.3 years
	Tetraplegia	37.9–41.7 years
	Paraplegia	46.3 years
	Intact motor function at any level	53.3 years
60 years	**No spinal cord injury**	**22.2 years**
	Ventilator assisted	3.1 years
	Tetraplegia	8.8–10.8 years
	Paraplegia	13.5 years
	Intact motor function at any level	18.3 years

Note. From National Spinal Cord Injury Statistical Center (2008 reports). Retrieved August 1, 2008, from http://www.spinalcord.uab.edu/show.asp?durki=19775&site=1021&return=19679 .

greater the level of functional impairment following SCI, the lower the life expectancy. Leading causes of death in SCI include pneumonia, other respiratory conditions, heart disease, subsequent trauma, septicemia, suicide, alcohol-related deaths, and cancer (Dawodu, 2007). The leading cause of death in tetraplegia is respiratory failure (McCrory et al., 2001).

- Predictors of mortality: Predictors of mortality following SCI include diabetes mellitus, heart disease, cigarette smoking, and the pulmonary function test of percent-of-predicted forced expiratory volume in the first second, with this final factor providing an indication of the influence of an individual's respiratory condition on health post-SCI (Brown, Di Marco, Hoit, & Garshick, 2006).
- Lifetime costs: The cost of care following SCI varies with higher costs associated with lower levels of physical independence. The hospital cost per day for patients with tetraplegia equates with the cost per day of a critical care bed. Ventilator dependency markedly increases costs during hospitalization and in the community. On return to the community costs associated with attendant care, equipment, and medical and allied health are ongoing.

CLINICAL MANAGEMENT OF TRAUMATIC SPINAL CORD INJURY

The management of SCI occurs in a number of stages, with multidisciplinary team involvement central to optimal patient outcomes across all phases of care. In 2008 the consortium for spinal cord medicine published clinical practice guidelines for the management of acute spinal cord injuries following a review of the research evidence. Hadley et al (2001) and the consortium concluded that clinical management in acute SCI was shaped largely by clinical consensus, rather than a high degree of clinical certainty since robust research evidence was limited. The following summary briefly describes typical clinical care for the SCI population. On retrieval from the scene of the SCI, the first priorities are to immobilize the spine during all procedures to prevent further damage, to achieve a satisfactory airway, and to maintain both breathing and vascular circulation. Use of immobilizing splints and handling procedures in cases of suspected SCI is mandatory in the emergency medicine practices of industrialized countries. An open airway will be established via endotracheal (ETT) intubation if necessary. If ventilatory failure is suspected, assisted ventilation may be provided with an emergency ventilator, and this procedure may require administration of medications to paralyze and sedate the patient. At this point, medical stabilization, assessment of the extent of injury to the spinal cord and vertebral column, and immobilization to prevent further trauma are the foremost clinical concerns.

At admission to the accident and emergency department, each individual will undergo a number of diagnostic assessments. These include a medical history, assessment of vital signs and blood work, physical examination, radiological imaging, neurological evaluation of brain and spinal cord function, and evaluation of the risk for ventilatory failure. Blood pressure management may require administration of fluids or medications. Insertion of a catheter as a precaution against urinary retention may be undertaken. Where emergency surgery is necessary, such as for patients with multitrauma (see Chapter 5), bed rest and a cervical collar (e.g., Philadelphia collar, Figure 3–4) may be applied to maintain spinal alignment. Admission to an intensive care, trauma or specialized acute SCI unit usually occurs following emergency interventions.

Identification of the extent of acute spinal cord damage is determined through diagnostic imaging and physical, medical, respiratory, and neurological testing. However, a full picture of the extent of impairment may not emerge until many weeks post-injury. A medical history detailing the mechanism (e.g., hyperflexion), circumstances of the SCI (such as a high fall), and any premorbid medical conditions can assist with diagnosing the

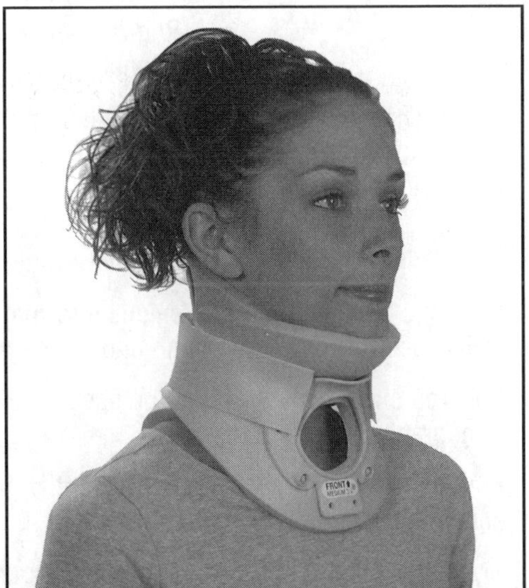

Figure 3–4. Philadelphia collar. Image provided courtesy of Ossur (http://www.ossur.com). Reprinted with permission.

nature and potential consequences of the SCI sustained. Physical examination detects signs of vertebral damage and multitrauma. During assessment of the patient's vital signs, medical interventions for the stabilization of an acute SCI are continuously reviewed, for instance, the presence of bradycardia (slow heart rate) and hypotension (low blood pressure) may point to an autonomic nervous system response to the SCI. However, these findings may also be due to other medical conditions, necessitating radiological and other examinations of the spinal cord and vertebrae prior to confirmation of a SCI (Table 3–8). Cardiovascular instability and respiratory insufficiency in the first 2 weeks after a cervical SCI are life

Table 3–8. Radiological and Other Techniques Used to Examine Spinal Cord Injury (SCI)

Assessment	***Information Obtained***
Magnetic resonance imaging (MRI)	• Used in the presence of suspected spinal cord lesions, ligament injuries, or other soft tissue injuries or pathology. • Used to determine location of the SCI and degree of spinal cord compression and detect hemorrhage, contusion, edema, and spinal cord disruption in acute and subacute SCI. • *Functional MRI* measures the anatomic/functional metabolic correlates of sensory motor activities in SCI. • *MRI diffusion weighted imaging* provides information on extent of axonal loss.
Computerized tomography (CT) and radiography	• CT and radiography provide information on the bony anatomy of the spine, specifically to identify vertebral abnormalities or fracture. • CT is able to detect small or fine fractures that cannot be seen on standard radiographic images.
Magnetic resonance (MR) spectroscopy	• Provides information on the biochemical characteristics of the brain and the damaged spinal cord.
Positron emission tomography (PET)	• Can be used to assess metabolic activity of the brain and spinal cord.
Intraoperative spinal sonography	• Used to identify gross pathology and spinal cord anatomy during surgery.
Myelogram	• Dye inserted around the spinal cord helps to locate the spinal cord injury and any areas of cord compression. After dye is inserted a CT scan reveals areas of injury.
Somatosensory evoked potentials	• Electric currents applied to the arms and legs allow measurement of how the current travels to the brain and are used to detect whether the spinal cord injury is complete or incomplete.

Note. Adapted from "Guidelines for the Management of Acute Cervical Spine and Spinal Cord Injuries," by M. N. Hadley et al., 2001, *Joint Section on Disorders of the Spine and Peripheral Nerves of the AANS/CNS.* Retrieved September 1, 2008, from http://www.spineuniverse.com/displayarticle.php/article2081.html .

threatening. Early ventilatory failure is a high risk in C1–C2 cervical injuries in particular. Intensive care monitoring and aggressive medical management of these problems have been shown to reduce mortality and morbidity and improve neurological outcome (Hadley et al., 2001). Medical interventions may include pharmacological therapies that aim to reduce edema and inflammation and offer neuroprotection, thereby improving neurological outcome post-acute SCI.

Findings from neurological examinations may be summarized within the ASIA scale (see Figure 3–3). In applying the ASIA rating, neurological reflexes and sensory and motor function are examined separately, one limb at a time, as sensory function and motor function may be retained differently on each side of the body. Over the first 72 hours of hospitalization neurological testing may be conducted several times, as spinal shock may alter the clinical presentation, and neurological changes may indicate a need to review management (e.g., should the SCI show signs of extending [worsening]).

Once immediately life-threatening conditions are managed, an optimal method of vertebral stabilization (e.g., a conservative versus a surgical approach, discussed later in this chapter) to limit secondary SCI is determined. Later, when the patient's condition has stabilized, tools that describe the day-to-day outcomes of SCI, such as the Functional Independence Measure (FIM) or Modified Barthel Index, shape rehabilitation plans. These and other tools (e.g., the Quadriplegic Index of Function [QIF], Walking Index for SCI [WISCI], Capabilities of Upper Extremity Instrument [CUE], Spinal Cord Independence Measure [SCIM], Canadian Occupational Performance Measure [COPM]) can assist injured individuals and their families to plan for the changes required to their physical surroundings (such as assistive devices and technology for computer access, mobility, and personal care), physical rehabilitation goals, carer support requirements and consideration of employment and social roles in preparation for the return to the community. Informal questionnaires that record a patient's own perceptions of adjustment to SCI can clarify for the team which aspects of rehabilitation are most relevant to each individual and their family.

Respiratory Function and Management

The mechanism of respiratory dysfunction in SCI differs from other at-risk populations. Respiratory muscle dysfunction due to SCI alone is classified as *extrinsic* lung dysfunction (i.e., due to muscle weakness) as opposed to *intrinsic* lung dysfunction that is the result of lung disease (e.g., emphysema), where exchange of oxygen and carbon dioxide is limited by damaged and congested alveoli. These different causes (intrinsic versus extrinsic) of ventilatory impairment require different respiratory interventions.

There is a high risk of both early and late ventilatory failure for individuals who have sustained a cervical SCI. Ventilatory impairment in SCI that is caused by weakness in the muscles of expiration (mainly the abdominals and intercostals) and inspiration (mainly the diaphragm) has the potential to cause first hypercapnia and then hypoxia (Bach & Goncalves, 2006). In cervical injuries, hypoventilation due to shallow breathing and atelectasis (alveolar collapse) caused by impaired airway secretions clearance is common, requiring a range of interventions (Bach & Goncalves, 2006; McCrory et al., 2001; Porth, 2005).

The respiratory consequences of a SCI correlate quite specifically with the neurological level and completeness of the injury. For example, Bach (1996) reported that a SCI between C6 and T6 will result in a 60% reduction in inspiratory muscle strength. In the cervical region, SCI may lead to temporary or permanent disruption to spontaneous ventilation. Table 3–9 contains a summary of the muscles involved in inspiration and expiration. Table 3–10 outlines the respiratory consequences of SCI following injury to different spinal cord levels. In addition to injury level, the extent of respiratory impairment is also dependent

Table 3–9. Pulmonary Function Following Spinal Cord Injury

Phase of Breathing	*Muscles*	*Spinal or Cranial Innervation*
Inspiration	Diaphragm	Phrenic nerve
	Intercostals:	Anterior branch of thoracic nerve
	• Levator costae	
	Accessory:	
	• Scalene	C4–C5 spinal nerves
	• Sternocleidomastoid	XI (accessory)
	• Trapezius	XI (accessory)
	Serratus anterior	Long thoracic nerve
	Serratus posterior inferior	Lower thoracic nerve
	Serratus posterior superior	T2–T3 spinal nerves
	Pectoralis major and minor	Anterior thoracic nerves
	Latissimus dorsi	Thoracodorsal nerve
	Subclavius and sternoclavicularis	Nerve to subclavius
Expiration	Abdominals:	
	• Obliquus abdominus externus and internus	T6–T12 and iliohypogastric nerve
	• Transverse abdominus	Thoracoabdominal, T7–T11, iliohypogastric, and ilioinguinal nerve
	• Transverse thoracis	Thoracic nerve
	• Rectus abdominus	T6–T12
	Intercostals:	
	• Intercostalis internus and dorsi	Thoracic nerve
	• Iliocostalis lumborum	Lumbar nerve
	• Serratus posterior inferior and subcostalis quadratus lumborum	Thoracic nerve L1–L3
	• Pectoralis major	Medial pectoral nerve

Note. Adapted from "Recognition and Management of Respiratory Dysfunction in Children with Tetraplegia," by S. C. Porth, 2005, *Journal of Spinal Cord Medicine*, *27*(Suppl. 1), pp. S75–S79.

Table 3–10. Respiratory Function Following Traumatic Spinal Cord Injury

Spinal Cord Injury Level	*Need for Assisted Ventilation Due to Spinal Cord Injury Factors Alone*
C1–C2	Lifelong
C3–C4	Initially Potential to wean to spontaneous unassisted breathing
C5–C7	Initially a majority will require assisted ventilation Eventually breathe independently Passive expiration
T1–T5	Weak cough Spontaneous unassisted breathing Quiet respiration affected
T6–T12	Weak cough Spontaneous unassisted breathing
L1 and below	No impairment

Note. Adapted from The Consortium for Spinal Cord Medicine. (1999). *Outcomes following traumatic spinal cord injury: clinical practice guidelines for health-care professionals. Paralyzed Veterans of America.* Retrieved June 27, 2008 from, http://www.pva.org/site/News2?page=NewsArticle&id=7655

on premorbid respiratory status and cooccurring injuries.

Respiratory Assessment and Monitoring

The life-threatening consequences of both acute and late onset ventilatory failure following cervical SCI necessitate monitoring via clinical, radiological, and endoscopic means throughout the acute care period, and whenever health deteriorates.

Respiratory clinicians and/or the patient's primary physician undertake clinical evaluation of the risk of ventilatory failure during sleep and wakefulness. Respiratory monitoring may be achieved through: close patient observation (e.g., effort of breathing); observation of the individual's ability to clear upper airway secretions; bedside monitoring of oxygen saturation (oximetry) and end tidal carbon dioxide (capnography) levels; laboratory studies of arterial blood gases; pulmonary function testing; and, less frequently, sleep studies (polysomnography) at the bedside. Imaging (diaphragmatic ultrasound and chest x-ray; see Table 3–8) may be utilized to evaluate lung health and the risks of ventilatory failure. Impairment and recovery in diaphragmatic function can be visualized using diaphragm fluoroscopy (Porth, 2005). Endoscopic evaluation of the airways (bronchoscopy) may be applied where an aspiration event or retention of airway secretions is suspected.

Assisted Ventilation

Spontaneous ventilation, described simply, is the unassisted movement of air into and out of the lungs. When this process becomes either temporarily or permanently disrupted, such as following high cervical SCI, assisted ventilation is required. A complete SCI sustained at C1–C2 (ASIA A; see Figure 3–3) necessitates immediate and lifelong assisted ventilation (see Table 3–10). In comparison, patients with lower complete and incomplete cervical injury (ASIA levels A, B, C, and D; see Figure 3–3) may require a period of assisted ventilation in the short term; however, there is the possibility of weaning despite some ongoing respiratory dysfunction. For individuals without cervical injury, assisted ventilation may not be required at all. However, in instances of advanced age, premorbid neurological and/or respiratory compromise, or for those individuals who present with multitrauma to the head, larynx, or chest and other relevant medical conditions, a period of assisted ventilation can be expected. For those SCI patients with premorbid respiratory disease, ventilatory support is understandably more protracted and complex.

Research has shown that 40% of patients with cervical SCI develop ventilatory failure within 12 hours to 7 days post-injury, and these individuals then proceed to assisted ventilation (Bach, 1996). The retention of airway secretions due to neuromuscular fatigue is often the prominent symptom of imminent ventilatory failure and may arise at any time. Other factors such as respiratory infection, episodes of acute respiratory distress, and pneumonia may also necessitate ventilatory assistance (Consortium for spinal cord medicine, 2005; De Vivo, Stover, & Black, 1992).

The management of assisted ventilation includes the use of pulmonary function tests that measure air flow volumes and forces during breathing maneuvers at various times (such as following respiratory therapies). Vital capacity (the maximum amount of air exhaled after a maximum inhalation) is one measure that is used to objectively describe an individual's effectiveness in spontaneous breathing. Vital capacity has been estimated to decrease significantly when an individual with a cervical SCI assumes a sitting position rather than lying down. Porth (2005) reports that flaccidity in the torso (due to impaired abdominal muscle innervation) leads to the abdominal organs "tugging" on the diaphragm (the primary muscle of inhalation) and thereby limiting diaphragmatic excursion during breathing. For this reason, patients may be returned to a supine position during ventilator weaning programs. In some individuals with cervical SCI, the neuromuscular fatigue of respiration is managed with nocturnal ventilatory support and assisted coughing techniques alone, effectively resting the muscles of respiration and thereby optimizing daytime spontaneous breathing.

A range of approaches to assisted or "mechanical" ventilation exists. The following sections have been designed to orientate the reader to key elements of assisted ventilation for the SCI population, including brief discussions of different ventilation methods (invasive versus non-invasive techniques, positive versus negative pressure ventilation), ventilation modes (e.g., assist control, pressure support ventilation), and ventilator settings (tidal volume, etc.). For more detailed information on assisted ventilation, the reader is directed to other sources (e.g., Dikeman & Kazandjian, 2003; on-line resources such as the Home Ventilation Guide, http://www.ventusers.org/edu/HomeVentGuide.pdf, accessible on the International Ventilator Users Network Web site, http://www.ventusers.org/).

Invasive and Non-Invasive Techniques. The ventilatory *method* refers to the way that breathing is assisted, whether through invasive or non-invasive delivery sys-tems. Invasive ventilation requires the insertion of an artificial airway (i.e., orotracheal, nasotracheal, or tracheostomy tube; Figure 3-5). Non-invasive ventilation (NIV) draws from a wider range of delivery devices or patient interfaces (Figure 3-6) that aid breathing and coughing. While used less

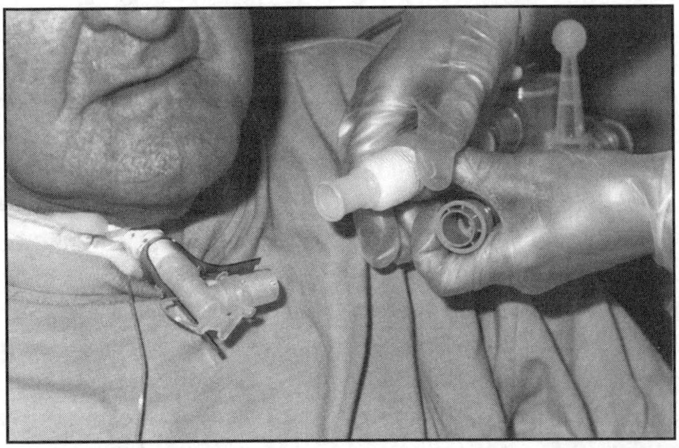

Figure 3–5. Tracheostomy ventilation where the ventilator circuit is about to be attached to the tracheostomy tube.

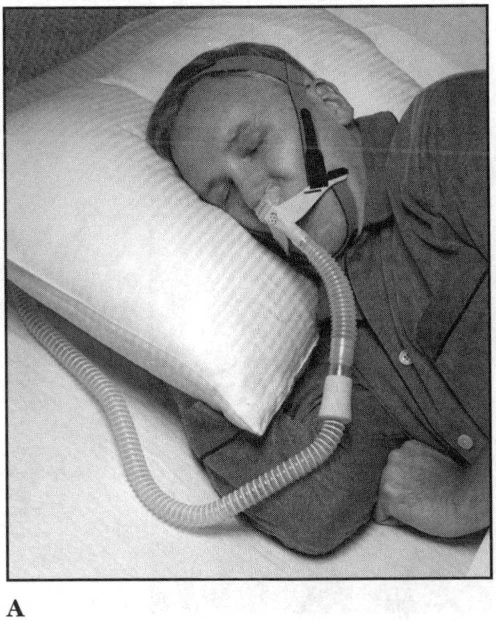

A

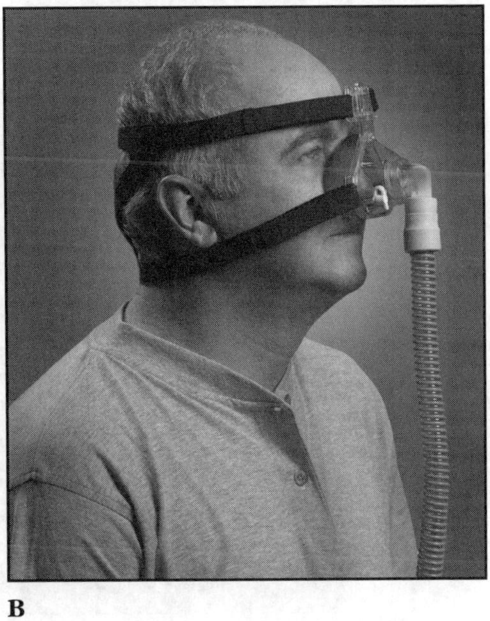

B

Figure 3–6. Examples of nasal pillows (**A**) and nasal mask (**B**). Images provided from Respironics (http://www.respironics.com). Reprinted with permission.

often than tracheostomy ventilation, NIV is reported to be effective for both acute and long term ventilation in the SCI population (McCrory et al., 2001)

Positive and Negative Pressure Ventilation. Negative pressure ventilators (NPVs) were developed before positive pressure ventilators (PPVs) and are in use in some European ICU settings. All NPVs assist breathing non-invasively and can be timed to reflect spontaneous inspiratory patterns. Thus, the usual physiology of breathing may be retained in the action of NPV. To achieve this, NPV typically involves the patient wearing a sealed "casing" around the chest and abdomen, or less commonly being placed in a 'tank'. An early example of NPV is the "iron lung," used extensively during poliomyelitis epidemics of the 1930s and in modified forms through to the 1960s. The iron lung is a form of 'body ventilator' that encases all of the body, except the head and neck, in a tank. Air is rhythmically sucked out and blown into the tank by a pump (a ventilator), thereby alternatively exerting and then relieving pressure on the chest and abdomen. When the chest wall and abdomen are exposed to subatmospheric pressure the chest will expand (be pulled/sucked outward), allowing intrapleural and alveolar pressures to also fall below atmospheric pressure. This change in pressure gradient allows the lungs to fill with air via the nose and mouth (as air moves from areas of higher pressure to areas of lower pressure). The reversal of these pressure changes assists exhalation. Other NPV devices such as the pneumobelt (Figure 3-7) use a more compact design, thereby enabling the patient to be more mobile. These more portable "body casings" are coupled with the ventilator type (pump) preferred by the patient and physician. Of the NPV devices, the iron lung is reported to be more effective than portable body ventilators, as the latter are limited by discomfort in wearing the device, requirement to be used in an upright position and the inability to

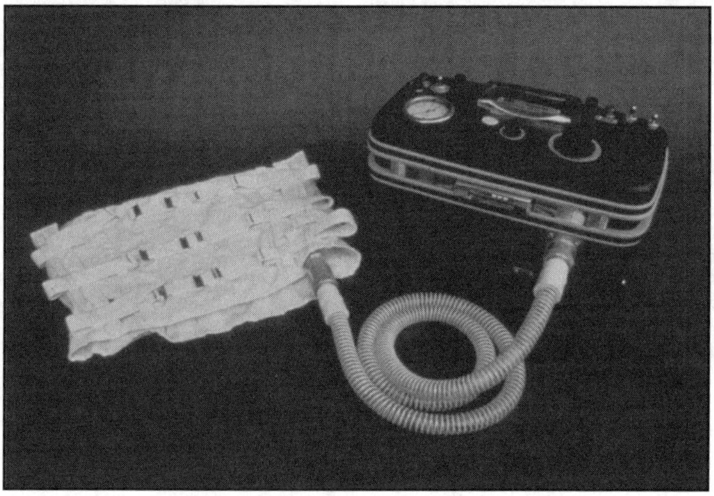

Figure 3–7. Pneumobelt. Image provided from Respironics (http://www.respironics.com). Reprinted with permission.

apply other therapies such as positive end expiratory pressure (PEEP; detailed further in the chapter).

PPV, in comparison, became possible with the development of materials suitable for endotracheal intubation and the advent of muscle relaxant medications for use during intubation. Unlike NPV, PPV may be delivered invasively (e.g. via tracheostomy or endotracheal tube) or non-invasively (e.g. mouthpieces, or nasal or facial masks). PPV involves the pumping of air into the patient's airway and thus alters the usual respiratory physiology. Volume cycled PPV involves the delivery of airflow ("inspiration") until a preset volume is met, whereas pressure cycled ventilation supports inspiratory flow until a preset pressure has been reached. Regardless of whether volume or pressure controlled, once the inspiratory cycle of PPV is finished, air is no longer pumped into the airways, and passive recoil of the chest permits exhalation. PPV is the most commonly used method of assisted ventilation in the SCI population.

Mode of Ventilation. Simply put, the *mode* of ventilatory assistance can be discussed in terms of the physician prescribed settings for the responsiveness of the ventilator to the patient's breathing efforts. The level of responsiveness ranges from full ventilatory support mode (referred to as controlled mode ventilation, CMV), in which the ventilator performs all the work of breathing regardless of attempts by the patient to take spontaneous breaths (e.g., may be applied in managing an unconscious patient or where assisted ventilation is required continuously day and night in a conscious patient), through to ventilatory modes that can support discrete changes in a patient's spontaneous breathing abilities or adjust to acute pulmonary conditions. The more commonly adopted modes of assisted ventilation for the SCI population have been outlined in Table 3-11. These may be combined with additional ventilatory therapies (such as PEEP and sigh breath; see Table 3-11) that refine the ventilator's program for lung health and patient comfort. The following is a brief explanation of these different assisted modes

- Assist control (AC) and synchronized intermittent mandatory ventilation (SIMV). Both of these modes have sensitivity to patients' breathing efforts. That is, the inspiratory time for each breath, the respiratory rate per minute, and the tidal volumes that the ventilator delivers at each breath will respond to spontaneous breaths "pulled" by the patient when these meet an inspiratory volume or pressure target. Consequently, any increase in breaths by the patient that reach target levels will reduce the number of breaths delivered by the ventilator. By synchronizing ventilator delivered breaths with patients' breathing efforts, hyperventilation risk is reduced. Despite the responsiveness of SIMV mode to the patient's ability to breathe, progressive ventilator free breathing programs have been described in the literature as a more effective approach to ventilator weaning in the SCI population (McCrory, 2001)
- Pressure support ventilation (PSV). Pressure support ventilation (see Table 3-11) is different from SIMV in that it doesn't provide any preset tidal volumes or breath rates; rather, each spontaneous breath taken by the patient is supported by a constant pressure delivered over the entire

Table 3–11. A Summary of Assisted Ventilation Modes and Therapies Regularly Used in Individuals with SCI

Ventilatory Modes and Therapies	***Type***	***Description***
Ventilatory modes	Assist control (AC)	Used as a full ventilation mode where patients can "trigger" a ventilator-assisted breath but are unable to inhale a sufficient volume of air or breathe reliably enough to always maintain adequate respiration. AC ventilation provides a preset pressure or volume for each breath taken by the patient. "Backup" breaths are provided if the patient fails to breathe.
	Synchronized intermittent mandatory ventilation (SIMV)	A mode where the respiratory rate and tidal volumes are prescribed by the physician. If the patient takes a breath within a preset time frame (between mandatory ventilator-delivered breaths), the ventilator-delivered breaths are synchronized with these. The difficulty of breathing through a tracheostomy and ventilator circuit may be offset with additional pressure support (PEEP; see below).
	Pressure support ventilation (PSV)	A ventilator weaning mode for patients who have some spontaneous breathing ability and variable endurance. In this mode the ventilator delivers a mandatory amount of positive air pressure during inspiration. The patient determines tidal volume. High levels of PSV reduce the work of breathing.
	Bilevel positive airway pressure	Also called *variable positive airway pressure*, bilevel ventilators allow different preset pressures to flow during inspiration (IPAP) and expiration (EPAP) in order to increase alveolar inflation.
Ventilatory therapies	Positive end expiratory pressure (PEEP)[1]	This ventilatory support improves oxygenation. This is achieved by preventing airway pressures from returning to atmospheric pressure or below at the end of exhalation and thereby promoting lung and alveolar inflation.
	Sigh[1]	This is a feature that may be programmed in to an assisted ventilation cycle. An assisted sigh periodically delivers a larger than usual inspiratory volume to expand the lungs and manage alveolar collapse.

[1]These ventilator therapies may be prescribed in addition to the mandatory assisted ventilation modes required by individual patients. For further detail, see Dikeman and Kazandjian (2003) and the International Ventilator Users Network Home Ventilator Guide at http://www.ventusers.org/edu/HomeVentGuide.pdf .

inhalation/inspiratory phase. This enables the patient to take a deeper and longer breath than he or she could without the pressure support. PSV is an alternative mode for ventilator weaning. Ventilator modes that respond to the patient's breathing efforts are increasingly available for use with invasive and non-invasive ventilation across acute care and long term settings.

- Bilevel positive airway pressure (BiPAP). BiPAP ventilation (see Table 3-11) provides assistance during both the inspiratory and expiratory phases of breathing. The level of pressure delivered can be varied during the phases of inspiration (inspiratory positive airway pressure, IPAP) and expiration (expiratory positive airway pressure, EPAP). For example, where neuromuscular disease causes difficulty in the inspiratory phase of breathing, the level of IPAP assistance may need to be higher than the EPAP http://www.ventusers.org/edu/HomeVentGuide.pdf, accessible on the International Ventilator Users Network Web site, http://www.ventusers.org/ .

Ventilator Parameters. There are also a number of ventilator parameters that are manipulated by the respiratory physician to optimize ventilation for each patient. Some of these parameters are particularly relevant for the SLP as modifications to some settings assist communication (Hoit, Shea & Banzett, 1994; Hoit & Banzett, 1997) and may alter swallowing, and these are outlined briefly below. It must be noted, however, that terminology varies between different models of ventilator, for example where one ventilator console displays an "i-time," that is inspiratory time in seconds, another ventilator may instead display an I-E ratio that, with some calculations, can be used to determine the same information. It is critical that the SLP consult with the ventilatory care team regarding the specific ventilator settings for each individual.

- Tidal volume. This setting determines the volume of air (in liters) delivered by the ventilator during the inspiratory cycle.
- Respiratory rate. This setting relates to the number of breaths per minute (bpm) provided by the ventilator. Normal adult respiratory rates fall within a range of 12 to 20 bpm.
- Inspiratory flow rate. Expressed in liters per minute (L/min), the inspiratory flow rate is the speed at which a preset volume of air is delivered during the inspiratory cycle each minute.
- Inspiratory to expiratory ratio (I:E ratio). This is the duration of inspiration in relation to the duration of expiration (usually measured in seconds). Typically, rates will be set where the expiratory phase is 1.5 to 2 times longer than the inspiratory phase (1:2); however, physicians may alter this ratio for patients with various lung disease conditions (e.g., COPD) that require longer expiration phases.
- Peak inspiratory pressure (PIP). The PIP relates to the setting that determines the highest permissible level of pressure in the airway during the inspiratory phase of ventilation (measured in cmH_2O).
- Inspiratory rise time. This measure indicates the time taken to reach the

preset inspiratory pressure (measured in seconds). Inspiratory rise time can be adjusted to compensate for leaks that occur with NIV interfaces, cuff deflation and to increase patient comfort.

- Fractional inspired oxygen concentration (FiO_2). Fractional inspired oxygen concentration (FiO_2). FiO_2 is the precent of oxygen in each breath that is inspired. Although oxygen concentration in room air is approximately 21%, FiO_2 supplemental oxygen delivered via nasal prongs, mask, or tracheostomy tube will increase this level.

Types of Assisted Ventilation in the SCI Population. While the sections above provide the reader with orientation to the "components" of assisted ventilation, the following sections discuss how these components are used in combination to provide assisted ventilation for the SCI population (e.g., PPV delivered via an invasive technique with assist control). Due to the high degree of individual variability in ventilator settings between patients, it is critical that the SLP becomes familiar with noting the ventilator settings and, in particular, the breathing conditions in which each dysphagia intervention occurs. The mode of ventilation and ventilation settings will change over time and such changes may impact on swallow function.

Invasive Ventilation: Tracheostomy Positive Pressure Ventilation. Tracheostomy positive pressure ventilation (TPPV) is by far the most common approach to acute and long-term assisted ventilation post-SCI, with incidence rates of TPPV occurrence across the wider SCI population reported to range between 11.2% in Denmark (Biering-Sorensen & Biering-Sorensen, 1992) to more recent estimates of up to 60% in Australia (Ross & White, 2003). With TPPV, the ventilatory support is referred to as continuous PPV (Table 3–12). In TPPV the patient's tracheostomy tube connects to flexible tubing, humidification devices (circuit; see Figure 3–5) and a ventilator unit, which pumps volumes and pressures of air according to prescribed ventilatory parameters to allow the patient to do more or less of the spontaneous breathing. For those patients with injuries consistent with the need for long-term ventilation, the typical period for endotracheal (translaryngeal) intubation of approximately 7 to 14 days prior to tracheostomy may be reduced due to the high predictability for ongoing reliance on TPPV. Tracheotomy procedures may be performed with a surgical or percutaneous approach; however, where the need for tracheostomization can be expected to be lifelong (e.g., ASIA level A; injury at C3 and above), a surgical tracheotomy may provide a more stable stoma and facilitate easier tube changes than a percutaneously formed stoma, which may "close down" more rapidly (although this clinical perspective has not been the subject of research to date).

With TPPV, ventilator settings are monitored daily in intensive care and a range of ventilatory therapies may be employed by intensivists to maintain optimum lung function while the patient's condition is yet critical. Ventilator settings may be reset for specific situations such as tracheostomy cuff deflation, following surgery, during weaning trials, upon the patient's transfer to a portable ventilator for rehabilitation and return to the home environment. For those patients using TPPV, secretion management is

Table 3–12. Invasive and Non-Invasive Ventilation Options for Patients with Spinal Cord Injury

Invasive or Non-Invasive	***Assisted Ventilation Method***	***Mechanism for Ventilation***	***Airway Secretion Management***
Invasive	Tracheostomy positive pressure ventilation (TPPV)	• Requires a surgical procedure to form an artificial airway (tracheotomy). • The inspiratory phase of ventilation is assisted as air is delivered directly into the lung via a tracheostomy. • The expiratory phase of ventilation relies on passive recoil of the chest and abdomen at the end of inspiration.	• Secretion management achieved via tracheal suction. • Spontaneous cough can be augmented with either a manually assisted cough or a mechanical insufflation-exsufflation (MI-E) device. • Intermittent positive pressure breathing (IPPB) and incentive spirometry may be used.
	Electrophrenic respiration (EPR)	• Requires a surgical procedure whereby electrodes are implanted into the phrenic nerves or diaphragm and are connected by leads to receivers in neck/chest. Patient wears an external transmitter. • Signals between the transmitters and receivers stimulate the phrenic nerves to trigger contraction of the diaphragm/intercostals and stimulate inhalation. • The expiratory phase of ventilation relies on passive recoil of the chest and abdomen at the end of inspiration. • A tracheostomy tube is usually retained.	• Secretion management achieved via tracheal suction. • Spontaneous cough can be augmented with either a manually assisted cough or MI-E. • IPPB and incentive spirometry may be used.
Non-Invasive	Respiratory muscle aids	• *Inspiratory* and *expiratory* phases of ventilation may be assisted non-invasively with respiratory muscle aids.	• No tracheostomy—patient must have adequate airway protection and must be low risk for aspiration of saliva.

continues

Table 3–12. *continued*

Invasive or Non-Invasive	***Assisted Ventilation Method***	***Mechanism for Ventilation***	***Airway Secretion Management***
Non-Invasive *continued*	Respiratory muscle aids *continued*	• One example of a respiratory muscle aid is an intermittent abdominal pressure ventilator (IAPV), which is an air-filled belt (e.g., pneumobelt). The IAPV applies compression to an individual's abdomen as the ventilator pumps air into the air-filled belt. This abdominal compression moves the diaphragm upwards, resulting in a forced exhalation. • When the cycle of pumping air into the IAPV device pauses and the device deflates, abdominal compression ceases. This pause allows inspiration to occur passively as the diaphragm and abdominal contents fall.	• Spontaneous cough can be augmented with both manually assisted coughing and MI-E. • IPPB and incentive spirometry may be used. • Proactive management of secretions by individuals/carers. • Glossopharyngeal breathing.
	Non-invasive positive pressure ventilation (NPPV)	• The *inspiratory* phase of ventilation may be assisted intermittently (IPPV) or continuously as a volume of air is delivered via a range of non-invasive airway interfaces including mouthpieces, nosepieces, and combination nasal and facial masks. • IPPV allows a patient to take the extra ventilator assistance when he or she feels the need (e.g., for a more effective cough). • In suitable candidates, oral and nasal interfaces can be used for continuous assisted ventilation overnight.	• No tracheostomy—patient must have adequate airway protection and must be low risk for aspiration of saliva. • Spontaneous cough can be augmented with both manually assisted coughing and MI-E. • IPPB and incentive spirometry may be used. • Proactive management of secretions by individuals/carers. • Glossopharyngeal breathing.

achieved primarily through tracheal suction; however, additional respiratory techniques (e.g., mechanical insufflation-exsufflation or intermittent positive pressure breathing, and assisted coughing detailed later in Respiratory and Ventilatory Treatments below) can be used to assist secretion clearance (see Table 3-12).

Invasive Ventilation: Electrophrenic Respiration. Electrophrenic respiration (EPR; see Table 3-12) requires a surgical implantation of devices that will electronically trigger movement in the muscles of breathing. EPR may be used for patients meeting certain criteria, specifically, where an injury results in a high tetraplegia (C3 and above) in the presence of intact phrenic nerves, normal lung function and adequate chest wall compliance: conditions often only present in young adults with SCI. For this reason, EPR, also called diaphragmatic pacing, is less common than TPPV in the general population. Phrenic nerve conduction studies are undertaken preoperatively to determine suitability for the procedure. EPR aims to replace use of a portable ventilator for at least part of the day. The EPR procedure can be carried out soon after a SCI or many years later.

A range of designs and implantation procedures for EPR exists. However, the general concept of EPR is to use electrical impulses to achieve inhalation. Signals are sent to electrodes implanted onto the phrenic nerves, intercostals, or diaphragm. The targeted muscles receive these impulses and contract in a way that mirrors normal inhalation. A tracheostomy is usually maintained for safety reasons (e.g., during sleep when upper airway collapse may occur or for the management of tracheal secretions). The presence of a tracheostomy allows secretion management via suctioning; the use of additional respiratory techniques can assist with secretion management (see details later in Chapter and Table 3-12).

Reported benefits of EPR over tracheostomy ventilation for the person with the SCI include easier mobility (freedom from a portable ventilator permits use of a smaller power chair), more spontaneous breathing time, reduced reliance on tracheal suctioning, improved sense of smell (due to nasal and upper airway airflow), improved appetite, and enhanced speech quality (Di Marco, Onders, Ignagni, & Kowalski, 2006; Hoit & Shea, 1996). In addition, favorable cost comparisons have been made for EPR, with a "one off" fee for the electrophrenic pacing procedure being more cost effective than the ongoing cost of portable home ventilators, associated consumable equipment, and attendant care (Di Marco et al., 2006). In addition to potential surgical complications, possible long-term nerve damage is a reported risk of EPR.

Non-Invasive Assisted Ventilation. Non-invasive assisted ventilation (NIV) is a specialized field within the domains of neurology, respiratory, and critical care medicine. It integrates a range of techniques to deliver either PPV or NPV and some patients use these in combination (see Table 3-12). Benefits of NIV include avoiding the risks associated with intubation (e.g., ventilator-associated pneumonia and tracheal stenosis) and greater ease in weaning when compared to tracheostomy ventilation. Limitations of this approach include skin breakdown from imperfect mask fitting (such as nasal skin pressure necrosis); air leaks; and abdominal distension. The use of NIV techniques in traumatic SCI in the acute phase of care is less common; however, some researchers advocate for its use in this population to augment ventilator weaning attempts (Bach & Goncalves, 2006; McCrory et al., 2001) and to avoid intubation (Bach & Goncalves, 2006).

When NIV PPV is prescribed, it can be delivered whenever the patient desires this kind of supplementation, which is referred to as intermittent PPV (IPPV), or in a continuous manner 24 hours per day. IPPV might be preferred by a patient who can breathe spontaneously during the daytime (if ventilator assisted at night) but requires the safety of a back-up ventilator breaths via a mouthpiece that also allows superior inhalatory volume and pressure to inhale more deeply and cough effectively, to speak at a greater intensity, and in longer phrases than is possible without IPPV.

The long-term adoption of a NIV approach requires the training of patients and caregivers in respiratory and ventilatory monitoring (Bach & Goncalves, 2006). The integrated regimen of techniques required for successful NIV includes: use of assistive breathing aids to achieve effective ventilation; undertaking active self-monitoring of respiratory condition; training in effective secretions clearance therapies (e.g., glossopharyngeal breathing and mechanical insufflation-exsufflation, which is detailed later in the Respiratory and Ventilatory Treatments section); and ensuring a leak-proof connection between the patient and the ventilator tubing (such as a facial mask). Non-invasive positive pressure ventilation (NPPV) delivers each inhalatory breath to the airways via the nose and/or mouth at a pressure greater than atmospheric pressure through the use of a range of interfaces. These interfaces include mouthpieces, nasal pillows, facial masks, nasal masks, and so on (see Figure 3–6) that must form a seal with the patient to prevent air leaks and are secured to the patient's head with adjustable Velcro straps (although recently some nasal connections have been designed that require no such harnessing).

Respiratory clinicians may determine that a particular patient can safely trial PPV delivered via a mouthpiece continuously (e.g., for sleep) or intermittently (IPPV) when alert. Mouth IPPV is possible when the ventilator circuit (tubing) is fitted with a mouthpiece (similar to spirometry mouthpieces, although designs can be customized with dental appliances and other approaches) and placed adjacent to the patient's mouth (such as carefully attached to the wheelchair) so that the patient can take extra breaths as desired independently. During the day an alert individual, with adequate bulbar function can hold the mouthpiece between the teeth and then form an airtight seal with the lips as breaths are delivered (Bach & Goncalves, 2006).

Nasal pillows or prongs are made of a range of materials (for example, thermoplastics) to allow insertion into the nostrils and may be angled for comfort and encased in a supporting sleeve before being strapped to the head for secure breath support during sleep or waking. Nasal and facial masks bear similarities to those SLPs will be familiar with for oxygen delivery, but are designed for greater durability, comfort and reliable skin seal. Each of these interfaces connects to flexible tubing that couples with the ventilator unit so that air can be delivered to the patient. NIV can also be achieved at least part-time with a range of body worn aids and tank ventilators that utilize negative pressure ventilation (see Positive and Negative Pressure Ventilation).

Bach and Alba (1990) reported on 25 adults requiring assisted ventilation following SCI. Based on their data, the authors advocate consideration of NIV in place of tracheostomy ventilation in this population where bulbar function and cognition are sufficient, even where an individual has very limited ability to breathe spontaneously. Twenty-three of the 25 patients who transferred from a tracheostomy to NIV perceived advantages in using this method (e.g., convenience, facilitation for speech and swallowing, appearance, and comfort). NIV may also yield the additional benefits of fewer respiratory complications and hospitalizations when compared to invasive ventilation and electrophrenic respiration (McCrory et al., 2001). Lead by the treating physician, and guided by research evidence into reintubation and mortality rates as well as length of stay findings (McCrory et al., 2001), the multidisciplinary team may consider use of NIV as a supportive therapy for tracheostomy decannulation, to facilitate clearance of secretions and prevent ventilatory failure. Whenever any change in ventilation methods are considered, protocols are established by the clinical team primarily to ensure that early signs of ventilatory failure are identified and appropriate steps are taken to restore satisfactory ventilatory performance. Where NIV was used this would involve establishing targets across a range of respiratory parameters. Speech pathologists working with NIV would benefit by participating in multidisciplinary education including the use of respiratory biofeedback, secretion clearance techniques, and glossopharyngeal breathing techniques. An awareness of how patients may apply glottic, pharyngeal, and oral control techniques to improve cough effectiveness and support spontaneous breathing efforts provides speech pathologists with knowledge that may be applied in the management of dysphagia associated with SCI. For a thorough description of NIV the reader is referred to Bach and Goncalves (2006).

Selection of Assisted Ventilation Method. Different ventilation delivery methods can be used during acute or long-term care. A patient may experience various forms of assisted ventilation as respiratory function evolves. Progression from short- to long-term assisted ventilation necessitates a discussion among medical and nursing staff, therapists, the individual, and often family to determine each patient's suitability for the use of invasive or non-invasive ventilation techniques. The choice of a particular approach to assisted ventilation is largely facility specific, but may also depend upon the local expertise and technical support available for each of the assisted ventilation methods. There are a number of patient-specific factors that must also be considered, including the patients' level of assisted ventilation dependence, bulbar neuromuscular control for both airway protection and ability to use non-invasive interfaces, cognition, finances, and personal preference (e.g., EPR is considered only for patients whose need for assisted ventilation is expected to be lifelong).

Respiratory and Ventilatory Treatments

Respiratory and ventilatory treatments for persons with SCI are prescribed by intensive care and respiratory physicians, respiratory care practitioners, and physiotherapists. These treatments have various purposes including: effective management of airway secretions in the presence of an impaired cough; maintaining the range of movement in the chest wall and lungs; providing an emergency form of respiratory support (like during a power failure in assisted ventilation); and educating patients in how to monitor their own ventilatory status in preparation for discharge from hospital. The following sections highlight techniques that may be relevant to dysphagia intervention.

Manually Assisted Coughing. This technique assists clearance of airway secretions by increasing the peak cough air flow, and is necessary for patients with a cervical SCI whose diaphragmatic impairment disables their cough effectiveness. Taught by nursing and respiratory clinicians, manually assisted coughing involves a maximal inhalation (either achieved spontaneously or ventilator assisted) followed immediately by a thrust to the abdomen with the hand or arm as the patient coughs on exhalation. The technique may be performed by individuals with SCI with spared arm movement. A trained caregiver or clinician can provide assistance to individuals with complete tetraplegia.

Mechanical Insufflation-Exsufflation. The aim of mechanical insufflation-exsufflation (MI-E) is to clear airways of pooled secretions when individuals cannot do this personally. MI-E requires the use of a device (Figure 3-8) to gradually increase positive pressure into the airway (insufflation) followed immediately with a shift to negative pressure within the airway (vacuum, delivered via the nose and mouth or tracheostomy) to create a forced exsufflation (cough). In non-

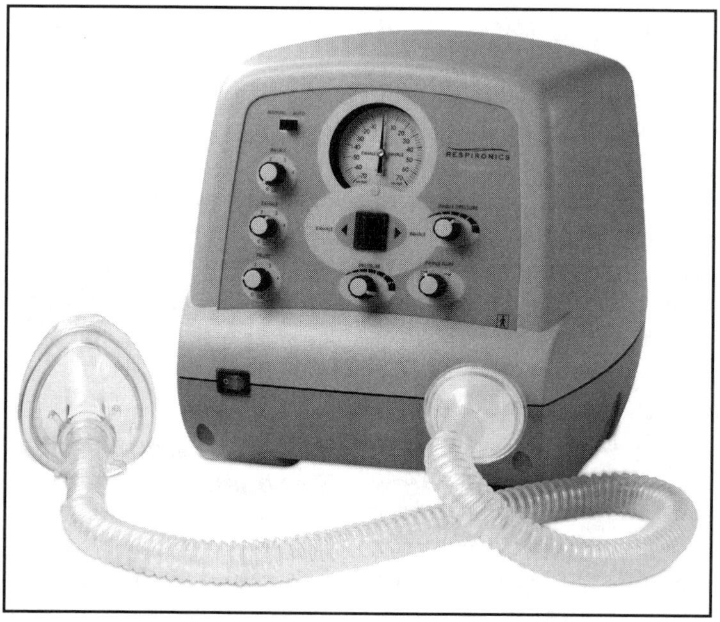

Figure 3–8. Manual insufflation-exsufflation (MI-E) device. Image provided from Respironics (http://www.respironics.com). Reprinted with permission.

invasively ventilated patients it replaces tracheal suctioning and is performed on an individual needs basis and proactively to avoid or treat chest infections. MI-E can be used with a face mask or mouthpiece or can be attached to a tracheostomy tube (and therefore can be used pre- and post-tracheostomy decannulation). MI-E advocates explain that its proper use can prevent the need for a tracheostomy where the tracheostomy is required only for suctioning retained upper airway secretions (e.g., where swallowing is unimpaired). Where dysphagia is present and causes persistent aspiration of saliva, MI-E would not be considered a substitute for tracheostomization. Non-tracheostomized patients using MI-E may have decided to avoid tracheostomization where possible. Such a decision could have been made with consideration to perceptions of cosmesis, concerns about infection (both respiratory and at the stoma), loss of speech quality, cost of consumables, and feelings about greater dependency on aids among, other factors (McCrory et al., 2001).

Glossopharyngeal Breathing. Glossopharyngeal breathing (GPB) is a modified breathing technique that patients with very limited spontaneous breathing ability may utilize. The majority of high-level tetraplegic patients can learn GPB sufficiently to maintain normal alveolar ventilation for a very limited period in the event of mechanical ventilator failure. The ability to use GPB is limited in the presence of a tracheostomy tube (and is impossible if the cuff cannot be deflated), or where bulbar function and cognition are not intact. GPB involves the repeated upward movement of the glottis to capture inhaled or oral residual air boluses in order to "stack" them in the lungs, thus enhancing inspiratory intake. For example one "breath" may consist of 6 to 9 gulps of 60 to 200 mL each that have been stacked. Patients are trained to use their oropharynx, glottis, and accessory muscles to trap boluses of air until sufficient reserve is attained to augment a voluntary cough and/or improve voice. With medical clearance, physical and respiratory therapists may train patients to use this technique to maintain spontaneous unassisted breathing for limited periods of time. The reader is referred to Bach and Goncalves (2006) for further detail. The SLP may consider the possible benefit of training non-ventilator-assisted mildly dysphagic patients in the use of GPB as an aid to improving oropharyngeal and laryngeal control for rehabilitative dysphagia maneuvers. Although there is no supporting research evidence on this technique to date, GPB may be an efficient way to reinforce swallowing maneuvers that require breath holding, vocal fold adduction, effortful swallows, specific tongue positioning, or maintenance of high larynx positions (e.g., Mendelsohn maneuvers).

Incentive Spirometry. Incentive spirometry is a breathing technique used to train longer, deeper inhalations. Patients inhale through the mouthpiece of the incentive spirometer (Figure 3–9) and receive feedback on the flow rate and depth of their inhalation. Multiple, repeated daily practice is advocated for achieving longer, deeper inhalations. Enhancing the volume of inhalation helps to assist with mucus removal and oxygenation and may facilitate weaning from the ventilator.

Intermittent Positive Pressure Breathing. Intermittent positive pressure breathing (IPPB) uses a device to deliver

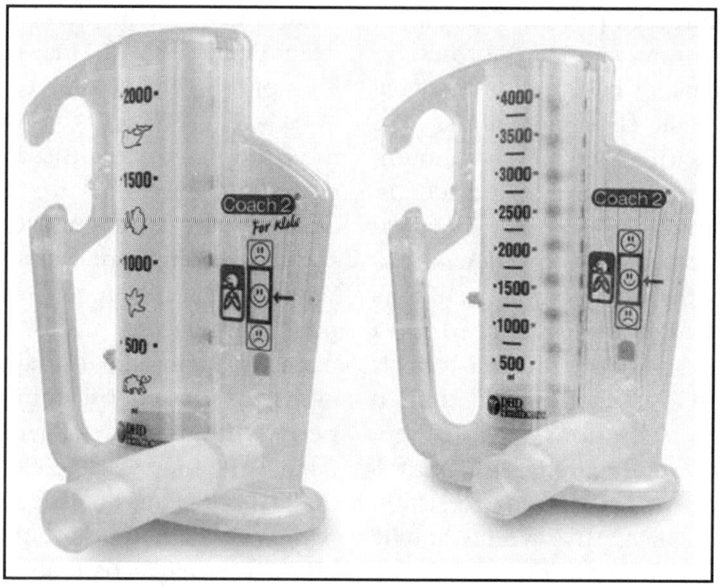

Figure 3–9. Incentive spirometer, adult and child models. Images courtesy of Smiths-medical (http://www.smiths-medical.com). Reprinted with permission.

increased pressure or volume of air during inspiration (Figure 3-10). It is a treatment technique used with intubated and non-intubated patients. It is designed to support deeper inhalations than incentive spirometry and spontaneous breathing alone, thereby preventing or treating atelectasis. Indications for use include those patients at risk for atelectasis, ventilatory failure, and reduced pulmonary function associated with a reduced cough reflex. Debate exists about the efficacy of this technique (Laffont et al., 2008). Patients requiring regular IPPB throughout the day are likely to have an unstable respiratory system, with fatigue and inconsistent swallowing coordination with breathing anticipated. Regular swallowing review will be required, and fluid and diet consistency may be modified to maintain swallow safety. For many patients, however, oral intake will cease and non-oral supplementation and hydration methods will be implemented until respiratory status improves.

Abdominal Binders. Abdominal binders are wide elastic belts worn by patients to improve blood pressure during the acute phase, and to support pulmonary function and cough effectiveness in patients with high cervical injuries. The abdominal binder may be removed once there is no further improvement in these functions. Binders are used with individuals who breathe spontaneously as well as those who require assisted ventilation. Respiratory muscle retraining, in combination with abdominal binders, can improve speech in SCI (Brown et al., 2006). Although no evidence exists as to the impact of abdominal binders on dysphagia, improvements in speech suggest that trial of an abdominal binder in a dysphagic patient (unless medically contraindicated) may have some impact on the shared

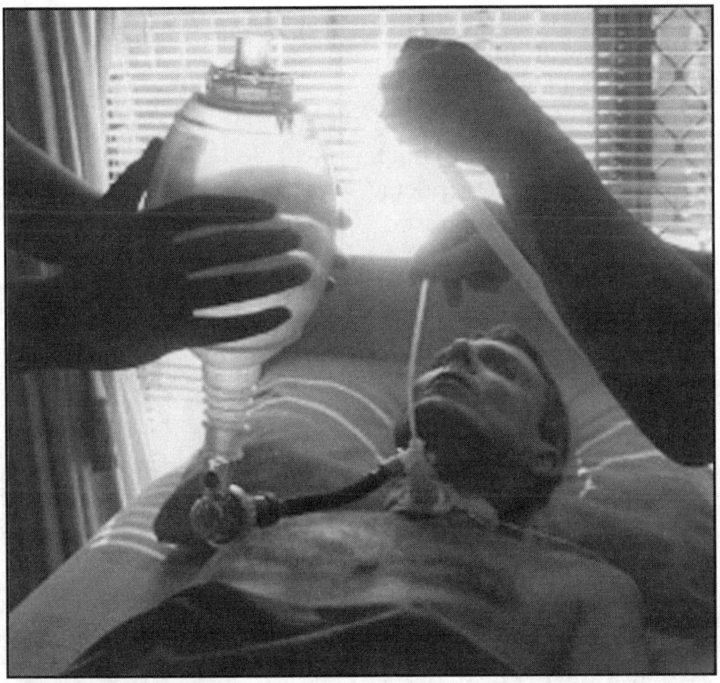

Figure 3–10. Intermittent positive pressure breathing (IPPB) provided manually with simultaneous tracheal suctioning to clear airway secretions.

physiology of speech and swallowing. In the acute phase of dysphagia treatment, it is important to determine whether a patient with dysphagia is using an abdominal binder and to monitor whether any changes occur in swallowing performance with its use or absence.

Respiratory Monitoring. Ongoing objective monitoring, including capnography, pulse oximetry, and arterial blood gas levels, can help identify early signs of ventilatory fatigue and indicate the need for intervention to prevent respiratory failure. Patients may receive training from respiratory clinicians prior to hospital discharge in how to self-monitor their respiratory function when at home. For example, respiratory clinicians may train patients to screen whether altered pulse oximetry levels are due to inadequate ventilation, retention of oral secretions, or intrinsic lung disease such as a chest infection and, if so, what action is required (e.g. urgent medical review or simply increasing the frequency of secretions clearance treatments).

Nonsurgical Management of Spinal Cord Injury

Movement of the injured spine has the potential to worsen spinal cord and spinal nerve root damage and therefore must be prevented or minimized. Traumatic injuries to the vertebral column that are stable and have minimal neurological injury are often managed conservatively. For example, conservative management of vertebral dislocation or subluxation may include a combination of bed rest, external fixation devices (such as traction and/or orthoses), and medications. Conservative management is not used where complete tetraplegia (with no expectation of recovery) has been diagnosed. Where neurological recovery is anticipated, acute stage management of soft tissue and ligament damage and stable fractures may involve the use orthoses (e.g., neck braces) and/or traction to immobilize fractures, decompress the spinal cord and nerves, avoid surgery, reduce pain, and in the case of orthoses, promote earlier mobility (for example, sitting in wheelchair, standing).

Cervical traction is a technique that applies a steady pulling force to the vertebral column to allow fragments to move into and maintain correct alignment during vertebral healing. In this way traction counteracts the effects of spinal cord compression, thereby reducing secondary neurological damage. Where this pulling force is maintained over a period of time, is it termed *traction* (e.g., a halo vest or tongs attached to weights and a pulley both provide traction). Where the pulling force is used briefly (such as during surgery or when fitting an orthosis under radiologic guidance), it is termed *distraction* or *reduction*.

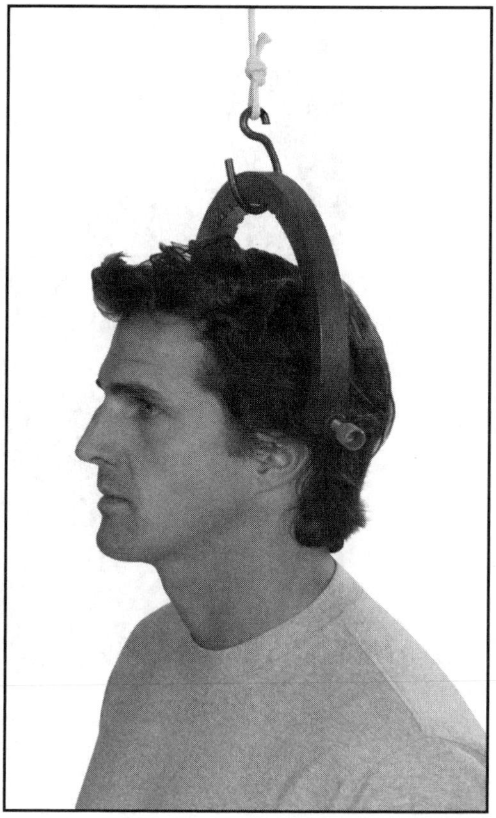

Figure 3–11. Cervical traction tongs. Image provided by Ossur (http://www.ossur.com). Reprinted with permission.

For cervical SCI, traction using skull tongs (Figure 3-11) is achieved by attaching metal tongs or calipers to the skull of the supine patient using spring loaded metal pins or screws that pierce the scalp to grip the skull. Traction is then applied with graduated force by the attachment of a pulley and free weights to the calipers/tongs for period of time (weeks), with alignment varying (extension or flexion), depending on the fracture being treated. As with many vertebral repair procedures, the spinal orthotist may apply a range of approaches and devices (for example, use of an additional chin sling or adjustment to the neck position). During this period the patient remains supine and must be turned regularly.

Cervical orthoses can be used while the patient is sleeping, seated, or mobile. An extensive range of custom-made and commercially available orthoses may be used to immobilize the cervical spine (Figure 3-12). Depending on the nature of the device, cervical orthoses limit both gross and fine vertebral movements to varying extents to support healing of the vertebral column and spinal cord,

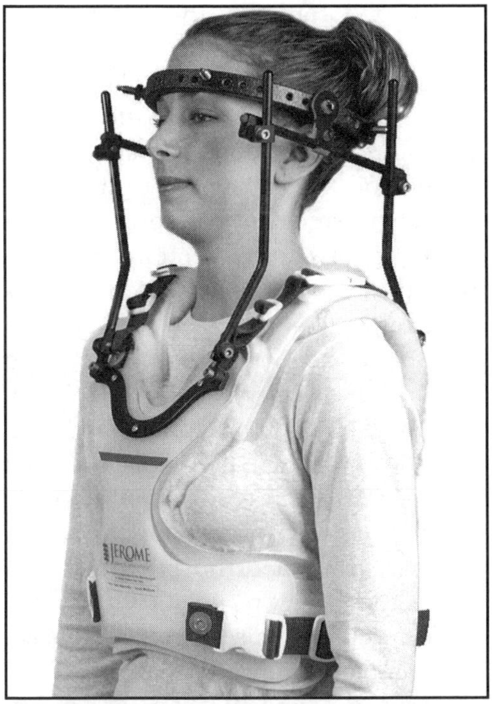

A

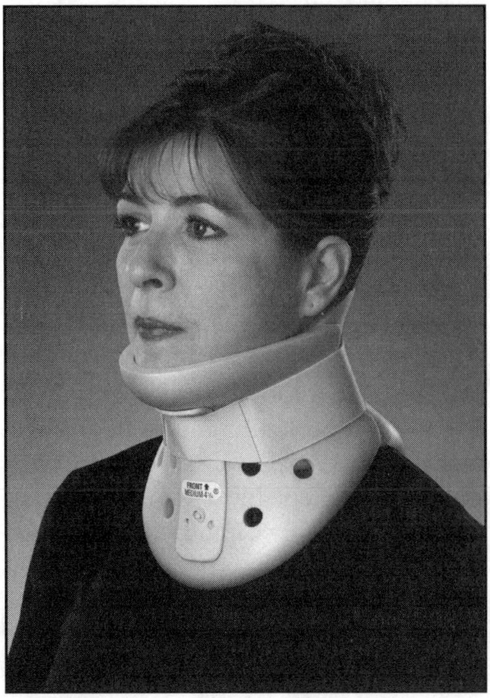

B

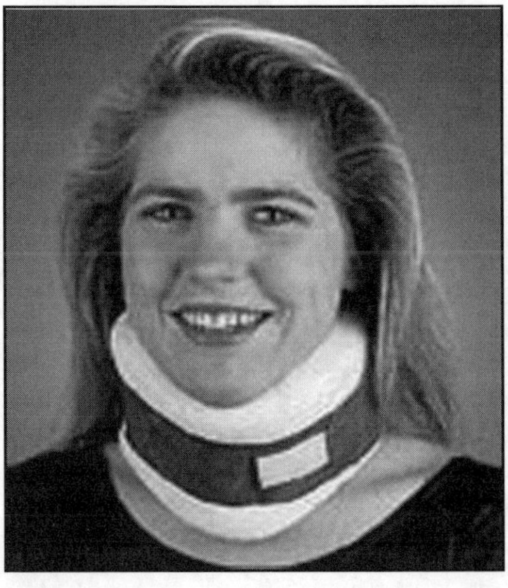

C

Figure 3–12. Examples of a halo brace (**A**), hard collar (**B**), and soft collar (**C**). Product images provided by Ossur (http://www.ossur.com). Reprinted with permission.

with allowances in cervical movement (e.g., extension, flexion) differing with each type. For example, soft foam collars allow a large amount of cervical movement and are generally applied to facilitate patient comfort and minor support. In contrast, hard collars limit flexion and extension. Throughout the recovery of vertebral stability, the patient may be refitted with a range of devices that respond to the vertebral healing process including a halo brace (named for its use of a metal support circling the head) (see Figure 3-12a), or a less restrictive hard neck brace followed by a soft collar (Figure 3-12b and c).

A halo brace involves a metal ring (halo) attached to the skull with four metal pins that is connected to a rigid plastic vest with four upright metal supports. It completely immobilizes the cervical spine (Figure 3-13) and requires skilled placement by a spinal orthotist, who confirms final alignment via radiography (Figure 3-14). In situations when an orthotist is unavailable, other devices (such as a sternal-occipital mandibular immobilizer brace, Figure 3-15) may be substituted, although these provide less restriction in movement.

It is important that the SLP be familiar with the types of different orthoses that may be used in their clinical settings, as some orthoses hold the cervical spine in positions that can inadvertently impinge on normal swallow physiology (e.g., chin extension). The presence of a cervical orthosis can, therefore, be a contributing factor to the swallow impairment due to the limitation of cervical movement and consequent changes in laryngopharyngeal mechanics (Han, Kim, Kim, An, & Lee, 2005). In acknowledgement of this potential complication the spinal orthotist asks the patient for feedback about ease of swallowing when fitting a cervical orthosis, and makes adjustments accordingly (where this does not compromise vertebral repair). For example, modifications may be made to a hard neck brace to allow for a mildly flexed chin tuck position for swallowing.

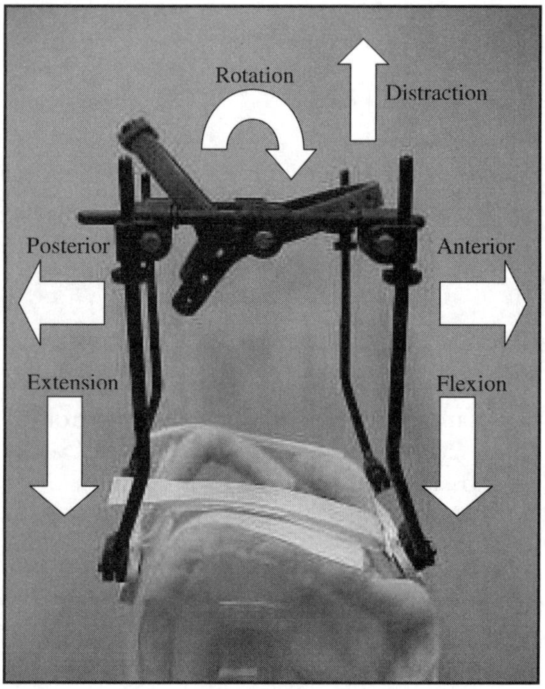

Figure 3–13. The halo brace applies cervical traction (*see distraction arrow*) and limits movement in all other planes indicated in illustration. Image provided courtesy of Mr. John Coffey, Spinal Orthotist, Princess Alexandra Hospital, Australia. Reprinted with permission.

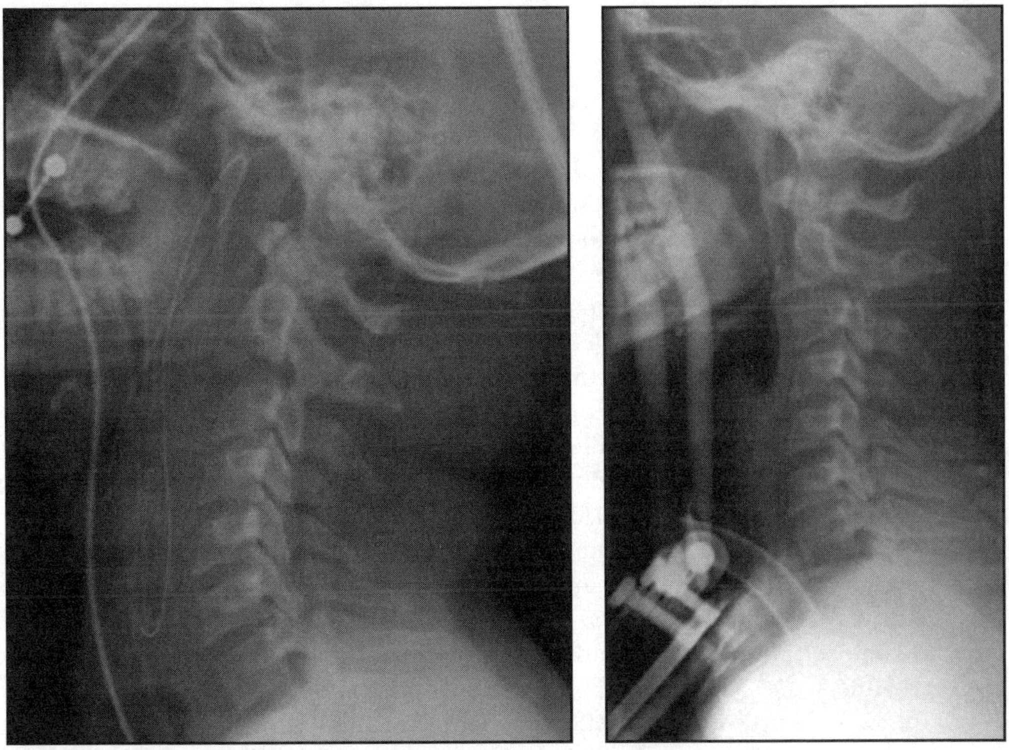

A B

Figure 3–14. Radiographic images of before (**A**) and after (**B**) halo thoracic brace fitting. Images provided courtesy of Mr. John Coffey, Spinal Orthotist, Princess Alexandra Hospital, Australia. Reprinted with permission

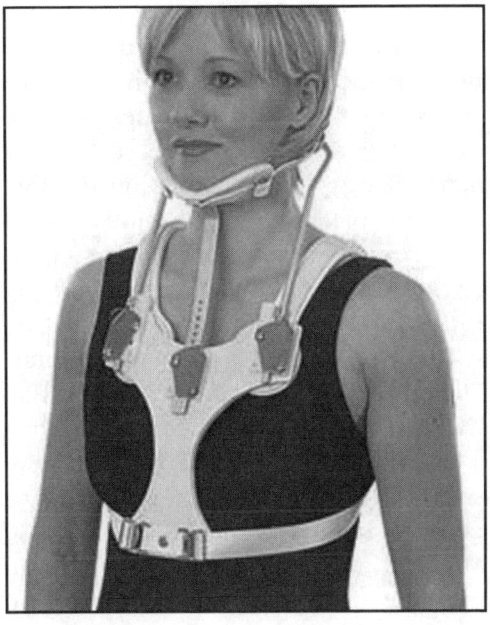

Figure 3–15. SOMI brace. Image courtesy of OPC Pty. Ltd. (http://www.opcpl.com.au). Reprinted with permission.

Any adjustment to a brace, however, requires medical approval.

Three studies have investigated the association between dysphagia and spinal orthoses in normal volunteers (halo vest: Morishima, Ohota, & Miura, 2005; soft neck collar, Philadelphia collar, and Minerva collar: Han et al., 2005; Philadelphia collar, sternal-occipital mandibular immobilizer [SOMI] brace, and halo thoracic vest: Stambolis, Brady, Kios, Wesling, & Hildner, 2003). Each study conducted videofluoroscopic assessments and found altered swallowing under the bracing condition compared to nonbracing in the majority of their volunteers. The extent of impact, however, depends on the type of device.

Of the cervical orthoses available, the halo thoracic brace limits cervical movement the most. In contrast, Philadelphia collars (see Figure 3–4) extend to the jaw anteriorly, occiput (posterior portion of the head) posteriorly, and upper thorax inferiorly, limiting neck flexion and extension to less than 30% of normal range of movement. SOMI braces (see Figure 3–15) are cervico-thoracic orthoses that can be used in place of a halo vest in situations where it is not possible to use the more invasive procedure of fixing the heavy metal halo to the skull (e.g., in the frail aged or palliative population). SOMI orthoses have a removable head strap to release the mandibular support during eating, thus providing only minimal restriction in flexion/extension movements. Like the SOMI, the Minerva cervico-thoracic brace is more lightweight than a halo brace and does not require "invasive" fixation (i.e., skull screws). In a comparison between soft collars, the Minerva, and the Philadelphia collar, Han et al. (2005) reported most alteration with the Minerva collar, where reduction in oropharyngeal diameter, decreased hyoid movement, increased residual volume, and a change in the initiation point of swallowing were evident.

Although the presence of an orthosis may alter the swallow process, it does not necessarily impair function or recovery for all patients. A study of dysphagia in high tetraplegia found that patients with and without a halo vest took the same amount of time (25 and 26 days, respectively) to return to a regular diet (Shem, Castillo, & Naran, 2005). However, where dysphagia is suspected, clinicians need to examine each orthosis for its potential to influence the biomechanics of the swallow. Collaborative review with the medical team and spinal orthotists at the bedside is essential to support vertebral repair and optimize swallowing function.

Surgical Management of Spinal Cord Injury

Although vertebral stabilization can be achieved through conservative methods for less extensive injury, more extensive spinal cord damage necessitates surgical repair of the vertebral damage to stabilize the fracture and decompress neural structures. Vertebral surgery is not without risk, with the potential for further neurological and/or tissue injury and infection associated with surgery. A number of surgical procedures may be undertaken to realign and stabilize damaged vertebral structures, and to relieve compression of the spinal cord and spinal nerves following a traumatic injury. The following sections outline the main surgical techniques used for patients following SCI.

Neural Canal Restoration

Restoration of the neural canal involves the removal of bone or disk fragments, blood clots, or foreign bodies from the spinal canal to restore the open diameter of the canal.

Reduction

Reduction involves realigning dislocated (i.e., where disruption in all ligamentous relationships to the joint can be demonstrated on imaging) or subluxed (partial dislocation) vertebrae into anatomic or near anatomic position. A closed reduction is nonsurgical and used when neurological injury is absent. An open reduction is a surgical intervention to relieve compression of the spinal cord.

Internal Fixation of the Spine

Goals of internal fixation include: stabilization of the vertebral column; maintenance of vertebral alignment; promotion of vertebral fusion; early rehabilitation; and avoidance of the use of a halo-vest brace. The process of attaching metal (such as titanium) rods, plates, or wires to the spine (individually or in combination) provides internal surgical stabilization of the vertebral column. In some cervical injuries, metal screws are implanted into the pedicles of the vertebrae as an alternative to the above materials and approaches.

Corpectomy

This procedure involves the removal of the vertebral bodies and the intervertebral discs at either end of the vertebra in order to decompress the damaged vertebral canal. One or more vertebral bodies are typically removed, and this defect is then restored with another material (a graft). An anterior approach for surgery is often used. The risks from this procedure include further SCI, bleeding, infection, spinal nerve damage, and graft damage.

Spinal Fusion

This process occurs following surgical removal of damaged vertebral structures. The aim of cervical discectomy and fusion is decompression of the spinal cord (that might arise from a range of processes including spinal cord swelling, disc herniation, and displaced bone fragments) where compression and neurological compromise are significant. In addition, surgical fusion is designed to restore intervertebral stability, augment natural vertebral fusion, allow earlier return to mobility, and reduce reliance on cervical orthoses. Different methods of spinal fusion are practiced and the devices implanted vary in their material composition, shape, and intended performance. In simple terms, spinal fusion restores intervertebral stability through the addition of a graft (often comprised of bone from the iliac crest of the hip if the patient is the donor or an allograft from the facility bone bank) or other material to the vertebrae. A cervical discectomy and fusion procedure may be undertaken with either an anterior or posterior approach. Anterior cervical discectomy and fusion (ACDF; discussed further in Chapter 5) has been reported in association with dysphagia for both nontraumatic (e.g., epidural abscess) and traumatic SCI at rates of between 2 and 60% (Lee, Bazaz, Furey, & Yoo, 2007). ACDF requires a dissection at the low anterior aspect of the neck (right or left side), and the larynx, pharynx, and esophagus are manipulated and retracted so that the anterior aspect of the cervical spine is exposed. The intervertebral disc(s) and any other sources of compression (such as bone fragments) are removed to allow examination of the compressed spinal nerves and/or spinal cord. A bone graft or other material is then placed between the vertebrae and a plate is screwed to the front of the cervical spine (Figure 3–16). In a prospective longitudinal study of 310 patients who underwent ACDF (following nontraumatic and traumatic SCI), dysphagia was more prevalent immediately post-surgery, with prevalence figures found to reduce over time from 54% at 1 month to 15.2% at 12 months and 13.5% at 24 months (Lee et al., 2007).

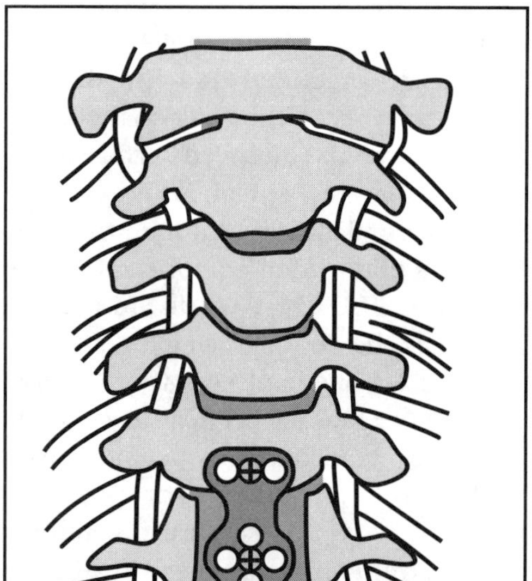

Figure 3–16. Schematic of the anterior view of an anterior cervical plate in situ.

Possible Surgical Complications

The surgical procedure itself, or hardware used during surgery, may result in surgery-related complications (e.g., migration of a screw from an anterior cervical discectomy and fusion repair). For example, damage to the pharyngeal and esophageal walls causing perforation may result in a mechanical pharyngeal dysphagia. Such complications are relatively rare, with Gaudinez et al. (2000) identifying just 44 instances of esophageal and/or pharyngeal perforation (EP/PP) in a series of 2946 patients. A patient with EP/PP may present with recurrence of spinal neurological deficits, dysphagia that is protracted or that deteriorates over a period of weeks, or a fever, or may have associated voice change and/or odynophagia. The SLP must alert medical team members if EP is suspected, as aggressive medical investigation may be required (Sahjpaul, 2007; Seidl, Niedeggen, Todt, Westhofen, & Ernst, 2007). Medical examination of posterior pharyngeal wall and esophageal integrity may be achieved with x-rays of the surgical repair, CT or MRI of the cervical spine, esophagoscopy, and/or VFSE. Radiological features that may indicate EP/PP include subcutaneous emphysema in the retropharyngeal space, loosening of screws, posterior esophageal diverticulae, retropharyngeal collection of gas and edema, widening of the mediastinum, pericardial or pleural effusion, and localized perforation. Serial radiographs of the migrated hardware through the gastrointestinal tract further confirm the cause of EP/PP in some cases (Gaudinez et al., 2000; Sahjpaul, 2007).

Once confirmed, EP/PP may be managed conservatively (e.g., medication and nil by mouth (NBM) with non-oral nutrition and hydration until esophageal fistula healing occurs) or with surgical repair (alteration of screw position). Where later complications occur (such as large perforations, extension to a cutaneous fistula, or abscess formation), surgical rehabilitation may be extensive and result in a protracted length of stay for the patient. The average length of stay was 253 days for patients with EP/PP compared to 125 days where no perforation occurred (Gaudinez et al., 2000).

Impact of Associated Conditions

For the majority of patients, factors in addition to the SCI will influence the course of care and recovery. Such factors may include the premorbid health of the patient, secondary injuries occurring with the spinal cord damage, medical/surgical trauma arising from aspects of acute care management, and long-term complications that accompany individuals with restricted mobility. Consequently, clinical management of this population requires consideration of not only the injured spinal cord but also of many concomitant factors, including the following.

Preexisting Medical Conditions

Conditions that may influence acute care interventions include poor lung health, advanced age, nutritional state (extreme overweight or malnutrition), sleep disorders, prior or comorbid neurological conditions, and/or degenerative changes to the spinal cord, for example, ankylosing spondylitis (a chronic inflammatory arthritis that causes calcification of the spine and adjacent structures and commonly progresses to eventual fusion of the involved joints)(Dawodu,2007).

SCI Syndromes

High cervical SCI syndromes affect facial, oral, pharyngeal, and esophageal functions variously due to damage to the spinal tract of the trigeminal nerve. These include Horner syndrome, which results from damage to the cervical sympathetic chain. The syndrome presents as ptosis (inability to open the eyelid), constriction of the pupil of the eye (miosis), and lack of sweating (anhidrosis). Posteroinferior cerebellar artery syndrome (PICAS) may arise following interruption of blood flow through the vertebral artery as a result of displacement of the cervical vertebral column. Symptoms of PICAS are diverse and may include dysphagia, dysphonia, hiccups, vertigo, vomiting, and cerebellar ataxia (Davenport, 2008).

Trauma

In addition to preexisting conditions, trauma that occurred with the SCI can complicate management. Hsu, Dreisbach, Charlifue, and English (1987) reported that where spinal cord injured patients experienced cooccurring injuries, 38% of these were head injuries, 21% chest injuries, 17% soft tissue damage to the neck, and 9% laryngeal fractures.

Impact of Trauma Intervention

Interventions required during acute care (e.g., during vertebral alignment and realignment) may result in further injury. For example, patients with cervical fracture must wear orthoses for vertebral alignment. Orthoses may minimize access to the upper airways and limit the patient's head and neck positioning, impairing the surgeon's ability to perform endotracheal intubation under ideal conditions, and laryngeal trauma may result. Laryngeal trauma may include vocal fold damage and, more rarely, arytenoid cartilage dislocation (Rubin, Hawkshaw, Moyer, Dean, & Sataloff, 2005).

Medications

Pharmacological management can have undesirable side effects, particularly for individuals who were dependent on multiple medications prior to their SCI. Some of these side effects may alter levels of alertness, orientation, and motor function.

Sleep Disorders

Many patients with SCI experience sleep disorder that may in turn be associated with diminished appetite, endurance, cognitive function, and mood (McCrory, 2001; Porth, 2005). *Sleep disordered breathing* is usually assessed by a respiratory physician using pulmonary function testing, sleep studies (polysomnography), clinical observation, and nocturnal oximetry and capnography. Treatment for sleep disorders in spontaneously breathing patients might include weight reduction, surgery, and/or nocturnal non-invasive ventilation. For daytime ventilator assisted patients, ventilator settings can be optimized for sleep.

Management of Pressure Areas

In SCI loss of muscle bulk below the level of the spinal cord lesion and inactivity place the patient at risk for the development of pressure areas and ulceration. Patients may remain in prone or supine positions for lengthy durations while tissues recover. In dysphagic patients, this may complicate swallowing as patients may be required to consume meals in these positions.

Altered Muscle Tone

Despite a lack of active movement in paralyzed limbs following SCI, affected muscles retain a low level of contraction or tone. Spasticity (increased muscle tone, spasms and tendon jerks as a consequence of hyperexcitability of spinal reflexes) is described as an upper motor neurone syndrome that may occur following SCI (Adams & Hicks, 2005). Nerve cells below the level of the SCI produce exaggerated reflex responses to pain, passive muscle stretch, and other stimuli throughout the body. Spasticity may range from a mild and infrequent occurrence to a severe and frequent problem. Without interventions (e.g., resting splints for the hands,), contractures of affected joints can arise from spasticity and lead to pain, loss of function, skin breakdown and deformity. Breathing ability may alter to some extent as initial muscle flaccidity is replaced with muscle spasticity. If distressed by symptoms of spasticity, patients may require systemic or locally injected medications, physical therapies and occasionally, surgery (Adams & Hicks, 2005).

Autonomic Dysreflexia

This is a serious complication following SCI. Patients with cervical spinal cord injuries are at greatest risk for autonomic dysreflexia. It occurs rarely for patients with injury below T6. Autonomic dysreflexia is an overreaction of autonomic nerves to noxious stimuli to the skin, bowel, or bladder (such as distended bladder, toenail infection) that the patient is unable to feel. In autonomic dysreflexia, an uncontrolled release of the hormone norepinephrine occurs. This hormone release triggers a dramatic increase in blood pressure and a slowing of the heart rate. The patient may experience an intense headache, profuse sweating, nausea, blurred vision, and goose bumps below the level of the injury. The condition can become chronic and recurrent, often in response to longstanding medical problems such as bowel and bladder irritation or pressure sores. The increase in blood pressure that occurs during autonomic dysreflexia can rapidly result in fitting, loss of consciousness, brain hemorrhage, or death. Medical assessment of autonomic function can be undertaken as a routine acute care evaluation to determine the risk for autonomic dysreflexia (Dawodu, 2007). Aggressive medical management is required when autonomic dysreflexia is suspected.

Psychological Adjustment to SCI

In this population of largely cognitively intact, previously active, young, and employed adults, significant psychological adjustment is necessary following spinal cord injury. Many patients will require referral to multidisciplinary specialists to support psychological adjustment during the acute phase of care. Early resumption of speech or other communication methods may have a positive impact on a patient's ability to cope with this adjustment (Tippett, 2000). Occasionally, the SLP might encounter patients and their families that express anger, anxiety or discouragement where tube feeding is recommended, or meal and fluid textures are downgraded. Patients may refuse dysphagia interventions. Such circumstances should be discussed within the multidisciplinary team. A majority of patients show great resilience in the face of the changes that a SCI demands of their lives beyond hospitalization. Regular involvement in multidisciplinary and family meetings enables SLPs to gain a broad understanding of the patient's psychological state and to then sensitively prioritize goals in dysphagia management. Clinical experience has shown that judicious involvement of a trained peer counselor (i.e. a carefully selected person with a spinal cord injury and a positive perspective on life following injury) may provide encouragement to patients and their families who consent to these visits.

DYSPHAGIA POST-SPINAL CORD INJURY

The assessment and management of dysphagia following SCI is influenced by factors that are particular to this clinical population. Each of these requires appraisal by the managing SLP to determine the likely impact, association, or causative relationship on swallowing function. Factors including the presence of preexisting conditions that increase vulnerability for dysphagia, the general medical state of the patient, positioning requirements, orthoses, surgical interventions, the need for assisted ventilation and/or a tracheostomy, the individual's need for the assistance of others during mealtimes, and the cognitive/emotional state require consideration at each intervention. Any planned changes in clinical management, such as changes to assisted ventilation status, the commencement of short trials of upright sitting, or a change in external fixation devices (e.g., cervical orthoses), may alter the patient's swallowing status and necessitate reevaluation of swallow safety under the changed condition(s). For this reason, decisions regarding aspiration risk, dysphagia severity, and management goals require frequent and ongoing review during rehabilitation post-SCI.

Importance of Multidisciplinary Care and Planning

The medically complex status of patients with SCI and the limited research evidence available supporting dysphagia interventions in this population present a challenge to even experienced clinicians. Where the SLP actively seeks communication with the patient and team members as to each patient's clinical path, he or she will be better able to facilitate interventions that respond appropriately to the total recovery process. A coordinated multidisciplinary approach to dysphagia management is recommended at all times. This approach ensures that SLPs maintain safe practice during swallowing assessment and treatment and are cognizant of broader rehabilitation frameworks and timelines. In addition close team work can enable timely use of instrumental assessments of dysphagia, which is of benefit as there is so little published research available to guide dysphagia practice in SCI. Table 3-13 provides some examples of situations when the actions of other team members may influence the direction of dysphagia management.

Table 3–13. Examples of Multidisciplinary Goal Setting and the Potential Impact on Dysphagia Management

Team Member	*Planned Activity*	*Opportunities or Implications for Swallow Management*
Medical Officer	Commencing trials of weaning from tracheostomy tube	Discuss dysphagia management priorities with treating physician and patient (e.g., instrumental swallow evaluation while tracheostomized to support weaning if this is expected to take weeks or months; or propose suspension of oral intake trials if tracheostomy weaning trials are imminent).
Medical Officer	Planning return to surgery: medical team decide to delay decannulation until recovered from surgery (weeks)	If tracheostomy is to be in situ long term, then SLP may propose use of a speaking valve (+/– ventilator settings adjustments) or specialized tube to support speech and swallowing rehabilitation. SLP may recommend nil by mouth for 24 hours post-tracheostomy tube change and until SLP swallowing evaluation post-surgery. SLP will request medical advice for timing of reevaluation of swallowing post-surgery.

Table 3–13. *continued*

Team Member	*Planned Activity*	*Opportunities or Implications for Swallow Management*
Medical Officer	Planned chest x-ray/ bronchoscopy	Opportunity to assess and discuss chest signs of aspiration or recovery from aspiration with treating physician.
Physiotherapist	Patient to commence sitting and mobility program	Indication that patient may soon be able to sit for oral intake (post-surgery and halo thoracic vest adjustment) and leave ward to attend physiological swallow assessment in radiology suite.
Physiotherapist/ Respiratory Therapist	Patient currently requiring active chest management	Discuss indicators for/against tracheostomy weaning including frequency and type of ventilatory therapies, effectiveness of spontaneous and assisted cough, and evidence of respiratory fatigue/aspiration during previous cuff deflation or oral intake trials (where these have been recently implemented).
Occupational Therapist	Readiness to trial voice recognition technology	Determine patient candidacy for trials of a speaking valve or "leak speech" (MacBean et al., 2008) in patients who are ready to access voice recognition software. Where speech trials are not possible, collaborate to establish access to communication technology.
Spinal Orthotist	Planned readjustment to traction and movement restrictions to be determined following cervical x-ray; cervical orthoses may be changed	Assess whether cervical orthosis fit alters patient control over swallowing. Access for palpation of laryngeal elevation and cervical auscultation is easier with a halo thoracic vest when compared to a hard collar (e.g., Philadelphia collar).
Registered Nurse	SP to seek brief review at each intervention to receive clinical update	Following chart review seek report on clinical changes and scheduled procedures that may influence dysphagia programs (for example, schedule dysphagia assessments during "optimal" positioning in patients with limited sitting endurance—discuss whether return to semirecumbent position is planned for all/some meals/medications/nasogastric feeding?)
Dietitian	Assess adequacy of caloric intake	Discuss ongoing requirement for supplemental feeding via nasogastric/gastrostomy tube. Removal may improve the mechanics of swallowing but maintaining adequate caloric/fluid intake may not be possible.

Prevalence, Predictive Factors, and Prognosis for Dysphagia Post-Spinal Cord Injury

The prevalence of dysphagia in SCI has not been systematically investigated, and therefore accurate data are not available. For those patients expected to be at the highest risk for dysphagia, such as those with high tetraplegia requiring acute care monitoring, dysphagia has been reported in 71 to 80% of cases (Shem et al., 2005; Wolf & Meiners, 2003). Further, in a study of 51 patients following SCI, half of the 80% of patients classified with swallowing difficulties at admission to intensive care were rated as having severe dysphagia (with a major aspiration risk). The remaining half were classified as having mild dysphagia, characterized by laryngeal edema, mild aspiration, and an effective cough response (Wolf & Meiners, 2003).

It is naturally anticipated that dysphagia prevalence would be higher among etiologies that result in both tetraplegia and associated multitrauma. Similarly, there is higher risk for elderly patients or where preexisting medical disorders complicate clinical management. Overall levels of functioning in terms of cognitive state, mobility, and mood are more commonly interrupted by medical problems, such as urinary tract infection, pneumonia, and confusion, in the aged patient when compared with younger patients with comparable SCIs. These medical vulnerabilities in the aged population can have a direct effect on swallowing ability and management.

A number of possible predictors for the presence of dysphagia following cervical SCI have been proposed; however, the relative value of these factors is debatable. Brainstem injury and ankylosing spondylitis were found to be predictive of dysphagia (Winslow, Winslow, & Wax, 2001), as were the presence of a tracheostomy and assisted ventilation with or without pulmonary complications (Abel, Ruf, & Spahn, 2004; Kirschblum, Johnston, Brown, O'Connor, & Jarosz, 1999; Shem et al., 2005). Despite the expectation of advanced age being linked to deterioration in swallow ability, age at injury was not found to be a predictor of swallowing function at admission to a SCI intensive care unit (Abel et al., 2004; Wolf & Meiners, 2003). Regarding level of injury, it has been reported that high and complete levels of SCI are more likely to be associated with dysphagia (Abel et al., 2004; Shem et al., 2005), whereas others have reported no association between dysphagia and level of SCI (Wolf & Meiners, 2003).

There is good prognosis for recovery from dysphagia in cervical SCI during the acute phase of care (Brady et al., 2004). Wolf and Meiners (2003) studied dysphagia in 51 patients consecutively admitted to a spinal cord injuries intensive care unit with tetraplegia (some of this cohort required assisted ventilation via a tracheostomy). Authors reported a statistically significant association between a higher level of SCI and a poorer dysphagia outcome on discharge. Overall dysphagia outcomes were excellent, however, with only one of the 51 patients not able to take any food orally at discharge.

Assessment of Dysphagia Following Traumatic Spinal Cord Injury

Injury to the cervical vertebrae may cause damage to prevertebral tissues and compression of the pharyngeal space as local tissue responses to injury such as inflammation evolve. In some circumstances cervical spinal cord injuries may progress to include the brainstem and cranial nerves (e.g., ascending edema) to result in a neurological dysphagia (Wolf & Meiners, 2003). Physiological and mechanical consequences of surgical management and other acute care interventions can also contribute to dysphagia severity. As such there is potential for impairment in all phases of swallowing and for each presentation to be unique. Systematic clinical and instrumental assessment of swallowing function for patients post-SCI is critical to identify aspiration risk and physiological targets for rehabilitation where treatment is appropriate.

Effective management of dysphagia and aspiration risk may assist successful weaning from assisted ventilation by helping to avoid pulmonary complications. Acute SLP management for the SCI population typically begins in intensive care or a high dependency trauma unit where the patient may be intubated and ventilated. Where a tracheostomy and/or assisted ventilation is in place, the SLP is urged to consider his or her own clinical competency and relevant departmental, facility, and professional clinical competency guidelines prior to providing services to patients with this level of respiratory compromise.

Importantly, early referral to SLP of acute tetraplegic patients at risk for dysphagia is supported by two small studies (Shem et al., 2005; Wolf & Meiners, 2003). Shem et al. (2005) found that patients assessed later by SLP developed pneumonia, whereas pneumonia did not develop in patients receiving an early SLP swallow evaluation. However, it is not known whether the group that developed pneumonia was referred later because a more severe clinical condition (and therefore at more risk of developing pneumonia from a range of causes) than the group that was referred earlier to speech pathology.

Where respiratory fatigue or failure is imminent, formal reassessment of swallowing safety is appropriate to prevent pulmonary aspiration of oral intake and oral secretions. Discussion within the multidisciplinary team may determine whether diminished respiratory function was a causal factor or a consequence of aspiration of oral intake and/or saliva. Deterioration in respiratory status, particularly in the acute phase of care, as signaled by high supplemental oxygen requirements, increased dependence on assisted ventilation, and more intensive secretions management or low oximetry readings, is a trigger for consideration of a nil by mouth order until (a) a physiological swallowing study can be undertaken, (b) an alternative cause is determined, and/or (c) the patient's condition improves. This cautious approach is necessary considering the high risk of further lung injury from aspiration of food, fluids, and oral bacteria in a patient with restricted mobility and a reduced ability to cough.

Although dysphagia assessment post-SCI largely follows the format of a standard clinical and instrumental assessment (as previously detailed in Chapter 1), population-specific considerations for the weaning or weaned patient will be discussed further below. Following this, specific issues relating to the assessment and management of the ventilated patient and the complex process of determining suitability for decannulation in the SCI population will be covered in the subsequent section titled "Assessment of the Ventilator Assisted and Tracheostomized Patient."

Clinical Swallow Examination

Consistent with a standard clinical swallow examination (CSE), the initial stage of the clinical assessment involves reviewing the existing medical history for dysphagia risk factors and factors limiting management decisions. It is strongly advised that the SLP undertake discussions with key medical, nursing, and other health staff, in addition to reviewing the medical notes, prior to patient contact in order to fully understand the complex medical state and rehabilitation process of the patient with SCI. In addition to the core information monitored for all patients with dysphagia, the following are population-specific issues that need review prior to dysphagia intervention with the SCI patient.

Injury-Specific Information. This includes the mechanism of SCI and the ASIA impairment scale rating, Glasgow Coma Score (see Chapter 2) on admission and at SLP assessment, and radiological findings of brain, spinal cord, and respiratory function. This data will inform risk for dysphagia and other key issues such as alertness, orientation, ventilatory needs, positioning and adequacy of respiratory support for swallowing.

Respiratory State and Management. History and current state of intubation and ventilation, including any weaning attempts, is needed. SLPs can observe oximetry and capnography patterns by recording baseline readings prior to their interventions. Any significant respiratory changes observed during SLP interventions must be relayed promptly to the nursing and medical team for review. Patients with a cervical or high thoracic SCI may have limitations in their ventilatory endurance, asynchronous spontaneous breathing patterns, difficulty clearing airway secretions and ventilatory fatigue. The SCI patient in acute care may sometimes experience pain (e.g., due to chest infection and intubation) during dysphagia assessment (when asked to cough, exhale, phonate, and swallow) and therefore not show as strong a response as might be possible. This can be determined by the SLP with relevant discussion, and can be accommodated for in dysphagia evaluation and treatment plans.

Chest Condition and Management. Clinicians need to familiarize themselves with the protocols for each patient regarding management of airway secretions (like suctioning regimens and/or use of any supportive respiratory maneuvers such as MI-E detailed previously in chapter).

Vertebral Restoration. Details of any surgical or conservative vertebral repair techniques that have been planned or undertaken should be noted and the resultant outcome for each approach.

Current Positioning Restrictions and External Fixation Devices. Patients managed by a conservative (nonsurgical repair) approach for vertebral fracture repair may need to remain supine, prone, semirecumbent, or in a side-lying position for a period of time with associated external fixation devices (e.g., traction/orthoses) fitted. For some patients this will mean that the SLP cannot assess swallowing in a preferred upright position as elevation beyond a surgically prescribed angle (often 30 degrees) may compromise spinal cord and vertebral healing. Specialized beds (like the Stryker frame or Rotorest bed) are designed to keep the fractured vertebral column stable yet enable staff to rotate patients into a limited range of positions (e.g., prone to supine or side to side) to promote lung health and skin integrity. Positioning limitations may continue for 6 to 12 weeks for patients who did not undergo surgery and for up to 6 weeks in patients following surgery. The SLP must therefore determine whether oral intake is safe in nonupright positions during this period. Although nonupright positioning is not optimal for oral intake, a significant group of patients will require nonupright positioning for many weeks, and consequently it is not appropriate to defer all dysphagia interventions. Patients may return to supine positions later in the clinical course for nursing management of skin pressure areas and ulcers. It is critical that the SLP seek medical consultation prior to considering any modification of patient position to optimize swallow safety. The effects of assuming supine positioning during swallowing have been the focus of two small studies (Barkmeier, Bielamowicz, Takeda, & Ludlow, 2002; Inagaki, Miyaoka, Ashida, Ueda, & Yamada, 2007). Both studies examined swallowing changes in normal adults assuming a supine position and revealed no significant differences in laryngeal function, though Inagaki et al. (2007) measured a mild decrease in swallowing duration in the supine position in comparison with more upright positions. However, given the inherent additional risks of dysphagia present for patients with a high spinal cord injury, where it is safe to do so, adjustment to a more upright position is recommended to promote a more controlled oral phase of the swallow and therefore a reduced risk of aspiration. The safety of eating and drinking in a nonupright position relies on thorough dysphagia evaluation, skilled carers/health team, accurate patient insight into dysphagia signs and consequences of aspiration, and close observations of the patient's chest and temperature status.

Psychological State. The majority of patients will undergo stages in the rehabilitation process when their emotional state and personal responses to their life-changing situation may impede or accelerate intervention effectiveness.

Outcomes of Any Previous Trials of Oral Intake. Depending on the clinical setting, referral to SLP may be made after other team members have observed signs of dysphagia on a screening examination or on initial trials of diet/fluids (administered by ward staff). The dysphagia observations of ward staff provide valuable information about current swallowing effectiveness, and mealtime strategies trialled to date that can guide subsequent assessment and treatment, as well as SLP dysphagia education to the multidisciplinary team.

Team Management Plan. Numerous events in the rehabilitation process will impact on dysphagia rehabilitation. For example, scheduled surgery, commencement of ventilator or tracheostomy weaning, and planned changes to positioning can all impact on the rate at which dysphagia rehabilitation will progress.

Once the patient's prior and current medical state has been determined, clinical examination can be undertaken. Issues for specific attention during oromotor examination of the SCI patient are in Table 3–14. Despite the expectation of an impaired voluntary cough in patients with a cervical SCI, the SLP should test voluntary cough strength and observe gag and

Table 3–14. Specific Considerations During Oromotor Examination Following SCI

Oromotor Component	*Cranial Nerve*	*Considerations for the SCI Population*
Lips	Facial (CN VII)	Typically preserved in SCI.
Tongue	Hypoglossal (CN XII)	Anterior tongue movements are usually preserved, but oral propulsion disorders occur in SCI, so thorough assessment of posterior tongue function is recommended. If impairment is suspected in lateral tongue movements required for cohesive bolus formation in chewing, this is best assessed via modified barium swallow in patients who may have impaired cough reflexes.
Jaw	Mandibular branch of trigeminal nerve (CN V)	Observations of range and strength of jaw movement will be made difficult where neck orthoses, tongs, or traction are used.
Larynx	Vagus (CN X)	Findings of dysphonia (with or without tracheostomy) in SCI may be due to: • Decreased respiratory support secondary to lack of innervation to accessory muscles of breathing, intercostals, and diaphragm • Laryngeal trauma secondary to endotracheal intubation (e.g., arytenoid cartilage luxation) • Tracheal damage limiting respiratory support for voicing (e.g., subglottic stenosis) • Organic laryngeal dysfunction (e.g., fixed vocal folds) secondary to damage to recurrent laryngeal nerve branch of cranial nerve X (vagus) • Generalized fatigue and fragile medical condition • Inadequate airflow around a deflated tracheostomy cuff (i.e., wide tracheostomy tube diameter in relation to patient's tracheal diameter) Where dysphonia is present and dysphagia risk is high, an endoscopic evaluation is warranted.
Cough	Vagus (CN X), phrenic nerves	Three phases constitute an effective cough: (a) inspiratory gasp (glottic opening and diaphragm muscle), (b) compression (glottic closure), and (c) expulsion (intercostal and abdominal muscles) (Porth, 2005). The degree of preservation of an effective cough post-SCI is largely dependent on the level of injury. A cough reflex may be present at the larynx when no bulbar damage is present, but is of limited function if the muscles of inspiration and expiration are no longer innervated. In patients who have a tracheostomy, the sensitivity of the trachea can be observed by the SLP when deep tracheal suction is needed. With severe desensitization, there

Table 3–14. *continued*

Oromotor Component	*Cranial Nerve*	*Considerations for the SCI Population*
		is no or limited reaction to the suction catheter on insertion deep into the trachea, where a violent coughing reflex would be expected.
Palate	Glossopharyngeal (CN IX), vagus (X), trigeminal (V), accessory (XI)	Examination of palatal elevation can be hampered by difficult visualization in patients with limited jaw opening due to cervical orthoses, etc. The presence of a wide gauge nasoenteric tube can also limit palatal elevation. Cranial nerve XI (accessory) is a motor nerve that has a cranial and spinal portion. The cranial portion supplies the uvula and the levator veli palatini muscles; therefore, damage to the cranial portion of the accessory nerve may limit velopharyngeal closure.
Gag Reflex	Glossopharyngeal (CN IX), vagus (CN X)	Although not a reliable indicator of swallowing function, the gag reflex can be an indicator of oral sensory protective reflexes. That is, a reflex that was initially present and is absent on a subsequent evaluation, in combination with other clinical signs of deterioration, may suggest a diminution in swallowing safety. In tetraplegic patients this sign may be important in indicating the progression of the SCI or rare complications of vertebral fusion surgery.

cough responses to invasive procedures (such as oropharyngeal and tracheal suctioning, if these are routinely performed) because some protective response can be expected despite being diminished in force. An absence of any protective response gives some indication of the state of laryngeal valving, sensory impairment, and aspiration risk. For some patients the preparatory swallowing examination (where no oral intake occurs) combined with consideration of dysphagia risk factors obtained during history taking may indicate a high probability of silent aspiration. Progression to an instrumental evaluation of swallowing (rather than a clinical trial of oral intake) under these circumstances may be the most judicious course in terms of patient safety and assessment efficacy.

Controlled trials of food/fluid boluses selected to minimize aspiration risk are conducted where silent aspiration risk is low. Food and fluid bolus trials should be delayed if a tracheostomy tube change is planned or has occurred within 24 hours; if management for respiratory distress or pneumonia is ongoing; if the patient is actively being weaned from assisted ventilation; where any acute deterioration is suspected; or if the patient is receiving parenteral nutrition only and nutritional absorption is impaired. In these instances, the SLP should advise the team on dysphagia risk based on the preparatory swallow assessment alone, recommending a nil by mouth order until the clinical status of the patient has stabilized.

When oral trials are appropriate, small fluid boluses (e.g., 3 mL) should be trialed initially (Figure 3-17). This is in keeping with safe practice whenever dysphagia risk is anticipated to be high and it is unknown what amount of aspiration can be tolerated before pulmonary status is compromised. Because oral preparatory phase impairments do not typically arise in SCI without a secondary injury (e.g., cranial nerve damage), assessment of this phase follows standard clinical assessment guidelines (see Chapter 1). One variation to this is the incorporation of straw drinking in initial evaluations of some patients to compensate for supine positioning or limited hand and arm control. It is still advised that 3 mL boluses not be exceeded initially, however, which the clinician can control by pinching the straw after each small sip. Oral propulsion phase deficits may occur in SCI, secondary to respiratory incoordination and/or loss of pharyngeal sensitivity. Oral propulsion deficits may be difficult to detect without a videofluoroscopic investigation and may be first indicated by multiple swallow attempts per bolus or an aspiration event.

The clinical assessment of the pharyngeal phase in SCI follows standard practices (see Chapter 1). During the acute phase of care, however, the SLP may be presented with unfamiliar equipment (e.g., traction, rotorest bed) and the presence of a hard or soft collar orthosis or tracheostomy tube, which can make the usual palpation of oral stage and laryngeal movements difficult (Figure 3-18). Where all other findings of the CSE indicate that oral intake may be safely trialed, the absent cough reflex in this population (C1-C3) should not be a barrier to

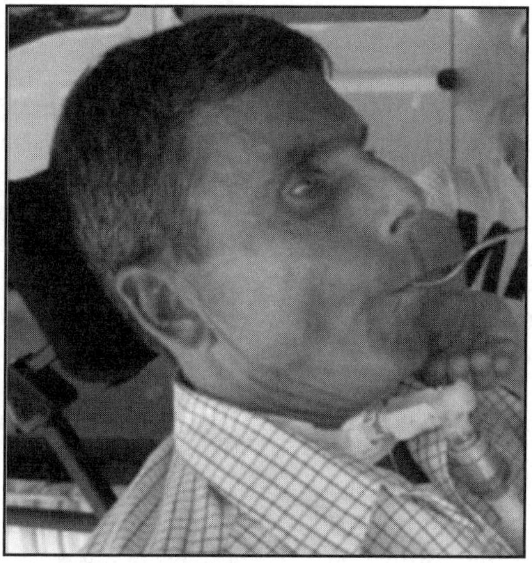

Figure 3–17. Small liquid boluses via spoon in a patient with tetraplegia.

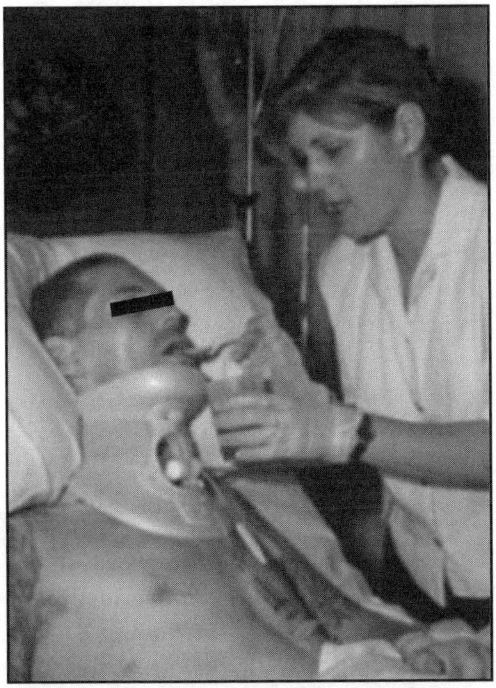

Figure 3–18. Illustration of the restrictions to head positioning for oral intake created by a hard collar in situ.

the delivery of limited oral trials (3 mL boluses) with SLP supervision, and clear guidelines for the cessation of oral intake trials discussed with the treating physician and documented in the medical record for the multidisciplinary team. When the cough reflex is absent, however, and assessment of the pharyngeal phase is difficult to conduct and/or interpret with CSE alone, an instrumental assessment of swallowing should precede the commencement of an oral diet, given the high risk of silent aspiration particularly in the acute phase of care.

Instrumental Swallow Examination

Early use of instrumental assessment is indicated for this population because of the high risk for silent aspiration and the lack of published research to guide SLPs in dysphagia practice for patients with SCI. Brady et al. (2004) conducted a retrospective study of 131 patients with both traumatic and nontraumatic cervical SCI. Clinical swallowing evaluations determined that 55% were dysphagic at the time of admission to a rehabilitation facility and, of these, 82% received subsequent instrumental swallowing evaluation.

The use of instrumental assessment has been reported to result in an earlier return to oral intake than CSE alone. In a study of 13 patients with high tetraplegia who had failed an initial CSE and a further patient who was suspected of dysphagia, 29% commenced regular diets following a videofluoroscopic assessment and 7% commenced a modified texture diet (Shem et al., 2005). In addition to diagnostic purposes, instrumental assessments offer a powerful tool for patient education. In this largely cognitively intact population, SCI patients can benefit from viewing the recordings from such assessments as a means of understanding their dysphagia and for conceptualizing the effect of therapeutic maneuvers. A number of factors must be considered, however, as regards the optimal timing and optimal instrumental procedure to be undertaken with each SCI patient. Discussion of these population-specific issues is outlined further in the sections below.

Videofluoroscopic Swallow Examination. Although both a videofluoroscopic swallow examination (VFSE) and an endoscopic swallow examination (ESE) have clinical application for the SCI population, reports of swallowing physiology in patients with tetraplegia have been largely compiled from VFSE assessments in the literature to date (Abel et al., 2004;

Brady et al., 2004; Ross & White, 2003; Shem et al., 2005). There are both staffing and procedural issues to be considered prior to instrumental assessment with the SCI population, and the need to maintain spinal alignment in unstable fractures (e.g., where halo brace is fitted) during any assessment cannot be overstated. Consequently, the SLP must be guided by the patient's physician regarding the safety of conducting a VFSE. In such instances, it may be difficult to achieve a full view of the oropharyngeal structures due to the presence of external fixation devices such as halo bracing. Where a patient's clinical picture is complex (for example, he or she is ventilator assisted, or there is deterioration in swallowing ability), VFSE interpretation by a radiologist will be required, rather than reporting by a radiographer and SLP alone.

Adoption of the patient's usual mealtime positioning for VFSE assessment is also of key importance for patients with high tetraplegia. Few patients with SCI are able to sit on the horizontal platform of the videofluoroscopy unit or grasp handles for stability. Consequently, assisted seating or semirecumbent positions may be necessary. For patients using wheelchairs, their wheelchair seating will have been custom fitted by the spinal injuries team or a specialist seating clinic. Some of the design features within a patient's own seating will have given consideration to headrest and seat angle adjustments to maximize the use of sip and puff, oral, and chin switch interfaces for access to technology and for comfort. In many instances a patient's customized wheelchair performs as an extension of that individual's body and enables significant gains in independence. Unfortunately, many of the new videofluoroscopy units are not wide enough for screening patient in their own wheelchair. In this case, patients need to be transferred to a VFSE chair. Commercially available VFSE chairs are useful for patients with lower SCI, while others with cervical and thoracic injuries are unlikely to feel stable in unfamiliar, nonprescription seating, and this may negatively influence swallowing performance. Nonetheless, commercially available videofluoroscopy units usually provide chest and head supports, so that with positioning guidance from the spinal physical therapist, these chairs enable patients to undergo assessment and gain valuable information. With medical approval and implementation of established protocols for minimizing aspiration risk and managing aspiration events should they occur, VFSE can be conducted in a supine position for those patients who must remain in this position for long durations of their recovery (Figure 3-19). Regardless of the situation, a team approach to positioning the patient is required, and this significantly increases preparation time for assessments.

Endoscopic Swallow Examination. ESE may be a more accessible tool than VFSE for the patient with a SCI during acute care, and its use with the SCI population has been described in a number of studies (Brady et al., 2004; Wolf & Meiners, 2003). Due to the clinical complexity of the SCI population, it is recommended that ESE is conducted jointly by an ear, nose, and throat (ENT) specialist and an SLP. In addition to the usual anatomical landmarks and functions explored in the initial stage of an ESE assessment, the clinician should ensure that they assess: the function and integrity of the posterior pharyngeal wall tissue at the site adjacent to anterior cervical fusion; effectiveness of the reflexive cough to

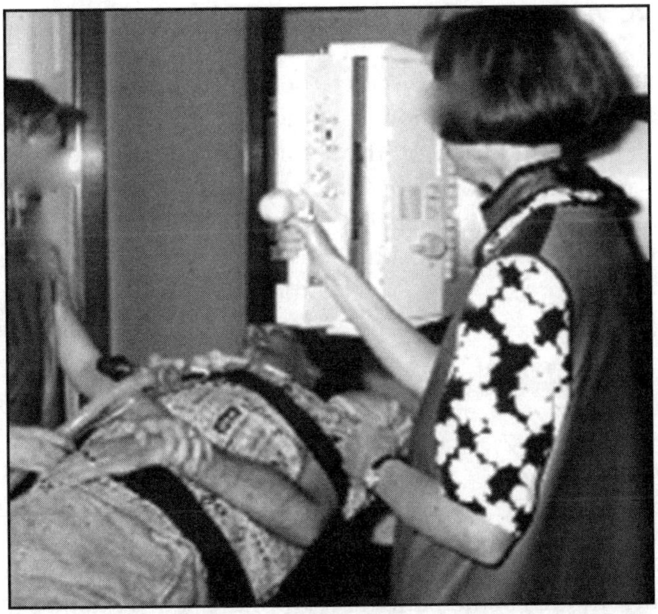

Figure 3–19. Conducting VFSE for a ventilator assisted patient while supine (positioning restrictions necessitated by the need for long-term pressure area management).

clear pooled or aspirated secretions; signs of vocal fold dysfunction (e.g., arytenoid dislocation); and signs of glottic stenosis and generalized edema. Moderate to severe laryngeal edema has been reported in patients with acute cervical SCI, and therefore the presence and extent of edema should also be documented.

ESE enables use of the patient's usual ventilator and seating, enabling a more valid evaluation of swallowing than would be provided with VFSE. As ESE assessment duration is limited only by patient tolerance (i.e., not limited by the risk associated with prolonged radiation exposure as with VFSE), it is possible with some patients to conduct more lengthy assessments, and gain greater insight into the impact of fatigue and so on. Alterations to physiology can be assessed under various ventilator and tracheostomy cuff conditions as required. ESE can also be used to help determine whether laryngeal sensitivity is impaired (see Chapter 1). Patients with SCI who have required a tracheostomy with an inflated cuff for 6 months or more are at greater risk of impaired laryngeal sensation due to the prolonged absence of subglottic airflow through the larynx and minimal stimulation of subglottic sensory receptors that influence glottic closure (Logemann, 1998). For these patients, laryngeal and tracheal sensitivity may be so diminished that no cough reflex is trigged even during deep tracheal suction. It is important for the SLP to differentiate between impaired laryngeal sensitivity and an impaired cough due to SCI at or above C5.

Wolf and Meiners (2003) reported contraindications for ESE in tetraplegic and respiratory compromised ICU patients, including *Klebsiella pneumoniae* (a bacteria found in the normal flora of the mouth, skin, and intestines that can cause pneumonia); methicillin resistant *Staphylococcus aureus* colonization of the respiratory tract; fractures of the facial bones; recent surgery to the nasal sinuses; dependence on ionotropes; disturbance of vertebral fracture healing; and risk of cardiac failure.

Clinical and Instrumental Assessment of the Ventilator Assisted and Tracheostomized Patient

Ventilator weaning is often protracted in SCI in comparison to the general critical care population. Although some patients are referred to SLP after they have been successfully weaned from both assisted ventilation and the tracheostomy, some patients referred for management may be in the process of weaning from ventilation, or will remain on ventilatory support (with or without tracheostomy) long term. In the wider population of TPPV users, some SLP services have adopted a policy of deferring trials of oral intake until patients have been decannulated; however, for patients with high cervical SCI who require lifelong ventilatory support, this is not an option.

The management of patients with SCI who require ongoing ventilatory support via a tracheostomy tube (TPPV) presents some of the most complex work undertaken by SLPs. Resumption of oral intake in ventilator users who are tetraplegic, alongside the loss of other body functions and social roles, is likely to influence quality of life perceptions in these patients (Tippett, 2000). Not all referrals to SLP for swallowing evaluation will be appropriately timed, particularly in the medically vulnerable group of TPPV users following SCI (e.g., if the patient is being actively treated for pneumonia) so the SLP may advise the team of indicators of patient readiness for dysphagia evaluation and defer SLP interventions until these indicators are present. Taking a role in educating the team on the risks and benefits of commencing oral intake in medically fragile SCI patients necessitates SLP acknowledgement of the lack of strong evidence describing dysphagia in the population of TPPV users post SCI. However, clinical practice guidelines are available for the wider population of adults who receive both acute and long-term TPPV, (Dikeman & Kazandjian, 2003; Tippett, 2000), and the SLP may use these as a very general guide for the population with SCI as discussed below.

Assessment of Aspiration Risk in the Ventilated Patient. Swallowing evaluation in the presence of TPPV must be authorized by the patient's physician, and should only be initiated once patients are medically stable, alert, and absorbing enteral feeds. Patients using TPPV who are referred to SLP for swallowing assessment fall into three groups: (a) those identified as being at high risk for dysphagia (such as cooccurring traumatic brain injury), (b) those who have demonstrated signs of dysphagia (e.g., non-SLP fluid trial has resulted in an aspiration event), and (c) those who have no demonstrated symptoms or risk factors for dysphagia (other than long-term TPPV use). Although the complexity of assisted ventilation technology, the fragile medical/respiratory condition of the SCI patient, and the lack of defined protocols for initiating and conducting dysphagia evaluations for the fully ventilated patient make conducting clinical swallowing evaluations of the ventilated patient particularly complex, cautious and judicious assessment can safely determine aspiration risk.

In assessing the risk for aspiration in the TPPV SCI population, it is relevant to note that the majority of spinal cord injuries do not result in dysphagia, and that the presence of ventilation does not automatically suggest dysphagia. Leder (2002) used ESE to study 52 patients with an acute illness requiring TPPV and concluded that more than two thirds swallowed safely. However, when aspiration did occur, it was largely silent in nature. Similar findings were reported by Elpern, Scott, Petro, and Ries (1994). Such evidence reinforces that, although some TPPV users can commence safe oral intake, this decision is best determined using instrumental assessment due to the risk of silent aspiration in approximately one third of the population. Indeed, a review of the literature pertaining to TPPV patients in general (Tippett, 2000) concluded that the CSE was inadequate for assessing the pharyngeal phase of swallowing and that instrumental assessment was recommended for a conclusive assessment. Instrumental assessment is therefore the most effective way of accurately determining aspiration risk and for developing early dysphagia management plans (McGowan, Gleeson, Smith, Hirsch, & Shuldham, 2007). If clinicians do not have access to instrumental investigations, it is suggested that several cautiously administered CSEs over consecutive days are required to make a dysphagia diagnosis and oral intake recommendations. Alternatively, if the patient is medically authorized to travel, then referral to a facility where an instrumental assessment can be conducted by an experienced team should be considered.

Aspiration of saliva is frequently reported in the tracheostomized patient with SCI and the possible causes for this are many. Up to 60% of patients with SCI have been reported to require frequent suctioning to manage "moderate to copious" secretions during their care (Hsu et al., 1987). Aspiration of saliva can be monitored and evaluated using a suction record form, designed to track the frequency of tracheal suction as well as the quantity and nature of secretions suctioned by nursing staff over a set period (typically 24 hours). New tracheostomy tube designs that allow above the cuff suction (e.g., Portex Suctionaid, Smiths Medical; see http://www.suctionaid.com) also facilitate such observations and allow clinicians enhanced ability to estimate of the amount of saliva aspirated, and from there to determine the relative risks and benefits of any dysphagia interventions.

It is prudent to couple the risk assessment for (a) the likelihood for aspiration of saliva (during cuff deflation trials) and (b) the impact any aspiration would have on the patient's well-being with the assessment of the potential for verbal communication in patients who are expected to require long-term TPPV. A team approach to the consideration of these risks is recommended. The SLP role in team management of cuff deflation in the SCI population is acknowledged in published protocols (Consortium for spinal cord medicine, 2005). Where tracheostomy cuff deflation is not possible, the SLP cannot gain vital information on laryngeal function. As such, the CSE is further limited, and only very general guidelines may be provided to the multidisciplinary team. As is true for spontaneously breathing nontracheostomized patients, the assessment of phonation and speech quality provides the SLP with essential information regarding aspiration risk. Patients using TPPV are advised, wherever it is medically safe to do so, to experience at least momentary periods of cuff deflation and voicing prior to a swallowing evaluation (Tippett, 2000). Indeed, when SLPs can "access the glottis" through tracheostomy cuff deflation, the quality of laryngeal function for phonation, coughing, or throat clearing during "decuffed" TPPV may suggest intact function in some instances and in other patients reveal laryngeal valving and airway protection issues that require more detailed swallowing and laryngeal investigations, including referral to an ear nose and throat surgeon.

A study of 12 tracheostomized patients who had recently weaned from ventilation reported that a deflated cuff (versus an inflated cuff) was associated with fewer and less severe aspiration occurrences as observed during VFSE studies of various bolus consistencies (Davis, Beras, Barone, Corvo, & Tucker, 2002). A decision to trial cuff deflation in TPPV users must be based on a prediction that aspiration risk is low. This prediction is based on a standard preparatory swallowing evaluation (no oral intake); examination of the amount of oral secretions suctioned (Dikeman & Kazandjian, 2003); the presence or absence of a cough or a discomfort reaction to tracheal suctioning (a lack of response is suggestive of depressed protective reflexes); as well as recording potential known risk factors for dysphagia in the individual, in the wider population of ventilator users and for the SCI population as a whole.

Should cuff deflation be considered an appropriate step in dysphagia management, the SLP must consult with the patient's physician and multidisciplinary team. Cuff deflation alters ventilation (creating a leak in a previously closed system), and in some ventilation modes, ventilator settings may need to be adjusted to accommodate the leak. The effects of cuff deflation on ventilation can be observed by monitoring the volumes and pressures displayed on the ventilator as well as respiratory measures (oxymetry and capnography) and patient comfort. Any significant deterioration in respiratory status during cuff deflation trials should be immediately noted and trials ceased. Depending on the patient, the effects of cuff deflation on assisted ventilation may be minimal or may trigger ventilator alarms (e.g., low pressure or low exhaled tidal volume alarm) that require a return to cuff inflation until new conditions for cuff deflation trials can be determined by the respiratory team. The possible reasons for marked changes in ventilation are many, ranging from the patient needing time and coaching to adjust to the return of airflow through the glottis, the presence of a mucus plug that requires immediate intervention (like deep tracheal suction) or an accidental disconnection of part of the ventilator circuit depriving the patient of the ventilator delivered breaths. Intact oropharyngeal and laryngeal valving assists in regulating exhalatory airflow during cuff deflation, and thereby maintains adequate ventilation. In patients with bulbar dysfunction, apart from dysphagia risk, ventilator adjustments may not be sufficient to compensate for the leak caused by cuff deflation, leading to chronic hypoventilation and precluding more than momentary cuff deflation, unless bulbar function recovers. As it is beyond the scope of SLPs' practice to interpret ventilator console readings or to recommend changes to ventilator settings, the patient's physician, critical care nursing, or respiratory clinicians should be present during cuff deflation trials to determine whether trials of greater duration may be undertaken. Patient safety considerations require that changes to ventilator settings for cuff deflation have been determined by the patient's treating physician, and that these settings, the duration of any trials, and the criteria for cessation of trials are documented in the medical record prior to commencing SLP intervention.

Where cuff deflation is permitted for patients using TPPV, the coordination between swallowing and the timed respiratory rate set during some ventilator modes may initially contribute to swallowing complications and aspiration risk, although this is yet to be extensively researched (Swanson, Schwartz-Cowley, & Dininny, 1991). Clinical experience suggests that in patients with mild or minimal dysphagia, this obstacle is rapidly accommodated if patients are encouraged to take the extra time needed to adjust to these respiratory changes during swallowing trials. As the acute dysphagia symptoms resolve, a proportion of patients who are ventilator assisted safely manage a soft/full diet and thin liquids without the need for supplementation, while their tracheostomy cuffs are deflated.

Once a consensus is reached by the multidisciplinary team to continue a cuff deflation program, one-way speaking valve trials can commence with the authority of the patient's physician. For many years the utility of one-way tracheostomy speaking valves in minimizing aspiration risk has been debated. No specific research is available in this area regarding patients with SCI. Current studies in other groups indicate a level of variability in patient responses to the use of a one-way speaking valve. Reduction in the frequency and severity of aspiration of thin fluids with the use of a one-way speaking valve in some spontaneously breathing patients using a tracheostomy tube has been reported (Elpern, Okonek, Bacon, Gerstung, & Skrzynski, 2000).

A study of patients receiving assisted ventilation following recently performed tracheostomies (Leder, 2002) concluded that aspiration rates were higher in older patients (mean age 73 versus 59 years) and was likely to be silent. This study did not discuss the influence of speaking valves or cuff status on swallowing ability; rather, it presented how swallowing can be influenced by each patient's "functional reserve" (or the ability to adapt to stress), the recency of the tracheostomy procedure, and the medical condition necessitating ventilation and tracheostomization. Specifically, the study reported a reduced functional reserve and ongoing medical condition may continue to cause dysphagia after tracheostomy decannulation and ventilator weaning. High silent aspiration rates in tracheostomized patients (with or without assisted ventilation) have led a number of authors to recommend instrumental assessment of the effects of cuff deflation or inflation and speaking valve use (Logemann, 1989; Suiter & Leder 2007).

The clinician may choose to supplement clinical assessment with other techniques such as the Evans blue dye test. Despite its use in this clinical population, the sensitivity of blue dye staining for the detection of aspiration of oral secretions or food and fluid boluses has not been established with large, well-designed studies for the ventilator assisted population. A study of 30 patients, however, reported 100% sensitivity in prediction of aspiration in a subgroup of ventilator assisted patients with use of a specific protocol for the modified Evans blue dye test (Belafsky, Blumenfeld, LePage,

& Nahrstedt, 2003). Blue dye testing serves as a quick screening tool in spontaneously breathing patients with a tracheostomy, where a positive result (i.e., blue dye present on tracheal suctioning) has been found to be more reliable than a negative result. The effectiveness of blue dye testing for microaspiration of oropharyngeal secretions, however, is reportedly limited (Donzelli, Brady, Wesling, & Craney, 2001; O'Neil-Pirozzi, Lisiecki, Momose, Connors, & Milliner, 2003).

Instrumental swallowing assessments can be employed with patients using TPPV where safety considerations can be met and sufficient time is allowed to ensure any additional intervention (e.g., tracheal suction) can be performed (Leder & Sasaki, 1999; Logemann, 1998; McGowan et al., 2007; O'Neil-Pirozzi et al., 2003). In the event that ESE is required while a patient is tracheostomized, the SLP can be guided by the protocol provided by Leder and Sasaki (1999), in which it is recommended that the larynx and pharynx be examined under the patient's usual cuff status initially. Few details are provided in this protocol, however, as to how the ESE should be altered for ventilator users or individuals post-SCI.

For patients with SCI who have retention of upper airways secretions with or without aspiration of oral secretions, visualization of the larynx during ESE may be obscured until these are suctioned. Suctioning may need to be performed via the oropharynx as well as the trachea. Even when it has been predetermined that cuff inflation will be maintained during oral intake, it may not be possible to use ESE unless momentary cuff deflation can occur to effectively clear secretions with simultaneous tracheal suction. Care must be taken to avoid aspiration of pooled secretions, and to this end, ideally above the cuff suction and pharyngeal suction should precede simultaneous partial cuff deflation and deep tracheal suction. A finding of persistent pooling of secretions in the oropharynx and larynx should alert the clinician to closely monitor overflow into the glottis (Leder & Sasaki, 1999). If gross pooling with glottic spillage is present, then the ice chip protocol is suggested as the safest option for proceeding with the ESE. Leder and Sasaki (1999) promote cuff deflation during swallowing trials (unless ventilator assisted) alongside brief digital occlusion of the tracheostomy with simultaneous phonation trials to determine the patient's effectiveness in clearing pooled secretions. If clearance of airway secretions is poor and aspiration of oral secretions is gross then the authors recommend that the patient is made nil by mouth. Where swallowing appears less compromised, the first consistency recommended is puree.

Use of the VFSE has been widely reported for patients with a tracheostomy (Logemann, 1998; O'Neil-Pirozzi et al., 2003); however, radiation exposure constraints limit the number and extent of swallowing behaviors that can be examined under fluoroscopy. Given the logistic constraints (e.g. SCI specialist staff attendance and equipment) for SCI patients attending VFSE clinic, careful preplanning of the food/fluid textures, swallowing conditions (e.g., tracheostomy inflated/deflated), and any compensatory or rehabilitation strategies to be examined is recommended to ensure efficient information collection within the radiation dosage limits. For patients with a tracheostomy tube, greater detail can be obtained on swallowing reflexes and laryngeal function when the tracheostomy cuff is deflated. The patient's ability to tolerate cuff deflation without compromise to ventilatory stability should be well established prior to the VFSE. Where cuff deflation and/or speaking valve trials are being evaluated, protocols for discontinuation should be determined by the SLP and medical team prior to the VFSE. Such cuff deflation and speaking valve discontinuation protocols would include, but are not limited to, clinical indicators of significant deterioration in baseline SpO2; triggering ventilator alarms (e.g., high- or low-pressure) that do not immediately respond to the interventions of the attending skilled respiratory clinician, registered nurse, or medical officer; patient discomfort; and more than trace aspiration of a test bolus. Such protocols may vary from facility to facility and should be individualized for patients.

Typically, the types of ventilators currently available in most critical care or intensive care units are not considered "portable" and have limited if any battery backup (though this is changing, with advances in technology producing sophisticated but portable units that can be used in critical care settings). As a consequence, in order to transport ventilated patients to the radiology department for VFSE, it may be necessary for the ICU team to transfer patients from their more sophisticated but nonportable ICU ventilator unit to a portable, emergency, and transport ventilator (Figure 3-20). This change to an unfamiliar ventilator can

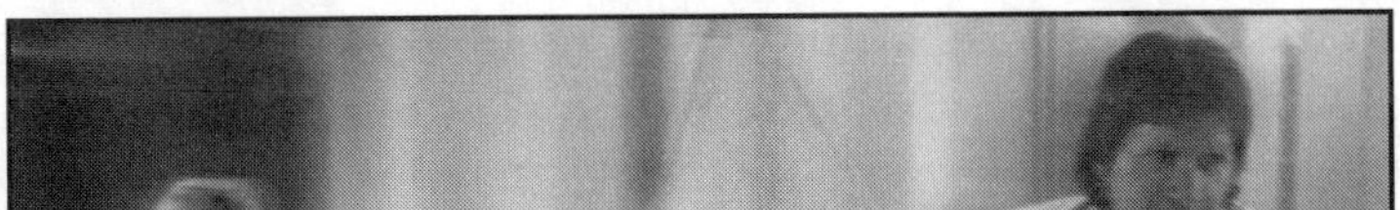

Figure 3–20. Portable ventilator units are necessary to transport fully ventilated patients to VFSE. Image provided from Respironics (http://www.respironics.com). Reprinted with permission.

create further discrepancy in swallow performances observed by the SLP under videofluoroscopy and on the ward. The patient may, understandably be apprehensive about the change and benefit from time to accommodate to the differences in ventilator styles. In the interests of achieving a reliable swallow investigation, the speech pathologist might raise this issue with the patient's medical team. In some circumstances, assisted ventilation plans may be reviewed by the team (i.e., transferring the patient to a portable home care ventilator, if this is an imminent goal, at least a week prior to instrumental assessment), so that the patient has time to adjust to the portable ventilator prior to a swallowing evaluation.

When taking patients who have a tracheostomy (with or without assisted ventilation) to the radiology department it is necessary to "take the critical care ward with the patient," and this requires advanced warning to the patient's ward, so that nursing or medical staff can attend the VFSE, and transfer respiratory monitoring and emergency ventilation equipment to the radiology suite. Each facility will have its own guidelines regarding obtaining medical authority for cuff deflation when absent from a patient's usual ward. SLPs should seek this information, and ensure that there are guidelines for checking and reporting on cuff and ventilation status at VFSE completion. An emergency plan for ventilatory failure is essential, and at very least must include the presence of a staff member throughout the VFSE who has clinical competency in administering manual ventilation and knowledge of how to manage ventilator technology. If this level of support and relevant equipment is not available, then it may be safer to defer the VFSE.

Suitability for Decannulation. Some patients post-SCI will always require a tracheostomy. However, for those patients with the potential to wean from ventilation and intubation, the SLP may be involved in the multidisciplinary decision regarding suitability for decannulation. Some key indicators of readiness for tracheostomy decannulation, such as the presence of an effective cough and ability to manage airway secretions over a 24 to 48 hour period of continuous cuff deflation (Thompson-Ward, Boots, Frisby, Bassett, & Timm, 1999), may never apply to some patients with a SCI, and yet decannulation may still be possible. Notably, patients with a complete injury at C5 and above will always lack an effective spontaneous cough. If a neurologically impaired cough can be augmented with assisted coughing techniques and there are no other dysphagia indicators, then the treating team and patient may consider that airway secretions can be safely managed without the need for tracheal suctioning.

Few studies have addressed the specific issues surrounding tracheostomy decannulation for patients with SCI. Ross and White (2003) reported the decannulation of four patients with SCI who were aspirating. Two of the patients had cervical injuries (one complete, one incomplete) and two had thoracic injuries (both complete). Each patient had undergone surgical fixation of their spinal cord injury. The maximum number of tracheostomy days was 101 and the minimum was 9. In this report of four cases, each patient was decannulated with return to verbal communication occurring immediately after tracheostomy removal and oral intake resuming within 4 days. The authors proposed procedures that aimed to safely facilitate decannulation trials in a very challenging clinical context, by anticipating possible adverse events of high-risk decannulation and using a multidisciplinary model as summarized below:

- SLP assessment of:
  - Presence or absence of aspiration of saliva through CSE and modified Evans blue dye test. If modified Evans blue dye test result is negative (i.e., no blue staining present) then further CSE is recommended in addition to physiological examination of swallowing, including a VFSE and/or endoscopic examination of swallowing.
  - Airway patency and vocal fold function assessment conducted by deflating the tracheostomy cuff and evaluating voice quality while the tracheostomy tube is briefly occluded manually and/or with a one-way speaking valve. Where voice quality is outside normal limits, ENT opinion is sought.
- Physiotherapy assessment of:
  - The patient's ability to cough secretions into the mouth (the patient must acquire the ability to perform an effective assisted cough to minimize the retention of airway secretions).
  - The risk of retention of secretions or respiratory muscle fatigue (second hourly assessment including an overnight service).
  - Forced vital capacity monitoring to identify signs of fatigue (fourth hourly).
- Nursing and medical management of:
  - Ensuring NBM during decannulation,
  - Tracheostomy tube removal early in the day and at the beginning of the week to increase the number of professional staff available to monitor patient for 24 to 48 hours post-decannulation.
  - Continuous pulse oximetry.
  - Patient observation each 30 minutes to determine need for suction or assisted coughing.
  - Considering insertion of a mini-tracheostomy tube immediately following decannulation to allow patient time to learn to perform an assisted cough effectively.

These procedures are implemented in addition to the tracheostomy management protocols of each health facility and the standard practices of obtaining medical practitioner authority for trial of decannulation; establishing agreed-upon criteria for reintubation; and bedside positioning of tracheostomy dilators and tracheostomy tubes of the same size and the size below the decannulated tube (Ross & White, 2003). Decannulation is usually considered once the patient is afebrile, able to sit up, breathing comfortably on room air, when vital signs are stable for at least twenty four hours and when blood gases and vital capacity are at acceptable values (Consortium for spinal cord medicine, 2005).

The role of a one-way speaking valve in the decannulation process has not been researched specifically for patients with a SCI, whose respiratory status is compromised. Ohmae et al. (2006), however, reported that valve use improved laryngeal clearance and reduced the incidence of laryngeal penetration during swallowing. Further, McCrory et al. (2001) and the consortium for spinal cord medicine (2005) list the use of speaking valves as a communication aid for tracheostomised patients with a cervical SCI. McCrory (2001) also detalied that hypocapnia (lower than normal end tidal carbon dioxide) due to cuff deflation during mechanical ventilation might be overcome with the addition of "dead space" (a section of the airway that does not provide gas exchange—such as ventilator tubing).

McCrory et al. (2001) and Bach and Goncalves (2006) also describe the use of mouth IPPV and other NIV modes as aids to tracheostomy removal in SCI. Bach (1996) outlined the utility of the respiratory functional measure "peak cough flow (PCF)" that can be tested in patients with a tracheostomy under consideration for decannulation. This measure is used as an indicator of ability to effectively clear airway secretions. PCF is the velocity of air emptied from the lungs in liters/second and can be measured during assisted coughing. Key barriers to generating adequate PCF include severe bulbar dysfunction; fixed upper airway obstruction (e.g., stenosis or granulation tissue), and severe lower airway obstruction.

An impediment to tracheostomy decannulation in the SCI population is the presence of a significant glottic and/or tracheal stenosis. Tracheal stenosis may occur at the stoma, the lower tracheostomy tip, and/or at the cuff. The respiratory consequences of tracheal and glottic stenosis may present with a tube in situ, or months after decannulation. For example, while a tracheostomy tube is in situ, a tracheal stenosis may occlude the lower tip of the tube, significantly increasing the work of breathing and risking respiratory arrest as the lumen through which the patient is breathing is severely narrowed. Patients who have been decannulated may be asymptomatic until they have an upper respiratory tract infection. Although the incidence of stenosis complications following tracheal intubation is reported to be the same in the spinal cord injured population as in the general population (1.2–2.0% or 13% of patients with SCI who are tracheostomized), patients with SCI are more vulnerable to the respiratory consequences of stenosis due to their underlying respiratory compromise (Hsu et al., 1987). Endoscopy (including bedside fiber-optic laryngoscopy or intraoperative rigid laryngoscopy and bronchoscopy) and computed tomography (CT) scanning are used to investigate tracheal and/or glottic stenosis.

Hsu et al. (1987) proposed that because the majority of SCIs occur due to motor vehicle accident, the rate of secondary traumatic laryngeal and tracheal injury would be high among those with SCI, but it may go undetected and untreated due to the higher priority to treat the primary SCI. The risk of development of stenosis may be minimized through a range of measures including: limiting the period of translaryngeal/endotracheal intubation to less than 10 days; ensuring adequate nutrition so that medical complications such as anemia are avoided and tissue health and healing are optimal; using a connection between the tracheostomy tube and ventilator tubing that minimizes stomal trauma during tracheal suctioning, cleaning, and movement (e.g., double swivel adapter); and close monitoring of cuff pressures, with regular cuff deflations to ensure healthy blood flow through the tracheal wall (Hsu et al., 1987). Treatments for stenosis range from observation in mild cases to permanent tracheostomization in more severe presentations.

A further impediment to decannulation may be the presence of ventilator assisted pneumonia (VAP). Critical care patients with SCI meet some of the criteria for patients at high risk of VAP. VAP arises from aspiration of the pathogenic microflora that colonize the oral secretions and dental plaque of critical care patients. By definition, VAP must occur at least 48 hours following intubation. Risk factors for VAP that typically apply to the SCI population include: immunocompromise following traumatic injuries; being dependent for teeth cleaning and oral care to prevent bacterial colonization of the oropharynx; being tube fed and nil by mouth, which may contribute to xerostomia; and supine positioning (such as where a conservative approach to vertebral stabilization is used) (Garp & Munro, 2004). New approaches to managing VAP are being developed due to the high incidence of this condition in the critical care population and its high mortality rate. Although research on VAP reduction is ongoing, some preventative measures of particular interest to SLPs include: upright positioning between 30 and 45 degrees unless contraindicated; daily lightening of sedation to assess readiness for extubation; second hourly mechanical (such as teeth brushing) and pharmacological oral cares; hand hygiene in health workers; and continuous clearance of pooled subglottic secretions. Many of these VAP prevention methods reinforce measures that also facilitate return to oral intake; however, the impact of VAP reduction measures on the application of SLP dysphagia protocols for patients using TPPV is yet to be determined. Concern over what level of tracheal aspiration of oral secretions gives rise to VAP in vulnerable patients raises issues relating to cuff deflation trials in tracheostomized patients. It may be prudent to defer cuff deflation and oral intake trials if VAP is diagnosed; this will require discussion with the critical care team.

Outcome Measures

A holistic approach to dysphagia management in SCI, where the physiological swallowing disorder and the lifestyle changes that swallowing disorder might cause are considered together, can be enhanced with the application of formal swallowing outcome measurements. Brady et al. (2004) applied the American Speech and Hearing Association National Outcome Measurement Scales (ASHA NOMS)–Swallowing Scale, Dietary Levels/Restrictions and Cueing to the SCI population as a means of comparing swallowing ability on admission to and discharge from speech pathology. Although no tools have been validated for use with SCI specifically, the ASHA NOMS and other assessments provide a breakdown of dysphagia features across each or some of the domains of impairment, activity limitation or disability, social integration, and quality of life/well-being. Implemented at initial assessment, at key intervals during rehabilitation, and on discharge from dysphagia therapy, swallowing outcome measures supply the dysphagia team with patient centered targets for dysphagia services.

Clinical and Physiological Characteristics of Dysphagia Impairment Post-Traumatic Spinal Cord Injury

Swallowing function may be intact in SCI, but this is less likely following complete cervical injuries. Where dysphagia is present in high cervical SCI, it is typically characterized by alterations in the oral transfer and pharyngeal phases of the swallow. Given that patients with cervical SCI are at greatest risk for swallowing impairment, the characteristics of dysphagia listed below are most frequently based upon findings from the cervical SCI group.

Oral Stage Impairment

Existing research reports of dysphagia in SCI do not provide characterization of oral stage impairments. The nature of oral phase impairment in SCI can be expected to vary with the neurological impairment(s) arising from SCI and associated comorbidities. Interestingly, no cases of isolated oral phase dysphagia were reported in a study of 73 patients with cervical SCI (Abel et al., 2004). Although 26 of the 73 were diagnosed as having dysphagia, 8 presented with both oral and pharyngeal stage disorders, and 17 had pharyngeal stage deficits only. Twice the number of patients had pharyngeal phase dysphagia only when compared to those with oral and pharyngeal phase disorders. Although the oral preparatory phase is usually preserved in patients with cervical SCI, an understanding of the pathophysiology of cervical spinal cord injury leads to the prediction that most disorders in the oral transfer phase of swallowing are likely to arise where a C1, C2, and/or C3 injury has been sustained in isolation or alongside multitrauma. Limitation in movements of the velum, base of tongue, and posterior oropharyngeal wall may indicate the involvement of cranial nerves X, XI, and XII, and direct nerve injury, or brainstem injury from a vascular event may be suspected. Where neurological involvement has been excluded, oral phase difficulties may be associated with fitting of external fixation devices (e.g., hard collar with chin extension), discomfort from compromised oral tissues (e.g. xerostoma and Candida Albicans) or ligamentous damage to the high cervical vertebrae with related problems in adjacent anatomy positioning or tissue health (including velum, mandible and base of tongue).

Clinically, these patients will have an adequate ability to maintain labial and anterior lingual control of the bolus. Anterior spillage of the bolus or saliva loss is seldom encountered with bolus cohesion typically maintained until propulsion into the pharynx. Oral transfer of the bolus to the pharynx, however, may be less well controlled and require multiple swallow attempts per bolus. In the absence of research evidence to define dysphagia characteristics, interpretation of clinical observations of dysphagic SCI patients suggests that this specific breakdown at the oral transfer phase with relative sparing of the oral preparatory phase is characteristic to the high cervical spinal cord injured patient during the acute phase of care. Because of these potential oral stage deficits, it is important to assess bolus control in each of the positions that the patient is likely to assume for eating (Figure 3-21). Supine positioning may or may not alter the patient's ability to form and control a bolus in the oral phase of swallowing.

Where the patient undergoes surgical management for SCI (e.g., spinal fusion), there are both transient tissue changes (for example, edema) and permanent structural changes that may also contribute to dysphagia. Where multilevel surgery is undertaken, post-surgical edema can cause changes in voice and swallowing functions. The edema and its associated physiological deficits typically resolve spontaneously. The surgical process of fixating the high cervical spine, however, results in permanent, albeit usually subtle, change in neck mobility, limiting to a varying extent anterior, posterior, superior, inferior, or lateral adjustments of the head in relation to the neck. This immobilization may diminish the natural

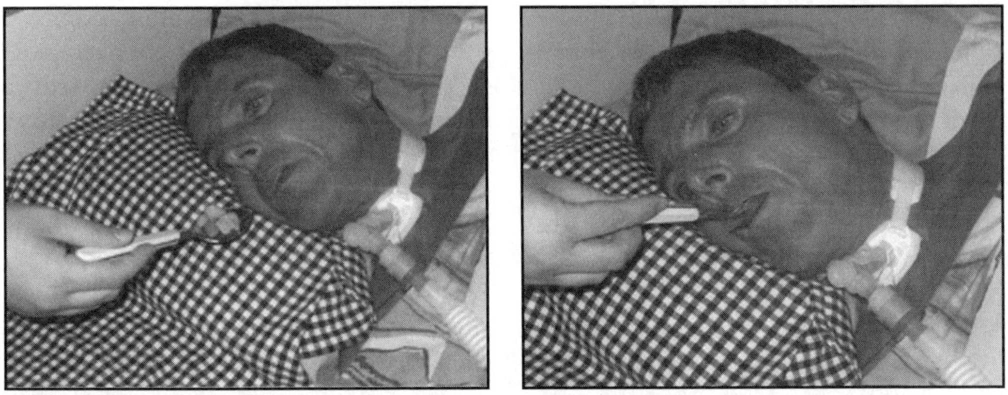

Figure 3–21. Following comprehensive assessment, some patients can resume safe oral intake in a side lying position.

head and neck adjustments that normally facilitate easy bolus transfer.

Pharyngeal Stage Impairment

In comparison to oral stage disorders, pharyngeal stage swallowing impairments are more prevalent in the SCI population (Abel et al., 2004; Brady et al., 2004), and are more variable in their presentation. This variability is due to the diverse etiology for dysphagia in this group, where disorder may arise from surgical and neurological events, local tissue breakdown, and/or the use of external fixation devices. A transient disruption to the pharyngeal phase of swallowing following cervical spine surgery has been reported in association with laryngeal edema, and descriptions of disorder in the pharyngoesophageal segment range from hyperactivity with normal coordination (Stewart, Johnston, Stewart, & Wilson, 1995) to hypotonicity (Brady et al., 2004). Neurological dysphagia in patients with tetraplegia may arise from damage to the vagus, accessory, and hypoglossal nerves and this damage can have a profound impact on the pharyngeal phase of swallowing. Beginning with a potential for impairment in the propulsion of the bolus into the pharynx (see Oral Phase section above), there may be multiple attempts to initiate the pharyngeal phase of the swallow. On clinical assessment, incomplete laryngeal elevation will be observed, with the patient making many attempts to clear the bolus through the pharynx. Clinical signs (e.g., wet breathing sounds, wet phonation) indicate pooling of the bolus within the pharynx.

On instrumental examination, pharyngeal stage deficits will again vary between individuals. The impact of sensory impairment, caused by prolonged use of a cuffed tracheostomy tube, may reduce awareness of the need to clear pooled and aspirated oropharyngeal secretions in high cervical injury. In particular, the loss of sensory awareness that accompanies C1–C2 injuries must be considered as a possible contributing factor to the severity of pharyngeal phase impairment in swallowing.

For the tetraplegic patient there may be no clinical indication of aspiration due to an absent/impaired cough reflex, since intact innervation to the diaphragm and intercostal muscles is required for the full functioning of the cough mechanism. Patients with complete injuries above C5 have a nonprotective reflexive cough and clinically require an assisted cough or suctioning to aid airway protection. Patients with injury below the level of C5 retain the ability to cough and may independently clear pharyngeal residue (Porth, 2005). In addition to the impact on cough function, injury to C1–C5 will also lead to a disruption of normal breathing patterns. This can influence the timing of the apneic period within the swallow cycle, placing the patient at further risk of aspiration.

Anterior cervical fixation (ACF) surgery can also have a negative impact on the pharyngeal stage of the swallow. Anatomical changes to the spine can be clearly visualized during a VFSE, and these may not be apparent when viewing the patient's neck position during CSE. The nature of dysphagia following ACF has been the focus of many studies. A case study of dysphagia in an elderly man following a subluxation of C5 on C6 is illustrative of the changes in the pharyngeal phase of swallowing that may arise following this procedure and the use of orthoses (Devitt, Delaney, Granell, & Walsh, 2001). Of note in this study, the acute phase of care was accompanied by two distinct phases of dysphagia: an initial neuromotor presentation thought to be due to surgery and then a later mechanical dysphagia due to the effect of a cervical orthosis. In addition to the subluxation, the subject of this study experienced a fracture of C5 and hematoma from C4 to C6. The subluxation was first managed conservatively (reduction with cervical tongs and stabilization with a halo vest). The subluxation recurred after a week and the halo vest was adjusted. This intervention failed with a further subluxation identified the following week. Anterior cervical fusion and discectomy at C5 was subsequently performed without operative complications and a Minerva collar was fitted. Aspiration was suspected on day 1 postoperatively during a CSE. Laryngoscopy on day 2 demonstrated normal vocal fold mobility. An initial VFSE revealed oral and pharyngeal phase disorders with aspiration occurring during the swallow in association with decreased effectiveness in laryngeal elevation, pharyngeal peristalsis, and aryepiglottic closure. Direct dysphagia therapy made no change in clinical symptoms by day 10. However, a further VFSE demonstrated a change in the dysphagia characteristics, with resolution of the neuromotor dysphagia (described above) and demonstration of a "mechanical dysphagia" (due to the effect of the Minerva collar). The mechanical dysphagia consisted of pooling at the cricopharyngeus, abnormal pharyngeal peristalsis, and aspiration post-swallow. Adjustment to the Minerva collar to allow more flexion greatly improved swallowing and the dysphagia was reported to have resolved by 3 weeks post-surgery (Devitt et al., 2001).

The above example of the changes in the pharyngeal phase of swallowing post-ACF reinforces the benefits of instrumental evaluation to guide treatment. Although ACF is highly beneficial, it can create changes in the natural movement of the pharyngeal constrictors, and it is associated with the complication of unilateral vocal fold palsy. In addition to potential laryngeal damage from surgical intervention, there is the potential for patients to have sustained traumatic laryngeal and tracheal damage during initial intubation.

As a consequence of efforts to avoid excessive flexion and extension of the neck and maintain spinal stability during intubation procedures, intubation can inadvertently cause trauma to the laryngeal structures. The possibility for organic changes to vocal fold function should be screened for during CSE where dysphagia is detected.

Management of Dysphagia

Published research and clinical guidelines for dysphagia management following SCI are scant, and any transfer of existing clinical guidelines for the general dysphagia population to the SCI population must be considered cautiously, because this population presents with particular challenges to standard dysphagia management practices. Simple safety precautions, such as delaying feeding until a patient can be positioned in an upright position, may not be relevant for some SCI patients due to long-term positioning restrictions. Therefore, the clinician must carefully weigh the risks of aspiration and pulmonary compromise against dysphagia rehabilitation progress, psychological and quality of life issues associated with unnecessarily delayed oral intake. It is advised that the SLP proceed cautiously in dysphagia management and with full support of the multidisciplinary team.

Non-Oral Supplementation

The use of non-oral nutrition in hospitalized patients with SCI is high. A significant change in metabolic function including an increase in energy requirements (hypermetabolic state) can be triggered by neurological injury and may lead to weight loss in the acute phase of care. Consequently, the aim of non-oral supplementation following SCI is to ensure that adequate nutrition and hydration are provided during this time of altered metabolism, as well as to enable reliable administration of medications.

Nasoenteric (i.e., nasogastric/nasojejunal) tubes (see Chapter 1) may be used for many weeks where the patient's level of consciousness is impaired, prognosis for dysphagia recovery is uncertain, or a paralytic ileus (absence of peristaltic movement in the gut causing fluid and gas accumulation in the small bowel) or gastroparesis (delayed gastric emptying) is present and contraindicates oral intake. Wolf and Meiners (2003) found 80% of tetraplegic patients in an acute SCI setting were managed exclusively with non-oral nutrition (NGT or PEG) at admission. The reason for extending a feeding tube beyond the stomach to the small bowel (i.e., postpyloric feeding with a jejunal or duodenal tube) is to reduce gastroesophageal reflux in patients with known gastroparesis or paralytic ileus. Despite these precautions, reflux aspiration is reported at a rate of 2.4% in this group (Pearce & Duncan, 2002). Parenteral nutrition (see Chapter 1), which bypasses the digestive tract with nutrition delivered intravenously, is often used in the short term for patients with bowel dysfunction. Acute bowel dysfunction in SCI may arise from a paralytic ileus, which typically resolves over a few days but can continue for weeks. Treatment may require free drainage via a NGT (gastric decompression), bowel rest, parenteral nutrition, intravenous fluids, nil by mouth status, and medication to restore gastric activity until bowel function is restored. Gastric emptying time for solid foods has been found to be significantly prolonged following spinal cord injury, both acutely and in the long term, particularly in tetraplegia.

Attainment of adequate hydration in the acute phase of care may be difficult to achieve without non-oral supplementation in patients with tetraplegia, not only due to dysphagia, but also due to reliance on others to provide assistance to bring fluids to the mouth, whole body positioning limitations, and fatigue. Ongoing assessment of nutritional adequacy by the dietitian/nutritionist is necessary. Tracking body weight alone is not considered a reliable measure of nutritional adequacy in SCI due to loss of muscle and soft tissue mass arising from neurological flaccidity. The absence of pressure areas over bony prominences, however, is a positive indicator for nutritional status in this population.

Although malnutrition can increase patient morbidity and mortality, treatments for malnutrition, including tube feeding, also carry risks. The SLP managing dysphagia in this population will benefit from close consultation with the dietitian/nutritionist and nursing team in developing a plan that not only supports adequate nutrition, but also aims for cessation of tube feeding as soon as the patient can meet his nutrition requirements orally. Wolf and Meiners (2003) reported that 80% of their subjects tolerated oral diets without supplementation at discharge, despite a majority of subjects requiring tube feeding at admission. Participants continuing to require non-oral nutrition at discharge were able to take food orally, with the exception of one patient who had confirmed findings of brainstem and cranial nerve injury. Interestingly, 13% of patients at discharge required supplemental tube feeding due to an inability to meet nutritional requirements orally in the absence of aspiration.

Compensatory Management

Findings of asymmetry in swallowing function during instrumental assessment can be acted upon with behavioral treatments. Where postural changes are indicated (e.g., head rotation to the weakened side for unilateral pharyngeal weakness), medical approval must be sought prior to implementation to ensure that maneuvers will not compromise vertebral stability at the injury site. The viability of postural modifications can be expected to be limited in some cervical and thoracic injuries where the presence of hard neck collars and surgical fixation may significantly limit the range of motion in the neck. However, where medical authorization has been provided, such maneuvers should not be discounted, as even a modified or limited completion of a maneuver may offer airway protection or facilitate a more efficient swallow.

Delivery of oral intake requires consideration in patients who have limitations in the fine control of hand function, such as in tetraplegia. Straw drinking in this group enables independence, reduces accidental spillage, and offers a rapid delivery of fluids to the mouth where desired. Flow rate can be moderated through tongue tip and/or lip control at the straw. Where patients return to supine nursing (e.g., for the management of pressure areas), straw drinking is the only feasible option apart from parenteral or enteral hydration. The benefits of straw drinking for those with tetraplegia necessitates earlier trial of thin (or straw suitable) liquids than might otherwise occur to support mealtime independence and adequate oral hydration. Where dysphagia is evident, the evaluation of compensatory and postural techniques under direct physiological examination may identify safe strategies for straw drinking. Specific positioning of drink containers when patients are straw drinking can facilitate more natural adoption of rehabilitative postures such as chin tuck or head rotation to the weaker side.

Where thickened fluids are recommended, the SLP must consider that oral intake of fluids may be limited to the point of needing non-oral supplementation, because delivery by spoon by others can be slow or unreliable, especially where patients are fatigued or nursed in supine. Documentation of thickened fluid intake volume in the patient's food and fluid charts is used to determine hydration adequacy (in addition to routine clinical measures such as urine output).

For the ventilated patient who presents with compromised laryngeal elevation, lessening the weight of devices and circuits that are attached to the tracheostomy hub (the opening at the neck) may be beneficial for swallowing (although this consideration must be guided by the treating medical officer). For example, if improvement in swallowing can be demonstrated, a trial of disconnecting in-line tracheal suctioning equipment to relieve "drag" at the stoma during swallowing may be recommended to nursing and medical team members. The decision to swap from in-line (i.e., always attached to the tracheostomy tube) to standard suctioning, however, carries costs in terms of staff training, extra time taken to use sterile gloves for each suction, and increased use of consumables. Alternately, ventilator tubing can be secured (taking care not to impede airflow) to an intravenous fluid stand, or the patient's bed or chair at a comfortable height, allowing some yield in the tube. Other solutions include different ventilator tubing (circuit) setups to distribute weight more evenly. A team approach to practical problem solving of these issues may provide simple and safe improvements in the ease of pharyngeal swallowing.

Active Rehabilitation

The cognitive abilities of patients with SCI are usually intact. Therefore, patients with SCI have the same cognitive capacity as the general population in order to master complex dysphagia maneuvers to enhance swallow safety or improve swallow physiology. Patients with respiratory complications may have reduced ability to perform swallowing maneuvers (see Chapter 1). Difficulty would be anticipated during voluntary breath holding beyond the reflexive apneic period of the pharyngeal swallow, for example, during the supraglottic swallow and the super-supraglottic swallow. In addition, the ability of the patient to monitor his performance of dysphagia rehabilitation tasks can be limited in cervical SCI by a number of factors. During acute care or where long-term ventilator assistance is required, background ventilator noise can mask the timing and quality of breathing sounds and phonation or airway clearance attempts. Further, an inflated tracheostomy cuff limits the sensory information available to the larynx.

The application of biofeedback modalities for dysphagia rehabilitation, such as surface electromyography, has not been reported in patients with SCI. However, biofeedback may facilitate this relatively young and largely cognitively intact patient group to better monitor their efforts and maintain motivation to complete dysphagia therapies. The risks of using these treatments while patients are simultaneously utilizing technology must, however, be carefully assessed.

ASSOCIATED SPEECH AND COMMUNICATION ISSUES

Following cervical SCI, patients can be at risk of altered or impaired speech production. Damage to the cervical spinal cord impairs respiratory function, with the severity and type of sensory and motor impairment dependent on level and degree of cord damage. In addition, there is potential for laryngeal injury/weakness to exist due to medical management such as intubation, prolonged assisted ventilation, and/or surgical repair of the injury site. For those patients with associated multitrauma, injuries to the brain, facial structures, and/or chest may also result in impaired cranial nerve function or structural changes to the speech production mechanism. Consequently, there is potential for impairments to exist in the respiratory, phonatory, articulatory, and possibly resonatory systems of speech production post-SCI. From the limited research conducted to date, speech characteristics of nonventilated SCI patients have been described as exhibiting inadequate loudness, monoloudness, short breath groups, slow inspirations, and a reduction in stress contrasts (Hixon & Putnam, 1983). In a study of a group of 10 male cervical SCI patients, Hoit and colleagues (1990) noted reduced loudness, imprecise articulation, long inspirations, altered breath groups, and voice quality variations including breathiness, hyponasality, and roughness. Using perceptual assessments of physiological function and speech production, MacBean et al. (2006) found impairments in the respiratory and laryngeal subsystems of speech production in their group of 24 participants, with some individual participants exhibiting impaired function of the articulators. Perceptually, mild deficits in prosody and phonation were evident in a substantial proportion of participants, with a few having perceptible deficits in respiratory support for speech, articulation, and resonance.

For those patients with high cervical spinal injury that requires ongoing assisted ventilation, voicing is disrupted until patients are able to tolerate cuff deflation (or a cuffless or fenestrated tube), enabling diversion of some airflow to the upper airways. This is referred to as *leak speech*, and it is only possible when there is sufficient airflow to generate adequate subglottal pressure to allow phonation (Hoit, Banzett, Lohmeier, Hixon, & Brown, 2003; Hoit, Shea, & Banzett, 1994). Such pressure is typically limited to the inspiratory and the beginning of the expiratory ventilator cycles (Hoit & Banzett, 1997). Consequently, this allows for voicing in only short bursts, corresponding to the rise and fall of tracheal pressure created by the ventilator cycle. Leak speech is described as low-volume or whispered speech of poor quality restricted to short phrases and long pauses (Hoit et al., 2003; MacBean et al., 2008; Manzano et al., 1997).

Once an individual can voice using leak speech, speech quality can be enhanced through the addition of positive end expiratory pressure (PEEP) or the use of a one-way tracheostomy speaking valve (Hoit & Banzett 1997; Hoit et al., 1994; Hoit et al., 2003). The addition of PEEP for speech purposes aims to lengthen the duration of adequate tracheal pressure for voicing into the exhalation phase and so reduce the rate of airway pressure change (Hoit et al., 2003). This has been shown to improve speech, specifically facilitating extended speech durations (increased syllables produced per ventilator cycle) (Hoit & Banzett 1997; Hoit et al., 1994; Hoit et al., 2003; MacBean et al., 2008).

The use of a tracheostomy speech valve is another means to reestablish communication for the ventilated patient once periods of cuff deflation can be tolerated. The speaking valve allows air to pass from the ventilator into the tracheostomy on inspiration, but prevents exhalation via the tracheostomy tube; rather, expired air must be exhaled through the glottis. This ensures that sufficient subglottic pressure is maintained during both the inspiratory and expiratory ventilator cycles for voice production. Using a speaking valve, patients are able to produce complete sentences with improved speech flow, volume, voice quality, and speech intelligibility (MacBean et al., 2008; Passy, Baydur, Prentice, & Darnell-Neal, 1993).

Reestablishing communication in ventilated patients can be a complex process, yet sometimes intelligible voiced speech is achieved at the first attempt. All aspects of assisted ventilation require consideration when a ventilator circuit that is usually closed (i.e., cuff inflated) is opened (cuff deflated) for speech. Under some ventilator settings (e.g., volume targeted ventilation), cuff deflation may result in a loss of volume that compromises alveolar ventilation, though the treating respiratory physician or intensivist can usually adjust ventilator parameters to accommodate for this (Prigent et al., 2003). The SLP can guide the ventilator team in understanding how ventilator variables (such as pressure support ventilation mode vs. volume cycled mode, inspiratory time, and PEEP) may influence phonation. It is very encouraging that with skilled ventilator adjustments, speech quality in fully ventilator assisted patients can be comparable to normal. However, the numerous factors that need to be considered for ventilator speech trials can only be managed within a skilled multidisciplinary team model. Readers wishing to learn more about this specialized area are referred to Dikeman and Kazandjian (2003) and the references detailed in the paragraphs above for further reading.

CONCLUSION

Traumatic SCI can have wide systematic impact. Particularly following cervical spinal cord damage, the risk of dysphagia during the acute stage of recovery is high due to complications of both the spinal injury and its management. On a positive note, long-term prognosis for dysphagia recovery is good. A number of population-specific issues, such as positioning restrictions and respiratory compromise, complicate dysphagia decision making and management. For this reason it is recommended that the assessment and management of dysphagia following SCI only be undertaken by clinicians with advanced clinical skills, working in a supported multidisciplinary team environment.

Acknowledgments. The authors would like to acknowledge the following individuals and teams: To Liz and Angela for sharing their knowledge and this opportunity; The Winston Churchill Memorial Trust of Australia for the resources to visit spinal cord injuries in the United States and the United Kingdom; John Coffey, Spinal Orthotist at the Princess Alexandra Hospital in Brisbane, for his ready contribution of images and expertise; David Riley for his generosity in providing insights into dysphagia following spinal cord injury and for being photographed for this chapter; Drs. Timothy Geraghty, Vernon Hill, Bill Davies and Craig Hukins, and the multidisciplinary team of the Queensland Spinal Cord Injuries Service for their openness to what speech pathology services might bring to patients; Damien Roberts and the Spinal Speech Pathologists Australia and New Zealand Interest Group for the supportive forum that members provide for learning; and Dr. Augusta Alba for her positive approach to rehabilitation possibilities and for accommodating budding "rehabilitationistas." Also heartfelt thanks to David for his support and immense patience along with Hugh, Liam, and Jean Solley for their love; and importantly to Brian and Elena for equipping me to do this work.

FURTHER READING

Dikeman, K. J., & Kazandjian, M. S. (2003). *Communication and swallowing management of tracheostomized and ventilator dependent adults* (2nd ed.). Clifton Park, NY: Thompson Delmar Learning.

REFERENCES

Abel, R., Ruf, S., & Spahn, B. (2004). Cervical spinal cord injury and deglutition disorders. *Dysphagia*, *19*, 87–94.

Adams, M. M. & Hicks, A. L. (2005). Spasticity after spinal cord injury. *Spinal Cord*, *43*, 577–586. Retrieved January 6, 2009, from http://www.nature.com/sc/journal/v43/n10/full/3101757a.html

Alpert, M. J. (2007). *Central cord syndrome*. Retrieved May 29, 2008, from http://www.emedicine.com/pmr/topic22.htm

American Spinal Injury Association (ASIA). (2006). Available at http://www.asia-spinalinjury.org/

Bach, J. R. (1996) *Pulmonary rehabilitation: The obstructive and paralytic/restrictive pulmonary syndromes*. Philadelphia: Hanley and Belfus.

Bach, J. R., & Alba, A. S. (1990). Noninvasive options for ventilatory support for the traumatic high level quadriplegic patient. *Chest*, *98*, 613–619.

Bach, J. R., & Goncalves, M. R. (2006). Pulmonary rehabilitation in neuromuscular disorders and spinal cord injury. *Revista portuguesa de pneumologica*, *12*(Suppl. 1), S27–S44. Retrieved 20 July, 2007, from www.sppneumologia.pt/download.php?path=pdfs&filename=RPP_2006_1_27_Pul.pdf

Barkmeier, J. M., Bielamowicz, S., Takeda, N., & Ludlow, C. L. (2002). Laryngeal activity during upright vs. supine swallowing. *Journal of Applied Physiology*, *93*(2), 740–745.

Belafsky, P. C., Blumenfeld, L., LePage, A., & Nahrstedt, K. (2003). The accuracy of the modified Evans blue dye test in predicting aspiration. *Laryngoscope*, *113*(11), 1969–1972.

Biering-Sorensen, M., & Biering-Sorensen, F. (1992). Tracheostomy in spinal cord injured: Frequency and follow-up. *Paraplegia*, *30*(9), 656–660.

Biering-Sorensen, F., Chalifue, S., DeVivo, M., Noonan, V., Post, M., Stripling, T., et al. (2006). International Spinal Cord Injury Data Sets. *Spinal Cord*, *44*, 530–534.

Brady, S., Miserendino, R., Statkus, D., Springer, T., Hakel, M., & Stambolis, V. (2004). Predictors to dysphagia and recovery after cervical spinal cord injury during acute rehabilitation. *The Journal of Applied Research*, *4*(1), 1–11.

Bridwell, K. (2007). Muscles of the Spine, Spine Universe, Retrieved July 27, 2008, from http://www.spineuniverse.com/displayarticle.php/article1272.html

Brown, R., Di Marco, A. F., Hoit, J., & Garshick, E. (2006). Respiratory dysfunction and management in spinal cord injury. *Respiratory Care, 51*(8), 853-868.

Consortium for spinal cord medicine. (2008). Early acute management in adults with spinal cord injury: clinical practice guidelines for health-care professionals. Paralyzed Veterans of America. Retrieved February 14, 2009 from http://www.pva.org/site/PageServer?pagename=pubs_main#CPG

Consortium for spinal cord medicine. (2005). Respiratory management following spinal cord injury: clinical practice guidelines for health-care professionals. Paralyzed Veterans of America. Retrieved June 27, 2008, from http://www.pva.org/site/PageServer?pagename=pubs_main#CPG

Consortium for spinal cord medicine. (1999). Outcomes following traumatic spinal cord injury: clinical practice guidelines for health-care professiona;ls. *Paralyzed Veterans of America.* Retrieved June 27, 2007, from http://www.pva.org/site/News2?page=NewsArticle&id=7655

Cripps, R. A. (2007). *2005-6 Spinal Cord Injury, Australia*. Research and Statistic Series Number 36. Adelaide, Australia: Australian Institute of Health and Welfare. Retrieved July 30, 2008, from http://www.nisu.flinders.edu.au/pubs/reports/2007/injcat102.php

Davenport, M. (2008). Fracture, cervical spine. *eMedicine.* Retrieved May 23, 2008, from http://www.emedicine.com/emerg/TOPIC189.HTM

Davis, D. G., Beras, S., Barone, J. E., Corvo, P. R., & Tucker, J. B. (2002). Swallowing with a tracheotomy tube in place: Does cuff inflation matter? *Journal of Intensive Care Medicine, 17*(3), 132-135.

Dawodu, S. T. (2007). Spinal cord injury: Definition, epidemiology, pathophysiology. *eMedicine.* Retrieved June 14, 2007, from http://www.emedicine.com/pmr/topic182.htm

Devitt, A., Delaney, F., Granell, M., & Walsh, M. (2001). Dysphagia following anterior cervical surgery. *Irish Journal of Orthopedic Surgery and Trauma.* Retrieved August 1, 2008, from http://www.iol.ie/~rcsiorth/journal/volume2/february/dysphag.htm

De Vivo, M. J., Stover, S. L., & Black, K. J. (1992). Prognostic factors for twelve-year survival following traumatic spinal cord injury. *Archives of Physical Rehabilitation, 73*, 156-162.

Dikeman, K. J., & Kazandjian, M. S. (2003). *Communication and swallowing management of tracheostomized and ventilator dependent adults* (2nd ed.). Clifton Park, NY: Thompson Delmar Learning.

Di Marco, A. F., Onders, R. P., Ignagni, A., & Kowalski, K. E. (2006). Inspiratory muscle pacing in spinal cord injury: Case report and clinical commentary. *Journal of Spinal Cord Medicine, 29*(2), 95-108.

Donzelli, J., Brady, S., Wesling, M., & Craney, M. (2001). Simultaneous modified Evans blue dye procedure and video nasal endoscopic evaluation of the swallow. *Laryngoscope, 111*, 1746-1750.

Elpern, E. H., Okonek, M. B., Bacon, M., Gerstung, C., & Skrzynski, M. (2000). Effect of the Passy-Muir tracheostomy speaking valve on pulmonary aspiration in adults. *Heart and Lung: Journal of Acute and Critical Care, 29*(4), 287-293.

Elpern, E. H., Scott, M. G., Petro, L., & Ries, M. H. (1994). Pulmonary aspiration in mechanically ventilated patients with tracheostomies. *Chest, 105*, 155-163.

Garp, M. J., & Munro, C. L. (2004). Preventing ventilator associated pneumonia: Evidence based care. *Critical Care Nursing Clinics of North America, 16*(3), 349-358.

Gaudinez, R. F., English, G. M., Gebhard, J. S., Brugman, J. L., Donaldson, D. H., & Brown, C. W. (2000). Esophageal perforations after anterior cervical surgery. Original articles and case reports. *Journal of Spinal Disorders, 13*(1), 77-84.

Hadley, M. N., Walters, B. C., Grabb, P. A., Oyesjku, N. M., Przybiski, G. J., Resnick, D. K., et al. (2001). Joint Section on Disorders of the Spine and Peripheral Nerves of the AANS/CNS. *Guidelines for the management of acute cervical spine and spinal cord injuries.* Retrieved September 1, 2008, from http://www.spineuniverse.com/displayarticle.php/article2081.html

Han, N., Kim, D., Kim, H., An, H., & Lee, N. (2005). Effect of cervical orthosis upon swallowing. *Journal of the Korean Academy of Rehabilitation Medicine*, *29*(6), 662-668.

Hixon, T. J., & Putnam, A. H. B. (1983). Voice disorders in relation to respiratory kinematics. *Seminars in Speech and Language*, *4*(3), 217-231.

Hoit, J. D., & Banzett, R. B. (1997). Simple adjustments can improve ventilator-supported speech. *American Journal of Speech-Language Pathology*, *6*, 87-96.

Hoit, J. D., Banzett, R. B., Brown, R., & Loring, S. H. (1990). Speech breathing in individuals with cervical spinal cord injury. *Journal of Speech and Hearing Research*, *33*, 798-807.

Hoit, J. D., Banzett, R. B., Lohmeier, H. L., Hixon, T. J., & Brown, R. (2003). Clinical ventilator adjustments that improve speech. *Chest*, *124*(4), 1512-1521.

Hoit, J. D., & Shea, S. A. (1996). Speech production and speech with a phrenic nerve pacer. *American Journal of Speech-Language Pathology*, *5*, 53-60.

Hoit, J. D., Shea, S. A., & Banzett, R. B. (1994). Speech production during mechanical ventilation in tracheostomized individuals. *Journal of Speech and Hearing Research*, 37, 53-63.

Hsu, S., Dreisbach, J. N., Charlifue, S. W., & English, G. M. (1987). Glottic and tracheal stenosis in spinal cord injured patients. *Paraplegia*, *25*, 136-148.

Hulsebosch, C. E. (2002). Recent advances in pathophysiology and treatment of spinal cord injury. *Advances in Physiology Education*, *26*(4), 238-255.

Inagaki, D., Miyaoka, Y., Ashida, I., Ueda, K., & Yamada, Y. (2007). Influences of body posture on duration of oral swallowing in normal young adults. *Journal of Oral Rehabilitation*, *34*(6), 414-421.

Kirschblum, S., Johnston, M. V., Brown, J., O'Connor, K. C., & Jarosz, P. (1999). Predictors of dysphagia after spinal cord injury. *Archives of Physical Medicine and Rehabilitation*, *80*(9), 1101-1105.

Laffont, I., Bensmail, D., Lartat-Jacob, S., Falaize, L., Hutin, C., Bomin, E. L., et al. (2008). Intermittent positive-pressure breathing effects in patients with high spinal cord injury. *Archives of Physical Medicine and Rehabilitation*, *89*(8), 1575-1579.

Leder, S. B. (2002). Incidence and type of aspiration in acute care patients requiring mechanical ventilation via a new tracheotomy. *Chest*, *122*, 1721-1726.

Leder, S. B., & Sasaki, C. T. (1999). Use of FEES to assess patients with a tracheotomy. In S. E. Langmore (Ed.), *Endoscopic evaluation and treatment of swallowing disorders* (2nd ed., pp. 188-200). New York: Thieme Medical.

Lee, M. J., Bazaz, R., Furey, C. G., & Yoo, J. (2007). Risk factors for dysphagia after anterior cervical spine surgery: A two-year prospective cohort study. *Spine Journal*, 7(2), 141-147.

Logemann, J. A. (1998). *Evaluation and treatment of swallowing disorders* (2nd ed.). Austin, TX: Pro-Ed.

MacBean, N., Ward, E., Murdoch, B., Cahill, L., Solley, M., & Geraghty, T. (2006). Characteristics of speech following cervical spinal cord injury. *Journal of Medical Speech-Language Pathology*, *14*, 167-184.

MacBean, N., Ward, E., Murdoch, B., Cahill, L., Solley, M., Geraghty, T., et al. (2008). Optimising speech production in the ventilator-dependent individual following cervical spinal cord injury. An examination of two cases. *International Journal of Language and Communication Disorders*, *iFirst Article*, 1-12.

Manzano, J. L., Lubillo, S., Henriquez, D., Martin, J. C., Perez, M. C., & Wilson, D. J. (1997). Verbal communication of ventilator dependent patients. *Critical Care Medicine*, *21*(4), 512-517.

Marino, R. J. (2002). International standards for neurological classification of spinal cord injury. Atlanta: American Spinal Cord Injury Association.

McCrory, D. C., Samsa, G. P., Hamilton, B. B., Govert, J. A., Matchar, D. B., Goslin, R. E., et al. (2001). *Treatment of pulmonary disease following cervical spinal cord injury. Evidence report/technology assessment Number 27.* (AHRQ Publication No. 01-E014). Rockville, MD: Agency for Healthcare Research and Quality.

McGowan, S. L., Gleeson, M., Smith, M., Hirsch, N., & Shuldham, C. M. (2007). A pilot study of fibreoptic endoscopic evaluation of swallowing in patients with cuffed tracheostomies in neurological intensive care. *Neurocritical Care, 6*, 90–93.

Morishima, N., Ohota, K., & Miura, Y. (2005). The influences of halo-vest fixation and cervical hyperextension on swallowing in healthy volunteers. *Spine, 30*(7), 179–182.

National Spinal Cord Injury Statistical Center. (2008). *2008 dated reports*. Retrieved August 1, 2008, from http://www.spinalcord.uab.edu/show.asp?durki=19775&site=1021&return=19679

O'Connor, P. J. (2005). Prevalence of spinal cord injury in Australia. *Spinal Cord, 43*, 42–46.

Ohmae, Y., Adachi, Z., Isoda, Y., Maekawa, H., Kitagawa, Y., Karaho, T., et al. (2006). Effects of one-way speaking valve placement on swallowing physiology for tracheostomized patients: Impact on laryngeal clearance. *Nippon Jibiinkoka Gakkai Kaiho, 109*(7), 594–599.

O'Neil-Pirozzi, T. M., Lisiecki, D. J., Momose, D. K., Connors, J. J., & Milliner, M. P. (2003). Simultaneous modified barium swallow and blue dye tests: A determination of the accuracy of blue dye test aspiration finding. *Dysphagia, 18*(1), 32–38.

Passy, V., Baydur, A., Prentice, W., & Darnell-Neal, R. (1993). Passy-Muir Tracheostomy Speaking Valve on ventilator-dependent patients. *Laryngoscope, 103*, 653–658.

Pearce, C. B., & Duncan, H. D. (2002). Enteral feeding. Nasogastric, nasojejunal, percutaneous endoscopic gastrostomy or jejunostomy: Its indications and limitations. *Postgraduate Medical Journal, 78*, 198–204.

Porth, S. C. (2005). Recognition and management of respiratory dysfunction in children with tetraplegia. *Journal of Spinal Cord Medicine, 27*(Suppl. 1), S75–S79.

Prigent, H., Samuel, C., Louis, B., Abinun, M., Zerah-Lancner, F., Lejialle, M., et al. (2003). Comparative effects of two ventilatory modes on speech in tracheostomized patients with neuromuscular disease. *American Journal of Respiratory and Critical Care Medicine, 167*, 114–119.

Ross, J., & White, M. (2003). Removal of the tracheostomy tube in the aspirating spinal cord-injured patient. *Spinal Cord, 41*, 636–642.

Rubin, A. D., Hawkshaw, M. J., Moyer, C. A., Dean, C. M., & Sataloff, R. T. (2005). Arytenoid cartilage dislocation: A 20-year experience. *Journal of Voice, 19*(4), 687–701.

Sahjpaul, R. L. (2007). Esophageal perforation from anterior screw migration. *Surgical Neurology, 68(2)*, 205–209.

Scott, A. (2001). Overview. In A. Nelson, C. A. Zedjlik, & L. Love (Eds.). *Nursing practice relating to spinal cord injury and disorders. A core curriculum.* (pp. 1-8). New York: Demos Medical.

Seidl, R. O., Niedeggen, A., Todt, I., Westhofen, M., & Ernst, A. (2007). Infrahyoid muscle flap for pharyngeal fistulae after cervical spine surgery: A novel approach—Report of six cases. *European Spine Journal, 16*(4), 501–505.

Shem, K., Castillo, K., & Naran, B. (2005). Factors associated with dysphagia in individuals with high tetraplegia. *Topics in Spinal Cord Injury Rehabilitation, 10*(3), 8–18.

Spinal Cord Injury Information Network. (2008). *Functional goals following SCI.* Retrieved July 30, 2008, from http://www.spinalcord.uab.edu/

Spinal Cord Injury Information Network. (2008). *Spinal cord injury facts and figures at a glance 2008.* Retrieved July 30, 2008, from http://www.spinalcord.uab.edu/show.asp?durki=116979&site=1021&return=19775

Stambolis, V., Brady, S., Kios, D., Wesling, T. F., & Hildner, C., (2003). The effect of cervical bracing upon swallowing in young, normal, healthy volunteers. *Dysphagia*, *18*(1), 39-45.

Stewart, M., Johnston, R. A., Stewart, I., & Wilson, J. A. (1995). Swallowing performance following anterior cervical spine surgery. *British Journal of Neurosurgery*, *9*, 605-609.

Suiter, D. M., & Leder, S. B. (2007). Contribution of tracheostomy tubes and one-way speaking valves to swallowing success. *Topics in Geriatric Rehabilitation*, *23*(4), 341-351.

Swanson, B. L., Schwartz-Cowley, R., & Dininny, D. H. (1991). Safe and effective oral feeding of ventilator-assisted trauma patients. *Panamerican Journal of Trauma*, *2*, 81-87.

Thompson-Ward, E. C., Boots, R., Frisby, J., Bassett, L., & Timm, M. (1999). Evaluating suitability for tracheostomy decannulation: A critical evaluation of two management protocols. *Journal of Medical Speech Language Pathology*, 7(4), 273-281.

Thurman, D. J., Sniezek, J. E., Johnson, D., Greenspan, A., & Smith, S. M. (1995). *Guidelines for surveillance of central nervous system injury.* Atlanta, GA: United States Department of Health and Human Services, Centers for Disease Control and Prevention.

Tippett, D. C. (2000). Swallowing, tracheostomy and ventilator dependence. In D. C. Tippett (Ed.), *Tracheostomy and ventilator dependency: Management of breathing, speaking and swallowing* (pp. 143-192). New York: Thieme Medical.

Winslow, C. P., Winslow, T. J., & Wax, M. K. (2001). Dysphonia and dysphagia following the anterior approach to the cervical spinal spine. *Archives of Otolaryngology-Head and Neck Surgery*, *127*, 51-55.

Wolf, C., & Meiners, T. H. (2003). Dysphagia in patients with acute cervical spinal cord injury. *Spinal Cord*, *41*, 347-353.

4 Burn Injury

ANNA F. RUMBACH, ELIZABETH C. WARD, CYNTHIA MCKINNON DUBOSE, AND NICOLA A. CLAYTON

INTRODUCTION

Medical and nursing management for burns has existed for over 3500 years (Barrow & Herndon, 2007), yet the discipline of speech-language pathology (SLP) has not played an active role within the management team until recent years (Ward, Uriarte, & Conroy, 2001). The need for SLPs to become more involved in the management of this population is twofold. First, advances in medical and surgical treatment have seen a substantial reduction in burn injury mortality. Reduced mortality results in an increase in burn injury survivors and, therefore, an increased demand for burn rehabilitation services. Second, there has been a greater acknowledgement of the importance of a multidisciplinary approach to care in this field in recent times. SLPs are now increasingly recognized as key members of the burn injury rehabilitation team for their role in prevention of contracture and hypertrophic scar formation of the oral and facial musculature, assessment and management of vocal cord function, and the assessment and treatment of dysphagia (Brooks & Hammond, 1986; Snyder & Ubben, 2003; Ward et al., 2001; Williams & Baker, 1992).

BURN AGENTS

Burn injury can result from a number of different types of agent, each causing different amounts of damage to the skin surface. The main categories of burn agent are thermal (e.g., flame), electrical (live wires), and chemical (acids, alkalis). Although there are similarities between the burn injuries resulting from different agents, there are a number of key differentiating factors that exist, as highlighted in the following sections. The most common cause of burn trauma is thermal injury (Pruitt, Wolf, & Mason, 2007), and patients' post-thermal burn injury (with or without concomitant inhalation injury) constitutes the majority of patients referred to SLP for dysphagia management.

Thermal

Thermal burns are caused by direct exposure to extreme temperature sufficient to cause injury to one or more of the three layers of skin (the epidermis, dermis, and the subcutaneous tissues). Most frequently, thermal burns are caused due to extremes of heat, but they may also result from extremes of cold. The extent and depth of damage is dependent upon the temperature of the agent and the duration for which the skin is exposed to the temperature extreme. The term *thermal burn* encompasses four subcategories, including flame, flash, scald, and contact thermal burns. Details of the common causes of each of these types of thermal burn are outlined in Table 4–1. When flame is the agent of thermal injury, the possibility for additional *inhalation injury* must be considered. If a thermal injury is caused by an explosion, particularly within a contained space, the risk for inhalation injury is substantially increased. The mechanism of inhalation injury consists of multiple factors, including upper airway injury due to the inhalation of hot air, steam, or gases; damage to the oxygen transport system through the inhalation of toxic gases, namely carbon monoxide and cyanide; and chemically-based lower airway injury resulting from the inhalation of smoke constituents (Knights, 2002; McCall & Cahill, 2005).

Table 4–1. Categories of Thermal Burn

Injury Type	*Common Causes*
Flame	• House fire • Careless smoking • Improper use of flammable substances • Vehicular accidents • Domestic incidents involving either self-immolation or assault by another individual
Flash	Explosions of: • Natural gas • Propane • Gasoline • Vapors of other flammable liquids
Scald	Contact with: • Hot water • Steam
Contact	Contact with: • Hot tar • Metals • Plastic • Grease • Glass

Electrical

Although at times considered to be a thermal burn, electrical injuries manifest with a complex clinical presentation, combining both thermal and nonthermal characteristics (Purdue, Arnoldo, & Hunt, 2007). Electrical burns occur when an electrical current is introduced to the body at a point of contact and travels through the body along the path of least resistance towards a natural ground, finally exiting through the earth contact (e.g., a child touching an electrical wire, where the entry point is the hand, and the exit point is through the feet). Heat is generated by the flow of electrical current through body tissue, with higher voltages creating higher temperatures and greater thermal injury (to both external and internal tissues). The severity of electrical burn injury is dependent on the voltage, path of current flow, duration of contact, and resistance of the tissue at the point of contact (Purdue et al., 2007). Although the local pathology of an electrical burn is less extensive (as only the entry and exit contact points with the electrical source show signs of visible skin injury), the deeper tissue damage caused by the electrical current passing through the body is often considerable and may be potentially devastating. All electrical burn injuries are full thickness and often damage underlying structures, necessitating radical reconstructive surgery. Electrical injury can also cause disruption of the body's normal electrical activities, leading to at least temporary neurological dysfunction in nearly all patients (Purdue et al., 2007). Transient nerve injuries resulting in temporary numbness and tingling are most common. In more severe injury, the impact of the electrical current also may affect cardiac and other systemic functions (such as renal and vascular).

Chemical

Although only 3% of all burn injuries are due to chemical exposure, 30% of all burn deaths are attributable to chemical injury (Luterman & Curreri, 1990). Examples of agents that commonly cause chemical burns include domestic cleaning agents, industrial acids and alkalis, cement, agricultural lime, phosphorus, and extravenously injected cytotoxic drugs (Cook, 2002a). Chemical injury may occur through direct contact with the body surfaces or via inhalation and ingestion. Principles of wound management for chemical burns correspond with those of thermal burns. Chemical burns, however, tend to be deep as a result of continued tissue necrosis caused by sustained and/or prolonged skin exposure. Rapid removal of the suspected chemical burn agent by copious irrigation (i.e., placing the burn wound under running tap water) is therefore the ideal immediate course of action. It is important to note that the mechanism of burn injury differs between acid and alkaline chemical damage. Acid causes burning via coagulative necrosis, whereas alkaline causes burning via liquefactive necrosis. As a result, alkaline burns may potentially result in a more severe injury. In addition to the primary or local injury and the physiological responses to the burn injury itself, additional systemic toxicity may also result from absorption/injection of the chemical material into the body. The severity of a chemical burn injury is dependent on the type of chemical, concentration (strength), quantity of the agent, duration of contact with the skin, and the chemical agent's mechanism of action (Cook, 2002a; Sanford, 2007).

EPIDEMIOLOGY OF BURN INJURY

Burn injury is recognized as one of the most devastating physiological and psychological insults. It is frequently associated with long periods of hospitalization, and with high rates of mortality (Duggan & Quine, 1995; Esselman, 2007; Locke, Rossignol, & Burke, 1990; McCall & Cahill, 2005). Approximately 60,000 to 80,000 people sustain burn injuries that require in-hospital care in the United States of America per annum (Pruitt et al., 2007). The nature and extent of injury are heterogeneous within the burn injury population, yet international studies have revealed relatively consistent patterns in relation to the age and sex of the typical burn injury patient, and the location, extent, and type of the most commonly occurring burns, as detailed in Table 4–2.

Table 4–2. Epidemiological Information for the Burn Population	
Age and Gender	• Research indicates a male predominance for burn injury (75.3% male).[1] • A population study of admitted patients indicates a median age of 30 years.[1]
Risk Factors for Burn Injury	• Factors placing a patient at risk for sustaining burn injury include: ◦ Presence of psychiatric disorders ◦ Very young or elderly ◦ Being on prescription medication ◦ Regular or excessive alcohol consumption ◦ Smoking ◦ Engaging in occupational activities pertaining to exposure to flammable liquids and gases or electrical equipment[2–4]
Burn Size and Mortality	• Determinants of death post-burn injury include: ◦ Larger percentage of TBSA burned ◦ Increasing age ◦ Presence of inhalation injury ◦ Absence of surgical treatment when surgical treatment is clinically indicated ◦ Female sex[5]
Burn Type	• Primary cause: thermal injury—accounting for ¾ of the burns population for both adults and children. Flame injuries account for almost half of all burn injuries in adults (flame injury 49.5%), whereas scalds are the most common cause for burns in children.[10] Other types of thermal injury account for approximately another third of the burns population (scalds 24.3%, contact with hot object 9.0%).[1–4,6–7] • To a lesser extent, burn injury occurs due to chemical (5.0%), electrical (6.8%), or friction (2.0%) agents.[1,6–7]
Location of Injury	• Most commonly burned areas include: the upper limb (45%), head and neck (25%), lower limb (16%), trunk (9%), and other areas (5%).[8,9]
Extent of Injury	• Most individuals receive between 11 and 20% total body burn.[2]

[1] *Royal Brisbane and Women's Hospital Burns Unit: 1972–2004 Mortality and Determinants of Death*, by J. Nicol and M. Rudd, 2004, Brisbane, QLD: RBWH Burns Unit, University of Queensland.

[2] "Burn Injuries and Characteristics of Burn Patients in New South Wales, Australia," by D. Duggan and S. Quine, 1995, *Burns*, *21*(2), pp. 83–89.

[3] "Adult Burns in Melbourne," by A. MacLeod, 1970, *Medical Journal of Australia*, *2*, pp. 772–777.

[4] "A Survey of Adults with Flame Burns at a Melbourne Hospital," by J. Masterton, T. Pressley, and G. Ramsay, 1979, *Medical Journal of Australia*, *1*, pp. 332–334.

[5] "Determinants of Death Following Burn Injury," by M. J. Muller, S. P. Pegg, and M. R. Rule, 2001, *British Journal of Surgery*, *88*(4), pp. 583–587.

[6] "Epidemiological, Demographic, and Outcome Characteristics of Burn Injury," by B. A. Pruitt, Jr., S. E. Wolf, and A. D. Mason, Jr., 2007, in D. N. Herndon (Ed.), *Total Burn Care* (3rd ed., pp. 14–32), Edinburgh, UK: Elsevier Saunders.

[7] "The Aetiology of Burns in Developed Countries: Review of the Literature," by O. van Rijn, L. Bouter, and R. Meertens, 1989, *Burns*, *15*(4), pp. 217–221.

[8] "Surveillance for Fatal and Non-Fatal Injuries—United States, 2001," by S. B. Vyrostek, J. L. Annest, and G. W. Ryan, 2004, *Morbidity and Mortality Weekly Report*, *53*(SS07), pp. 1–57

[9] "Burns of the Head and Neck," by R. F. Edlich et al., 1984, *Otolaryngologic Clinics of North America*, *17*(2), pp. 361–388.

[10] *Emergency Management of Severe Burns [EMSB] Course Manual*, by Australian and New Zealand Burns Association [ANZBA], 2008, Brisbane, Australia: The Education Committee of the Australian and New Zealand Burns Association Limited.

ANATOMY AND PHYSIOLOGY OF THE SKIN

Despite the high degree of heterogeneity within the burn population, a loss of skin integrity is a common feature between patients regardless of etiology (Johnson, O'Shaughnessy, & Ostegren, 1981). Although clinical assessment of the wound is the responsibility of the experienced burn specialist, all members of the multidisciplinary management team require a basic understanding of skin biology. Referred to as the integumentary system, the skin is the body's largest organ, occupying a surface area of approximately 1.8 m^2 for the average adult (Cook, 2002b; Trofino & Braun, 1991). The skin is a highly complex organ system that serves a number of functions, including:

- Protection from environmental elements
- Immune response
- Perception of stimuli
- Fluid and electrolyte balance
- Thermoregulation
- Cosmetic appearance

Structurally, the skin is made up of two distinct histological areas: the epidermis and the dermis (Figure 4–1), which are separated from underlying bone and muscle by a subcutaneous interface of areolar and adipose tissue (Cook, 2002b; Johnson et al., 1981). The epidermal layer varies in thickness, ranging from 0.05 mm thick on the eyelids to over 1 mm thick on the upper back and soles of the feet (Pham, Gibran, & Heimbach, 2007; Trofino & Braun, 1991). In contrast, the dermis is estimated to be at least 10 times thicker

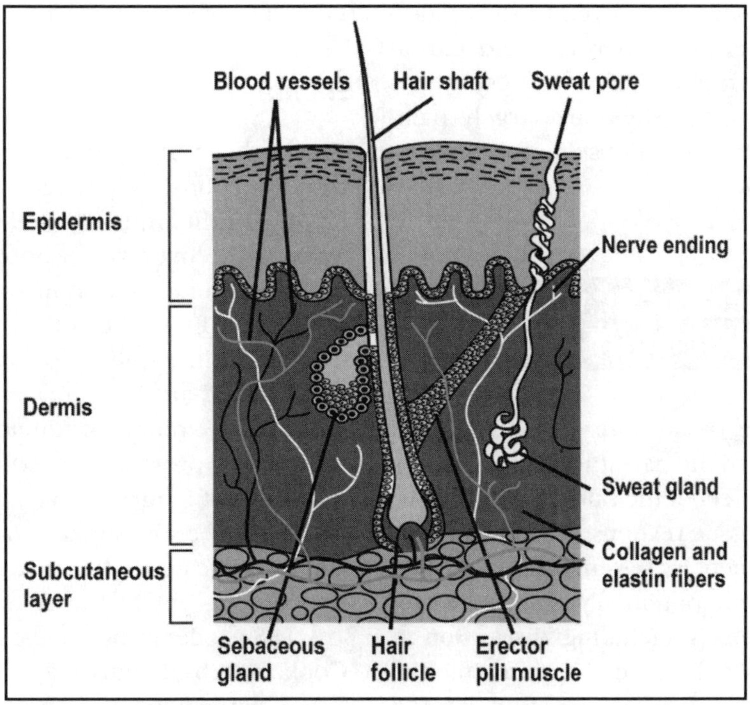

Figure 4–1. Anatomy of the skin.

than the epidermal layer (Pham et al., 2007). Similarly, the dermis also varies in thickness, and is typically thickest on the dorsal aspects of the body and on the lateral aspects of the extremities (Cook, 2002b). Given this variation in thickness, exposure to an injurious agent of the same temperature and duration will lead to burns of different depths at different locations on the body (Trofino & Braun, 1991).

The dermis is primarily composed of fibrous connective tissue rich in collagen and elastic fibers that provide the skin with its strength and elastic properties (Cook, 2002b; Johnson et al., 1981). The dermal layer also contains the appendages of the skin, that is, sebaceous glands, sweat glands, and hair follicles. Sensory nerve endings are embedded within the epidermis, dermis, and the underlying subcutaneous tissue. These nerve endings contribute to the pain associated with burn injury when skin integrity is compromised to the levels of the epidermis and dermis (superficial and partial thickness burns). Full thickness burns (i.e., the wound sites) are largely painless, as all layers of the skin and its derivatives are lost.

PHYSIOLOGICAL RESPONSE TO BURN INJURY

The visible tissue injury resulting from contact with the harmful agent is merely the *local* effect of the burn. In addition to this local tissue response, disturbance to the integumentary system leaves the body susceptible to potentially life-threatening *systemic effects*, including: disruption to homeostasis, an induced hypermetabolic state, increased risk of infection, altered sensation, and pain, all of which can pose additional threat to patient recovery and survival. Consequently, it is important that clinicians have an understanding of degree of injury severity (as defined by depth and area) and the resultant physiological responses to burn injury, as these factors invariably influence management decisions, and the prognosis or healing potential of the patient (Pham et al., 2007).

Tissue Response to Injury

Burn injury causes cell damage or death and deranges the functions of the skin resulting in pathophysiological tissue changes. These pathophysiological responses occur within minutes of a burn being sustained and occur in both the tissues local to the burn as well as systemically over seemingly unaffected areas. The magnitude of these changes depends on the extent of damage to the integument.

Edema

When a burn injury occurs, the inflammatory response is initiated within a few minutes of the injury. A well-recognized entity is the massive tissue edema that ensues within 8 to 24 hours after injury (Demling, 2005; Edlich et al., 1984). Due to changes in capillary permeability in the damaged areas, edema concentrates beneath the injury, producing copious amounts of protein-rich exudate (fluid discharge). If a burn is smaller than 30% of the total body surface area (TBSA), edema is localized to surrounding the injured area, yet in burns greater than 30% TBSA, edema becomes generalized (Cook, 2002b). Edema may also be manifested by the need for considerable fluid resuscitation. Fluid resuscitation is the process by which the patient receives additional fluids, usually intravenously. Large amounts of fluid resuscitation are required within the first 24 hours of sustaining a severe burn injury in order to combat evaporative loss from the burn wound and to prevent decreased plasma volume, which may in turn lead to intravascular hypovolemia. If untreated, intravascular hypovolemia precipitates organ system failure, predominantly renal failure (Australian and New Zealand Burn Association [ANZBA], 2008). In most cases, swelling subsides over the first 3 to 4 days after the injury (Cook, 2002b; Pankhurst & Pochkhanawala, 2002).

Tissue Death and Damage

Exposure to extreme temperatures, incompatible with cell life, results in tissue destruction and impaired skin function at the direct site of contact and to surrounding tissues. Conceptually, this phenomenon is expressed by classifying the burn wound as having three zones: the zone of coagulation, zone of stasis, and zone of hyperemia, all of which are three-dimensional (Dyer & Roberts, 1990). The *zone of coagulation* (also known as the zone of necrosis) is concentrated in the center of the wound, where nonliving tissue is situated. This includes the eschar, the area of dead surface skin. The *zone of stasis* is located deeper and peripheral to the zone of coagulation, and it consists of viable tissue; however, this tissue is still at risk of further damage from ischemia due to decreased perfusion. Around the zone of stasis is the *zone of hyperemia*, the outermost part of the injury. This consists of normal tissue or cells with minimal injury, and is characterized by increased blood flow (vasodilation) due to the inflammatory response to the injury.

Tissue Regeneration

The ability of the skin to repair itself depends on the depth of damage. Wound healing processes and medical management will differ between burn types, with many burns being a combination of varying depths. Generally, superficial burns heal within 7 days without scarring, and some partial thickness burns have the potential to heal spontaneously with minimal scarring within 14 days. This is possible given that islands of viable epithelium remain intact around the skin appendages, each being a source of regeneration. Deep partial thickness burns may take up to a month to heal, and surgical intervention may be warranted. A burn that destroys all remnants of the integumentary system (full thickness burn injury) will necessitate surgical intervention as there may be damage to the underlying muscle, bone, or tendon. Even in the event where re-epithelialization occurs, it will typically be slow, and result in poor-quality, thin skin. These wounds heal by granulation and contraction processes that prolong the healing time to months, resulting in undesirable cosmetic outcomes such as scar and contracture formation, as discussed in the following section.

Scar, Contracture, and Stricture Formation

Deep dermal burns that are allowed to close spontaneously typically result in hypertrophic scarring (Bayat, McGrouther, & Ferguson, 2003). The hypertrophic scar consists of hypercellular and disorganized connective tissue. At the commencement of skin healing, occurring 3 to 24 days after the initial injury, cells begin to proliferate. Cells called fibroblasts begin to produce collagen, the main component of connective tissue. Early production of collagen is irregular and this precipitates the physical appearance of the burn scar. This collagen scaffolding supports fragile new capillaries that make up granulation tissue. With the completion of cell proliferation, the wound is filled by granulation tissue. This may give the appearance of being healed, yet the skin will remain red, raised, and itchy. Wound maturation can take up to two to three years, with the scar being extensively remodeled during this period. It is during this time that there is a progressive decrease in vascularity, and with the use of pressure garments the pattern of collagen fibers flattens, consequently resulting in scar flattening and softening, leading to improved scar flexibility and esthetic appearance.

Given that large wounds will contract over time, the healing process must be monitored to facilitate a positive functional and cosmetic outcome. Dougherty and Warden (2003) highlight that all scarring and free grafts shrink with tissue maturation, unless influenced by an opposing force. Contractures are therefore considered common sequelae after extensive burn injury. Contraction can begin as early as 4 days after injury. Full thickness wounds appear to shrink as the surrounding skin is pulled together as a result of the forces generated by the proliferation of differentiated fibroblasts (Bessey, 2007). Contraction of the burn wound may result in either *contracture* or *stricture* formation. Both are the result of the same process, but a narrowing of a tube or canal (e.g., esophagus) is referred to as a stricture, whereas the term contracture refers to the shortening of the muscle, skin, and other soft tissue. Both can lead to a decline in functional abilities if they remain untreated throughout the acute and rehabilitation stages of burn management.

Disruption to Homoeostasis

The skin plays a major role in thermoregulation of our body. Approximately 97% of the heat from the body is lost through the skin. Thermoregulation is controlled by modulating the amount of blood flowing through the vessels within the dermis. As the body produces more heat, the capillary network within the skin becomes dilated, increasing the temperature of the skin and producing excess sweat. Excess heat is able to be dissipated through a number of ways; patients may need to be cooled further (for example, by use of additional fans). The production of excess sweat leads to copious water, sodium, and chloride loss. Under these conditions, the body's heat loss may exceed heat production; thus, energy must be supplied by increasing the room temperature to 28°C or more. For the reasons described above, it is imperative that a patient's body temperature is monitored closely for signs of hypothermia, particularly during the early stages of treatment, during dressing changes, and in the operating room.

Hypermetabolic Response to Burn Injury

Severe burn injury is followed by dramatic metabolic alterations. The cause of post-burn hypermetabolism is not yet well understood, but it is thought to be predominantly due to hormonal changes in response to the physiologic stress caused by loss of skin integrity (Atiyeh, Gunn, & Dibo, 2008; Demling & Seigne, 2000). The intensity of the metabolic response is dependent on the extent of the injury, body weight upon admission, the presence or absence of sepsis, and the time from injury to excisional surgery (Norbury & Herndon, 2007; Rose & Jordan, 1999; Wilmore, Long, Mason, Skreen, & Pruitt, 1974). In the initial 12 to 24 hour period after a burn injury is sustained, there is a reduction in a person's metabolic rate—commonly known as the *ebb* phase. This is followed by a gradual increase in metabolic rate, plateauing around 5 days post-injury, that can persist through acute admission for up to a year (Pereira, Murphy, & Herndon, 2005; Pham et al., 2007). This hypermetabolic or *flow* phase leads to an overall increase in energy expenditure. During this phase it is important to meet the body's nutritional demands in order to prevent excessive weight loss, preserve muscle tissue, promote rapid wound healing, and support immunocompetence. Optimal nutrition via oral intake can be difficult, especially if the patient has dysphagia. Alternative methods for delivering nutrition during the early phase of recovery are commonplace, especially in adult patients who have sustained deep partial or full thickness burns to more than 20% TBSA, despite the presence or absence of dysphagia. For the adult patient who has sustained a deep burn with surface area exceeding 20% TBSA, the caloric requirements are approximately double what the patient would usually require on a daily basis without the burn injury (ANZBA, 2008). High-calorie nasogastric feeds coupled with normal oral intake has been suggested as the most expeditious way to normalize the hypermetabolic response (Sologub, Zaets, Tarasov, Mordkovitch, & Yu Yashin, 1992).

Infection

Infection is a common and serious complication of major burn injury. Burn injury causes the loss of the epithelial layer of the skin, the natural protective barrier that prevents microorganisms from entering the body. In addition, infection is further promoted by malnutrition induced by the hypermetabolic response to injury and a generalized post-burn immunosuppression. Despite the use of antimicrobial agents, the eschar is rapidly colonized by microorganisms within a few days post-burn and can lead to invasive burn sepsis (the presence of various exudate-forming and other pathogenic organisms or their toxins, in the blood or tissues), given that it occurs in the presence of a compromised immune system. Infection may also potentially lead to burn wound conversion, where the initial burn wound depth converts to a deeper burn wound as a result of the body's inability to effectively utilize the appropriate defense mechanisms to combat invading pathogens.

Impaired Sensation and Pain

Hearing the word *burn* for almost any individual conjures up vivid images of unbearable, unrelenting pain and suffering. However, no two people will react to a burn injury in the same way, experience the same level of physical or psychological pain, or endure the same process of recovery (Faucher, 2003; Meyer, Patterson, Jaco, Woodson, & Thomas, 2007).

The spectre of pain experienced after burn injury is due to stimulation of the sensory nerve endings that transverse both layers of the skin and the underlying subcutaneous tissues (Johnson et al., 1981; Pham et al., 2007). Every burn injury is painful, yet a greater degree of discomfort will be experienced when the nerve endings in the skin survive, such as following superficial or partial thickness burns. Full thickness burns can also be painful even though all components of the skin have been eradicated, as they often receive nociceptor (pain receptor) input from surrounding undamaged or less severely burned areas, because wounds are rarely uniform.

Pain experienced by the patient with burn injury varies on a minute-to-minute, hour-to-hour, and day-to-day basis. The presence of severe pain can complicate, or altogether hinder, a patient's recovery (Patterson, Tininenko, & Ptacek, 2006). It is important to remain cognizant of potentially painful experiences during activities of daily living (ADLs), clinical examination, and treatment. If adequate pain relief is not provided, patients may begin to anticipate pain (even when the forthcoming experience may not be painful), resulting in poor compliance with treatment processes.

PSYCHOLOGICAL RESPONSE TO BURN INJURY

Treatment of the burned individual includes the recovery of optimal functioning in all areas of life. Burn survivors experience a multitude of traumatic assaults, yet many individuals do not look past the physical appearance to the patient's psychological morbidity. Knowledge gained through clinical observations, patient self-report, and empirical studies suggests that burn care that incorporates psychosocial management can facilitate more positive psychological adaptation in response to the challenges of recovery and rehabilitation (Blakeney & Meyer, 1994; Sheridan et al., 2000). Manifestations of psychological distress may present differently throughout the stages of burn management. Extensive psychology and psychiatry involvement is commonplace for the treatment of sleep disturbance, depression, body image dissatisfaction, and acute and post-traumatic stress in this population (Cromes, Holavanahalli, Kowalske, & Helm, 2002; Ehde, Patterson, Wiechman, & Wilson, 1999, 2000; Fauerbach et al., 2000; Wiechman et al, 2001; Yu & Dimsdale, 1999). It is crucial that all members of the multidisciplinary team provide constant reassurance and encouragement to assist in reducing patient anxiety and to facilitate patient motivation and cooperation.

CLASSIFICATION OF BURN INJURY

Burn classification serves as a foundation for description of the burn for diagnostic purposes, for prognostic and therapeutic decisions, and as an outcome measure to analyze the efficacy of treatment protocols (Johnson et al., 1981). Traditionally, burns have been classified on the depth of the tissue damage at the time of injury, usually indicated as one of three degrees of severity. Correlations between greater areas of TBSA burned and higher mortality rates led to the addition of this measurement to the description of burn depth. Today, the severity of burn injuries is determined by taking into account a range of variables, including the area and depth of injury, as well as other influencing factors including patient age, prior medical history, the presence of concomitant injuries, and the location of the wound itself. Each of these aspects will be described in turn below.

Depth of Injury

Depth of injury is an important prognostic factor, as it is well recognized that the greater the depth of the burn, the poorer the prognosis. The degree or depth of injury is dependent upon two variables: the intensity or concentration of the burning agent and the duration of exposure to the agent (Dyer, 1988). For example, in thermal injuries, the depth of injury will be influenced by both the level of heat generated by the burn agent and its duration of contact. Depth of the burn wound is assessed using the following clinical indicators: color, presence of blisters, capillary refill response, sensation, and healing properties (ANZBA, 2008). It is important to consider that the burn wound is heterogeneous and its appearance and characteristics may change with time. Consequently, first aid and medical techniques must be carefully considered before being applied at each stage of change, as a one size fits all approach will not be appropriate.

In current clinical practice, the depth of burn is described based on the level of destruction of the skin surface. There have, however, been recent changes to the terminology used to classify depth of burn. The terms superficial, partial thickness, and full thickness burn are now used in most clinical settings. Explanation of these three levels of classification has been outlined in Table 4–3.

Area of Injury

The area of injury is typically described as a percentage of total body surface area (%TBSA) burned. This measure is not only an important clinical indicator of burn severity, but it is a determinant used in a number of management decisions (e.g., whether the patient requires transfer to specialized burn unit, requirement for fluid resuscitation, need for enteral nutrition), and is an important prognostic indicator for long-term form and function of the affected areas. Consequently, it is critical that an accurate assessment of TBSA burned is made. An exception to this rule is the use of TBSA to determine severity of electrical burn injury. Due to the fact that there may be only a small extent of surface tissue damage at the contact point of the electrical burn (and therefore small TBSA), this measure fails to account for the extensive underlying tissue damage.

Throughout history, various methods of calculating burn area have been adopted, each being modified and later replaced by more objective methods (Klaus, 2004). Two formulas are currently used in specialized burn facilities worldwide: the rule of nines (Wallace, 1951) for an estimate of extent; and the technique of Lund and Browder (1944) for more accurate assessment.

Clinically, the rule of nines is considered a useful assessment tool for evaluating the extent of burn injury in an emergency setting, such as in disaster areas or at the

Table 4–3. Clinical Depth of Burn

Current Nomenclature (Old)	***Depth of Integument Damage***	***Color***	***Blisters***	***Capillary Refill***	***Sensation***	***Healing***	***Example***
Superficial thickness (first degree)	Loss of epidermis	Pale pink	Small blisters	Present	Painful	Within 1 week	Bad sunburn Brief contact
Partial thickness (second degree)	Loss of epidermis and superficial-mid-portions of dermis	Dark pink	Large blisters	Present but sluggish	Reduced sensation. May have areas that are painful and areas that are insensate	1–3 weeks May need surgical intervention May scar	Flash burn Scald
Deep–full thickness (third degree)	Loss of epidermal and dermal layers, potentially down to subcutaneous tissue	Blotchy red, white, waxy, or charred appearance	Absent	Absent	Absent	Will not heal in <3–4 weeks Requires surgical intervention Will scar	Scald Flame burn Friction

Note. Adapted from Australian and New Zealand Burn Association [ANZBA], 2008, *Emergency Management of Severe Burns [EMSB]—Course Manual*, p. 44, Brisbane, Australia: The Education Committee of the Australian and New Zealand Burn Association Limited.

site of the accident (Klaus, 2004). This method divides the body into standardized segments, with each segment grossly corresponding to multiples of 9%, with the exclusion of the perineum, which accounts for 1% (Figure 4-2). For example,

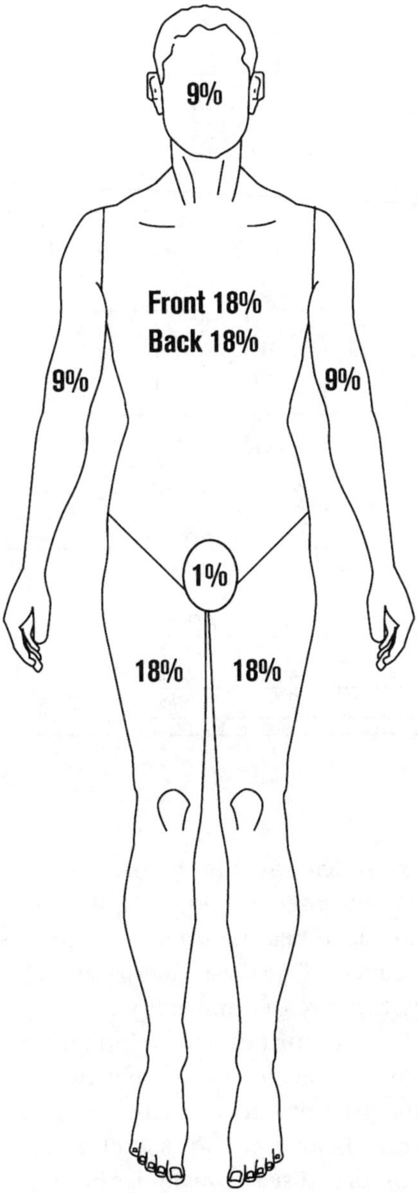

Figure 4–2. Rule of nines.

a circumferential burn to the left arm, including the hand, would be classed as 9% TBSA. Although this method has proved to have clinical utility in some situations, it is not used widely in burn centers largely because it does not account for the variability of body proportion with age. A modified version of this algorithm (the pediatric rule of nines) should be used in the pediatric population, as the child has different body proportions to the adult (i.e., the head is proportionally bigger to the rest of the child's body).

The method proposed by Lund and Browder (1944) relies on the accurate drawing of the burn onto a standardized chart. The areas are then added together using the specified percentage of body surface area (Figure 4-3). For example, shading on the palmar aspect of the left hand and the anterior aspect of the left thigh in an adult indicates a TBSA burned of 6.25% (1.5% + 4.75%). The Lund and Browder (1944) chart is used in most burn facilities worldwide, as it accommodates for the changes in body surface area accounted for by growth.

Other Influencing Factors

There are a number of characteristics that have significant bearing on the survival of a patient with burn injury. It is universally agreed that TBSA burned and age of the patient (discussed below) are the two most important factors that contribute to mortality. It is acknowledged, however, that there are a variety of other influencing factors that may assist in defining the patient's prognosis (Tejero-Trujeque, 2000). These factors include:

- Age. Prognosis is worsened in patients under the age of 2 years and

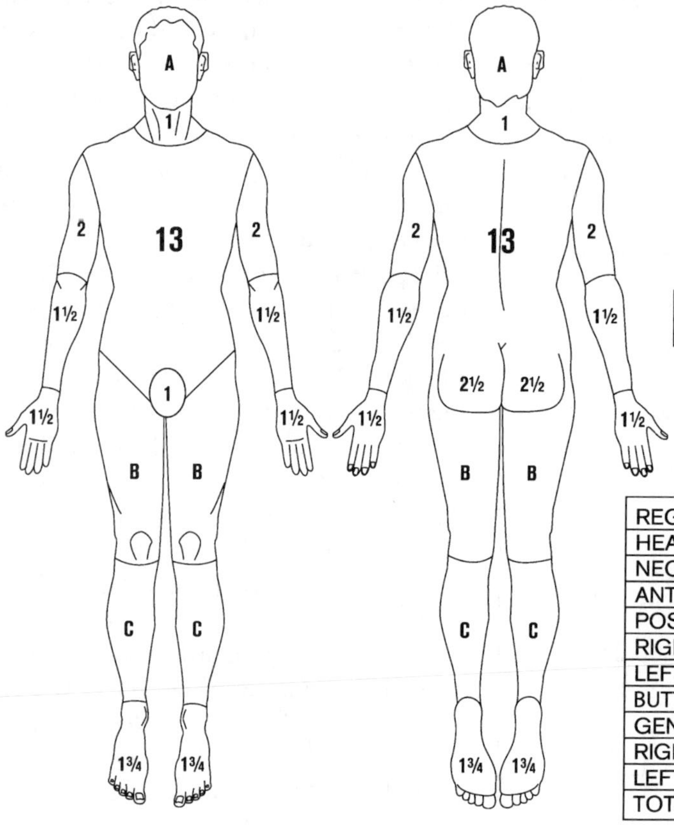

Ignore simple erythema

Partial thickness loss (PTL)

Full thickness loss (FTL)

	%	
REGION	PTL	FTL
HEAD		
NECK		
ANT. TRUNK		
POST. TRUNK		
RIGHT ARM		
LEFT ARM		
BUTTOCKS		
GENITALIA		
RIGHT LEG		
LEFT LEG		
TOTAL BURN		

Relative percentage of body surface area affected by growth

AREA	AGE 0	1	5	10	15	ADULT
A = ½ OF HEAD	9 ½	8 ½	6 ½	5 ½	4 ½	3 ½
B = ½ OF ONE THIGH	2 ¾	3 ¼	4	4 ½	4 ½	4 ¾
C = ½ OF ONE LEG	2 ½	2 ½	2 ¾	3	3 ¼	3 ½

Figure 4–3. Lund and Browder chart.

over the age of 60 relative to other age groups suffering from a similar size injury (Cook, 2002a). This difference is due to the fragility of skin in these age groups: if an elderly person is exposed to a burning agent for the same time as a middle aged adult, the elderly patient will suffer a deeper injury due to the differences in their skin structure.

- Medical History. A number of preexisting medical conditions can complicate wound management and the healing process, as well as having a crucial bearing on an individual's chance of survival. Factors associated with increased mortality post-thermal burn injury include heart disease, sickle cell anemia, diabetes mellitus, atherosclerosis, chronic renal failure, cirrhosis, collagen vascular disease, malignancy, use of steroids, leukopenia secondary to chemotherapeutic agents, and states of immune compromise (Cook, 2002a; Trofino & Braun, 1991).

- Concomitant Injuries. Injuries sustained simultaneously with the burn injury may markedly influence an individual's survival and the course of their recovery. Those patients who may have sustained their injuries in accidental situations may have related trauma such as head, chest, and/or abdominal trauma, spinal cord injury, and associated orthopedic injuries requiring attention. In the circumstance of a more serious concomitant injury, the burn wound may be assigned as a low treatment priority (Trofino & Braun, 1991).
- Presence of Inhalation Injury. A report of the patient's circumstance at the time of injury can aid in determining if an inhalation injury should be suspected. Approximately one third of all individuals admitted to burn treatment facilities present with inhalation injury (Clark, 1992a). Specifically, inhalation injury is defined as an "injury to the epithelial lining of the lower tracheobronchial tree and the lower airway" (Muehlberger, Kunar, Munster, & Couch, 1998, p. 1003) and has been correlated with decreased rates of survival (Bayley, 1991; Muller, Pegg, & Rule, 2001). Inhalation injury is typically described as being either above or below the glottis, yet patients are not limited to either type of injury in isolation (Knights, 2002). Indicators for the presence of inhalation injury include: signs of respiratory failure, patient unconsciousness, exposure to smoke or heat in an enclosed space, singed facial hair, dysphonia, erythema or soot in the oral or nasal areas, and carbonaceous sputum (Grunwald & Garner, 2008; Muehlberger et al., 1998). The presence of inhalation injury increases a patient's risk of mortality by up to 40% when compared to patients with similar cutaneous burns without inhalation injury (Bayley, 1991). If pneumonia transpires, the mortality rate may increase to 70% (ANZBA, 2008).
- Site of Injury. A number of anatomical locations, specifically the face, feet, hands, and perineum, are considered to signal more severe burns regardless of the extent and degree of injury. This is because burns to these regions are prone to infection, may result in functional deformities if not correctly treated, and may lead to an increased incidence in pulmonary compromise (Hartford & Kealey, 2007; Trofino & Braun, 1991).

MEDICAL MANAGEMENT OF BURN INJURY

The National Hospital Ambulatory Medical Survey conducted within the United States of America found that in 2005, 593 of every 100,000 emergency room visits were for injuries sustained from fire, flame, or hot substances (Nawar, Niska, & Xu, 2007). Of the patients that present for burn treatment in the emergency departments of hospitals worldwide, many cannot be admitted due to the sheer number and the demand on specialized services (Hunt, Arnoldo, & Purdue, 2007). With Australia having an estimated 100,000 people suffering burn injuries on an annual basis (Medicine Australia, 2006), it is no surprise that the cost and labor demands prevent specialized burn treatment centers throughout the nation from accommodating the patient with a less severe burn as an inpatient. Therefore, these individuals are successfully treated with outpatient intervention.

There has been a drive towards access to and efficiency of health care for the more severely affected individuals in this population; thus, criteria for burn center admission have become necessary. Despite differences in international health care practices, the criteria specified by both the Australian and New Zealand Burn Association (2004) and the American Burn Association (American College of Surgeons, 2006) to support patient transfer to a specialized burn care unit are largely consistent and have been outlined in Table 4–4.

For patients admitted for inpatient care, management of burn injury is typically complex. Although there is extreme heterogeneity in treatment, with each patient requiring a different level of medical intervention depending on the area and depth of the burn as well as other influencing factors, there are a number of medical and surgical procedures that are routinely required and are detailed below.

Intubation and Ventilation

Direct thermal injury to the orofacial region with subsequent swelling of the tissues may result in obstruction of the external nasal passages and mouth, rendering the patient unable to maintain a patent airway. If prophylactic intubation has not been successfully performed by emergency services in the field or on hospital admission, tracheostomy may be necessitated to relieve upper airway

Table 4–4. Australian and New Zealand Burn Association (ANZBA) Endorsed Criteria for Burn Injuries Requiring Transfer to a Specialized Burn Facility

Criteria for Specialized Burns Treatment
• Burns greater than 10% of total body surface area (TBSA)
• Burns of special areas—face, hands, feet, genitalia, perineum, and major joints
• Full thickness burns greater than 5% of TBSA
• Electrical burns
• Chemical burns
• Burns with an associated inhalation injury
• Circumferential burns of the limbs or chest
• Burns in the very young or very old
• Burns in people with preexisting medical disorders that could complicate management, prolong recovery, or increase mortality
• Burns with associated trauma

Note. From Australian and New Zealand Burn Association (ANZBA), 2004, *Burn Injuries Requiring Transfer to a Burns Unit.* Retrieved July 9, 2008, from http://www.anzba.org.au/ . Reprinted with permission.

obstruction. Upon admission, fiberoptic bronchoscopy may be performed to investigate damage to the airway. Alternatively, nasendoscopy can be used to examine mucosal integrity of the nasal passages and upper airway.

Prophylactic intubation is often performed on patients who are suspected to have sustained airway damage, but the use of this technique for managing and maintaining airway patency in the early stages after thermal injury is not without controversy. Knights (2002, p. 115) states, "If in doubt, intubate!" Although this treatment approach has been accepted within many burn facilities, the literature has not yet identified a definitive diagnostic set of indicators for intubation and ventilatory support (Madnani, Steele, & de Vries, 2006). The decision to intubate should be made with consideration of the risk of sustaining further damage to the larynx and subglottic regions (Muehlberger et al., 1998; Prater & Deskin, 1998; Valdez, Desai, Ruhl, & Nigri, 2006). Other reasons that may indicate the need for intubation include medical instability or severe pain requiring a large amount of medications, which may cause suppression of the respiratory system.

Generally in the burn population, tracheostomy is reserved for those who are unable to undergo translaryngeal intubation secondary to edema, those who require prolonged mechanical ventilation in excess of 2 weeks, or those who fail extubation (Barret, Desai, & Herndon, 2000; Calhoun et al., 1988; Jones, Madden, Finkelstein, Yurt, & Goodwin, 1989). Tracheostomy may also be beneficial in the burn patient requiring lengthy or radical facial reconstruction. Although previously considered to be an indicator for increased mortality (Eckhauser, Billote, Burke, & Quinby, 1974), authors have now refuted this belief (Palmieri, Jackson, & Greenhalgh, 2002; Saffle, Morris, & Edelman, 2002), stating that tracheostomy is safe and that it may promote increased comfort levels in this patient population. There have, however, been noted increases in aspiration, dysphagia, respiratory infection, and tracheoesophageal fistula following adoption of tracheostomy in this field (Barret et al., 2000; Calhoun et al., 1988; Coln, Purdue, & Hunt, 1998).

Surgical Repair and Reconstruction

Early surgical excision and closure of the burn wound has repeatedly been shown to decrease mortality and length of hospital stay, minimize risk of infection, and help modulate the hypermetabolic response (Hart et al., 2000; Hart et al., 2003; Herndon et al., 1989a; Muller, Gahankari, & Herndon, 2007). During the acute, intermediate, and late phases of burn management, a number of different surgical procedures may be required to facilitate functional and cosmetic healing potential of the wounds. These procedures are briefly outlined below.

Escharotomy

Escharotomy is a surgical procedure performed to relieve compression caused by constrictive burned tissue known as eschar (Pruitt et al., 2007). Following full thickness circumferential burns, the tough eschar limits elasticity or skin stretching. The lack of ability for the skin tissue to stretch, particularly when edema sets in, may result in vascular compromise to extremities if a limb is circumferentially burned, or respiratory compromise if the torso is circumferentially burned. The procedure involves making an incision through the eschar to expose the subcutaneous tissue below. Residual tissue pressure will often cause the opening to widen substantially. This procedure may be necessary to release restriction of a limb or the chest wall to improve circulation and ventilation (Mlcak & Buffalo, 2007).

Debridement

Debridement is the surgical removal of foreign material or debris and dead, damaged, or infected tissue from a wound (Bessey, 2007). Wound cleansing and debridement in the early stages of hospital admission can occur daily during dressing changes, either in the operating room or on the ward. Debridement is necessary to facilitate dermal regeneration and to provide a clean wound bed prior to laying a graft.

Skin Grafts

Skin grafts are applied after the wound has been cleansed and debrided. During the grafting procedure, donor skin is excised using a specialized instrument called a dermatome that is used to produce thin slices of skin (split thickness skin graft) from a donor area. Commonly used donor sites include the limbs, buttocks, back, chest, abdomen, and scalp. Patients with large burns may have a restricted amount of donor skin available. In these cases, skin may be taken from donor sites considered to be less preferable, such as the neck and perineum. Furthermore, cover with allografts (cadaver or live donor) or xenografts (porcine skin) may be required. The split skin graft can be applied as a sheet (unmeshed) or can alternatively be meshed using a dermacarrier (mesher board) to allow the donor skin to be expanded to cover a larger surface area. The donor skin is then secured to the graft site using a combination of fibrin glue, staples, sutures, Steri-Strips, gauze, splints, and secure dressings. All viable skin grafts should heal within 5 days, with donor sites taking approximately 14 days to heal (Bailie & Wilson, 2002). It is imperative that the patient participate in an individualized contracture management program (see later in chapter) once grafts have healed sufficiently.

Cultured epithelial autograft (CEA) is another treatment used to achieve wound closure. In this technique, a biopsy is taken from the patient, and skin epidermal stem cells are isolated and grown within a laboratory setting. These skin cells can then be harvested into a suspension that is applied to the patient's donor sites or burn wound utilizing a "cell spray" technique with meshed grafts, in order to facilitate more rapid wound healing.

Contracture and Stricture Release

To prevent or limit contracture formation, anticontracture positioning, splinting, and a range of movement exercises are important to maintain soft tissue length during the acute and rehabilitative phases of recovery. Although anticontracture positioning may not facilitate the greatest degree of comfort for the patient, it is necessary to prevent soft tissue shortening and to maintain range of movement.

In some cases, contracture formation cannot be prevented. This is particularly apparent for structures that are not anatomically fixed in position or around a joint (e.g., the mouth, eyes, and neck). Where the extent of contracture is too great to allow functional mobility, or nonsurgical methods of intervention have failed, surgical intervention to release the tissue is required. Release of contractures can occur during the acute, intermediate, and late phases of treatment. Releases that are performed when the scar tissue has matured, however, tend to often have better functional and cosmetic outcomes. It is the goal of surgery to release tension so that good functional and cosmetic outcomes can be facilitated. An extensive range of surgical techniques exists for achieving contracture release, including Z-plasty and split skin and full thickness skin grafts. For more detailed information regarding the range of techniques used in stricture/contracture management the reader is referred to Donelan (2007), listed in the Further Reading section at the end of this chapter. A popular surgical technique for releasing contracture at the lateral oral commissures is the mucosal advancement flap. Care must be taken not to dissect the orbicularis oris muscle when conducting surgical mouth angle release; otherwise, oral incompetence will ensue. In severe cases, a free flap or pedicle flap may be required in order to achieve maximal functional outcome with lower risk for secondary contracture. It is also important to understand that, although the patient may feel immediate benefit from surgical contracture release, ongoing exercise, splinting, and positioning are essential to prevent repeat contracture.

Strictures isolated to the esophagus are corrected with substernal colon bypass, substernal colon interposition, or esophagectomy. Esophageal dilation may be the procedure of choice for less severe strictures; however, there is a chance of restenosis (Shikowitz, Levy, Villano, Graver, & Pochaczevsky, 1996). Laryngeal and tracheal stenoses may occur when edematous mucosa from inhaled gases and heat is scarred from irritation of an endotracheal or tracheostomy tube. In these instances, tracheal stenting and resection may be required to promote adequate oxygenation (Gaissert, Lofgren, & Grillo, 1993). For the patient with severe burn injury caused by inhalation or ingestion, multiple complex surgical interventions are often necessary. For example, pharyngoesophageal strictures that occur as a result of chemical ingestion can require extensive surgical intervention. Hoseok, Shim, Son, Kim, and Choi (2006) describe two patients who both required end to end pharyngocolostomy with supraglottic partial laryngectomy and pharyngoplasty due to an oropharyngeal stricture that extended the entire esophagus, combined with a laryngeal stricture in which the pyriform sinuses were stenosed.

Reconstruction and Flaps

Surgical reconstruction may be necessary in cases of severe burn injury that result in either complete destruction of anatomical structures including the underlying muscle, or disabling contractures that render the patient functionally incompetent. In these situations, multidisciplinary preoperative planning is mandatory in order to facilitate optimal patient outcomes. The site from which the flap is harvested is carefully selected by the surgeon with the view to enhance functionality and cosmetic appearance. For these reasons, flaps are usually harvested from a site with tissue of similar color and texture to the defected tissue region. The flap procedure is advantageous in that the risk for contracture is reduced, although this may be at the expense of normal sensory function. Figure 4–4 illustrates pedicle, rotational, and local tissue advancement flaps to reconstruct a patient's nose, chin, and philtrum, respectively (Clayton, Ledgard, Haertsch, Kennedy, & Maitz, 2008a).

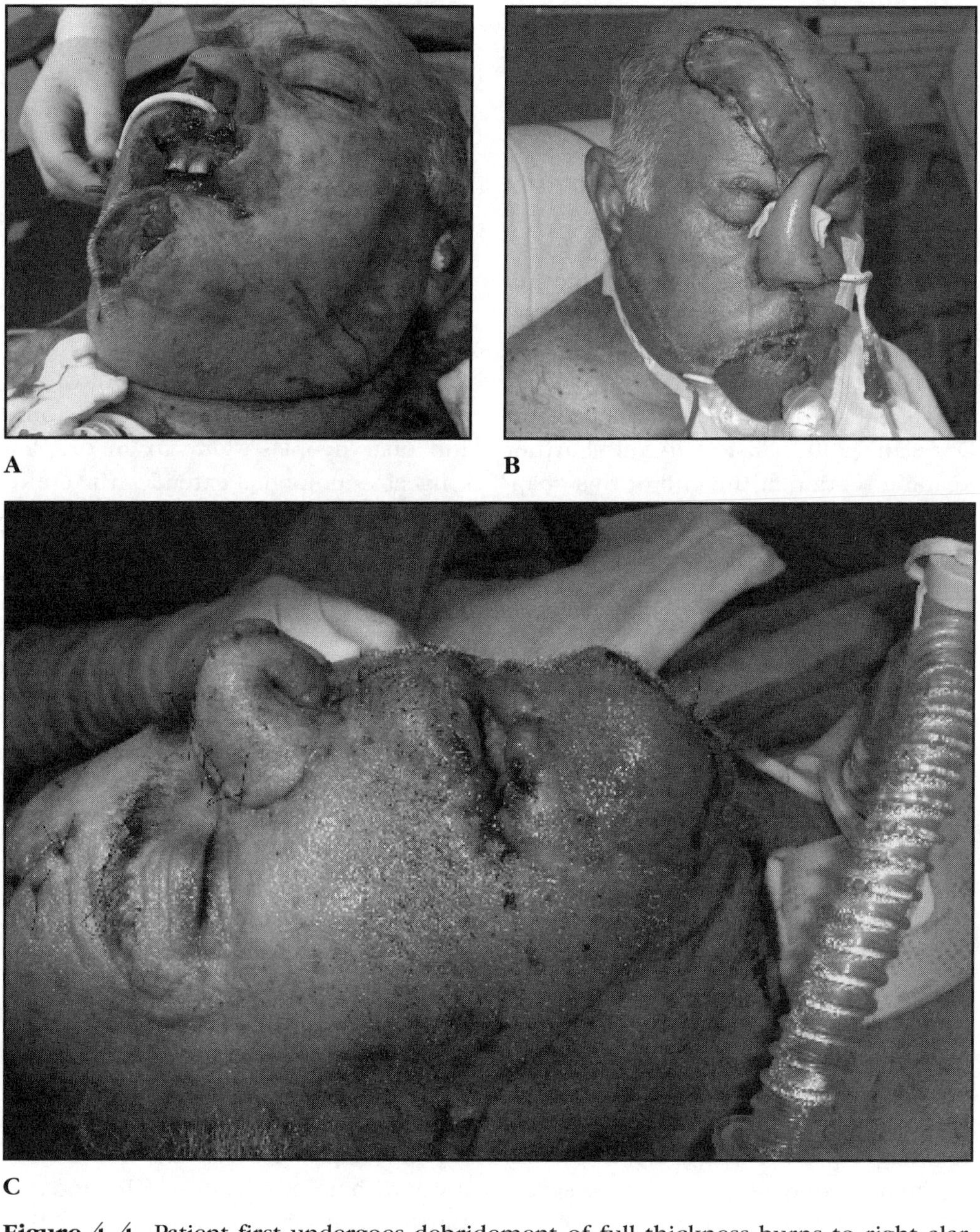

Figure 4–4. Patient first undergoes debridement of full thickness burns to right alar, philtrum, and chin (**A**), and then a pedicle flap is used to recreate right alar, a rotational flap to recreate chin, and local tissue advancement to recreate philtrum (**B**), with the final stage of reconstruction being disconnection of pedicle and revision of chin flap (**C**).

Pain Management

Pain management is complicated in the burn population as the pain experienced by the patient varies from hour to hour and day to day (Choiniere, Melzack, Rondeau, Girard, & Paquin, 1989). Effective and coordinated pain management is of the utmost importance for facilitating patient comfort, cooperation, and participation in active rehabilitation. Administration of opioids is one the foundations to effective management of severe burn pain (Abdi & Zhou, 2002; Faucher & Furukawa, 2006). Intravenous opioids (e.g., morphine), however, are often administered as only part of a comprehensive pain management plan (Gallagher, Rae, & Kinsella, 2000). Further pharmacological intervention includes administration of analgesia or sedatives as typically delivered via oral and/or intravenous routes. The presence of oropharyngeal burns and/or dysphagia should be considered by the medical team when developing a comprehensive pain management program for the individual. Delivery of certain analgesics that cannot be manipulated in form may be limited if the patient is unable to take medications orally.

Consistent reports of central nervous system (CNS) side effects from certain medications are presented throughout a wealth of pain and pharmacology literature. Given that swallowing is under complex neurological control, many of the medications prescribed for use within the burn population may significantly influence both the patient's swallowing function and their suitability for assessment and treatment of oral intake difficulties. Although analgesics and sedatives may be added in addition to the key opioid management regimen, opioids (and benzodiazepines) also inherently have both analgesic and sedative properties (Abdi & Zhou, 2002). Drugs with analgesic or sedative properties may result in extrapyramidal side effects, manifesting as impaired brainstem regulation, and consequently have the potential to delay cricopharyngeal relaxation (Broniatowski et al., 1999). A decreased level of alertness consequent to medication side effects is a common clinical scenario for those patients receiving specialized burn care and other clinical populations accessing SLP services. The list of medications used to manage pain in the burn patient is extensive and ever growing, yet those CNS-depressant medications in current and common use may increase the likelihood of synergistic compromise in swallow safety (Buchholz, 1995).

DYSPHAGIA POST-BURN INJURY

Dysphagia has anecdotally been reported as a common sequela following severe burn injury. At present, however, a systematic research base to support the prevalence, anticipated severity, or the patterns of recovery and resolution of dysphagia in this population is lacking. For this reason, current literature will be referred to where it is available, and the remaining content is derived from our clinical experience with this population.

Prevalence and Predictive Factors

There is an absence of literature reporting on the prevalence of dysphagia across an entire cohort with burn injury. Studies have reported on the number of burn patients referred to SLP during a certain period (Edelman, Sheehy-Deardorff, & White, 2008; McKinnon DuBose, Groher, Carnaby Mann, & Mozingo, 2005; Ward et al., 2001); however, these samples are naturally biased due to the tendency to receive referrals for only those patients with more severe injury or complicated recovery. Two of the current chapter authors (Rumbach & Ward) and colleagues are presently conducting a large-scale longitudinal study involving dysphagia screening of all patients admitted to a major statewide burn unit. Although data collection is incomplete, evidence from the first 200 admitted patients suggests a dysphagia prevalence rate of approximately 10%. Patients presenting with dysphagia were admitted with an average TBSA burn of 27% (ranging from 4 to 66.5% TBSA), with 52% of the patients suffering concomitant inhalation injury. McKinnon DuBose and colleagues have also completed an unpublished prospective observational study where data related to dysphagia and nutrition were collected on 122 consecutively admitted burn patients. Results from this study revealed a dysphagia prevalence rate of 18%. Risk for dysphagia appeared to be higher for the older, more severely burned patients who required mechanical ventilation and tracheostomy.

Like most of the trauma population, the burn population is highly heterogeneous, with no two individuals presenting with the same injury. No reliable clinical indicators have been systematically defined to help identify which burn patients are at greatest risk for dysphagia. Some clinical patterns and similarities can be observed in the populations of dysphagic patients described in the literature, including the presence of inhalation injury, high percentage TBSA burn, and/or facial burns; patients requiring intubation and ventilation and often a tracheostomy; and long admission within critical care units (Table 4-5; Edelman et al., 2008; McKinnon DuBose et al., 2005; Ward et al., 2001). However, although overall similarities are reported in this group data, it is important to note that there is a high degree of individual variability in this population; for example, TBSA has been reported to vary immensely within samples (7 to 85%; Ward et al., 2001). Future research will hopefully help to elucidate whether any of these parameters can be used to reliably predict whether a patient will go on to develop dysphagia post-burn injury. It is possible that not a single clinical factor will predict dysphagia, but rather that an interaction between multiple factors, such as the location of the injury and the patient's overall medical and psychological stability, will influence the patient's ability to swallow safely and efficiently (Ward et al., 2001).

Two unpublished studies by Clayton and colleagues (2006, 2008b) have identified associations between endotracheal intubation, tracheostomy, and dysphagia in the burn population. One study examined the effect of endotracheal intubation on swallowing function and reported that 78.72% of patients intubated for greater than 48 hours demonstrated some degree of dysphagia post-extubation. Positive correlations were also identified between the number of hours the patient was intubated and the following variables: size of the burn injury, days to commence oral intake, and days to achieve premorbid diet consistency with or without supplemental enteral feeding (Clayton, 2006). A second study evaluated the effect of a tracheostomy tube on dysphagia recovery. Severe burn injury patients who had

Table 4–5. Comparison of Current Evidence of Dysphagia Following Thermal Burn Injury

	Ward et al. (2001) N = 30	***McKinnon DuBose et al. (2005) N = 29***	***Edelman et al. (2008) N = 11***
Mean TBSA	50%	35%	36%
Patients with inhalation injury	33%	57%	64%
Patients on mechanical ventilation	100%	96%	100%
Mean duration of ETT	15 days	13.7 days	8 days
Patients with tracheostomy	80%	71%	100%
Mean duration of tracheostomy	(Reported total duration of intubation [ETT + tracheostomy] of 47 days)	42.2 days	Unstated
Mean days to SLP consult	20 days	46 days	54 days
Mean days to oral intake	30 days	46 days	63 days
Mean duration of supplementary feeding	50 days	Unstated	Unstated
Mean length of stay	84 days	66 days	44–85 days
Modified diet at start of oral intake	100% (30% fluids only; 70% food and fluid intake) Consisting of: Fluid: 40% full thick, 23.3% half thick, 36.7% thin Food: 56.7% puree diet, 13.3% soft mechanical diet	79%	73%
Normal diet at start of oral intake	0% food; 11% fluid	7%	9%
Normal diet at discharge	90%	39.3%	45%
Modified diet at discharge	10%	36%	55%
Nil by mouth at discharge	0%	25%	0%

Note. ETT = endotracheal tube; SLP = speech-language pathology; TBSA = total body surface area. Data from "Bedside Assessment of Swallowing Is Predictive of an Abnormal Barium Swallow Examination," by E. A. Edelman, D. A. Sheehy-Deardorff, and M. T. White, 2008, *Journal of Burn Care and Rehabilitation*, *29*(1), pp. 89–96; "Pattern of Dysphagia Recovery after Thermal Burn Injury," by C. McKinnon DuBose, M. G. Groher, G. S. Carnaby Mann, and D. W. Mozingo, 2005, *Journal of Burn Care and Rehabilitation*, *26*(3), pp. 233–237; "Duration of Dysphagic Symptoms and Swallowing Outcomes after Thermal Burn Injury," by E. C. Ward, M. Uriarte, and A.-L. Conroy, 2001, *Journal of Burn Care and Rehabilitation*, *22*(6), pp. 441–453.

a tracheostomy for an extended duration were likely to have a larger area of burn injury and were found to take longer to commence oral intake and to achieve their premorbid oral diet (Clayton, Kennedy, & Maitz, 2008b).

Assessment of Dysphagia Post-Burn Injury

Referral processes are acknowledged to differ between clinical settings; however, referral to SLP for an initial dysphagia assessment typically occurs when the patient has achieved a level of medical stability appropriate for trialing or commencing oral intake. Although for some patients this point may be achieved towards the end of their admission to the critical care unit, for the majority, initial dysphagia assessment will occur after discharge from the critical care or intensive care unit. Depending on the severity of injury, SLP referral practices, and subsequent medical management, the duration to initial dysphagia assessment may range between 20 and 54 days after hospital admission (Edelman et al, 2008; McKinnon DuBose et al., 2005; Ward et al., 2001). Retrospective analyses of SLP involvement in one burn facility showed that on initial SLP assessment, 3.3% of patients still required mechanical ventilation, 56.7% were in the process of weaning from mechanical ventilation, and 40% had been weaned from mechanical ventilation (Ward et al., 2001).

Referral criteria to SLP may differ between individual sites, yet larger organizations such as ANZBA have attempted to unify service provision across facilities by developing principles and guidelines for SLP management of the burn patient. These referral criteria are outlined in Table 4–6.

Both clinical and instrumental assessment tools are used to assess dysphagia in this population. As with other medically complex patients, instrumental assessment allowing better visualization of the pharyngeal phase is strongly recommended to guide decision making for the burn population. Frequent reassessment is often required, initially due to their fluctuating medical status and later in order to monitor ongoing change in functional swallowing recovery. Although both clinical and instrumental assessment techniques have been described in general in Chapter 1, the following contains a discussion of specific issues that should be considered when conducting dysphagia assessment with the burn population.

Table 4–6. ANZBA Speech Pathology Referral Criteria

- Endotracheal tube longer than 48 hours
- Inhalations burns (requiring intubation)
- Ingestion of chemicals
- Facial and/or neck burns
- Presence of a tracheostomy tube
- Concern expressed by patient, family, or team members about aspects of swallowing, communication, or orofacial contracture management in the burn patient

Note. From Clayton, N. A., Whitney, S., O'Loughlin, G., Crouch, A., & Patterson, M. (2005). Speech pathology. In D. Edgar (Ed.), *Burn survivor rehabilitation: Principles and guidelines for the allied health professional* (pp. 74–88). Brisbane, Australia: Australian and New Zealand Burn Association. Reprinted with permission.

Clinical Swallow Examination

A clinical exam is part of a standard dysphagia assessment battery; however, for some burn patients it can provide limited useful information regarding swallow safety, for example, where severe burns and subsequent contracture formation preclude oromotor capabilities from being adequately assessed, or where wound dressings/contracture formation may make laryngeal palpation and cervical auscultation challenging. In these cases, aspiration risk should be determined from oral intake trials performed during an instrumental assessment, most likely an endoscopic swallowing examination (ESE).

The following specific information should be obtained prior to conducting a clinical assessment with a patient with burn injury:

- Prior medical history, including:
  - Preinjury health status and psychosocial history that may influence prognosis and recovery of burn wounds
- Severity of burn injury:
  - %TBSA and depth of burn
  - Location of burn, specifically, the location of any head and neck burns
  - Presence or absence of inhalation injury and the extent of damage to the oral and pharyngeal mucosa
- Associated medical conditions and management:
  - Concomitant injury, including the possibility of hypoxic brain injury from prolonged exposure to smoke
  - Respiratory status and details related to mechanical ventilation and tracheostomy
  - Pain management; pain medications and their impact on cognition/alertness
  - Current nutritional status and nutritional requirements; issue of hypermetabolism
  - Plans for medical/surgical interventions (i.e., timing of debridements and grafting and plans for release of contractures)
  - Timing of daily routine wound care—including pain management and patient's physical and mental state before and after
  - Other therapeutic interventions, e.g., timing and targets of physiotherapy and occupational therapy treatment programs
  - Psychological state

During the acute phase of injury, the clinical assessment is most helpful in determining readiness for oral intake and the timing of instrumental assessment(s). While conducting the clinical assessment, the following issues should be taken into consideration:

- Patient report of pain and response to pain at the time of assessment. Painful experiences in ADLs may lead to increased anxiety and unwillingness to participate in the dysphagia evaluation. Poorly managed background and procedural pain may render the patient unable to perform the fundamental actions required during clinical swallow examination and consumption of meals (Faucher, 2003; Jones, 2002). Pain can be quantified using either a visual analogue scale (VAS; 10 cm line with one end representing no pain and the other end representing worst pain possible) or a numerical rating scale (NRS; for example, a 0–10 scale, with 0 indicating no pain and 10 indicating worst pain possible).

- Timing of assessment. Daily wound cleaning and patient care activities can result in periods of extreme fatigue, which often heighten the presence of pain and exacerbate features of dysphagia. All clinical decisions must be made within the context of the patient's current functional status, and depending on whether that status is stable or fluctuant (e.g., presence of fatigue) throughout the day.
- Extent of tissue injury and stage of recovery. As edema subsides over the initial weeks after admission, range of movement (ROM) will typically recover, resulting in improved function of the oral, pharyngeal, and laryngeal mechanisms. In parallel with improved edema, however, the formation of scar tissue and contractures may become a new source of movement restriction. ROM of the mouth should be measured throughout the acute and rehabilitation phases of treatment. A paper measuring tape can be used to make objective measurements in both the vertical (superior surface of lower lip to inferior surface of upper lip) and horizontal (distance between oral commissures) planes upon full active ROM. Ideal dimensions are a ROM greater than 50 mm in the vertical plane and greater than 60 mm in the horizontal plane.
- Patient's ability to maintain appropriate positioning. The presence of a burn injury may significantly alter an individual's ability to accomplish and maintain a normal body position. Poor positioning and anticipated deformity from the presence of burns to the head and neck can have a substantial impact on the patient's level of functioning, affecting the ability to safely consume food and fluid orally and causing a disruption to the ability to self-feed. The patient with severe burns to the upper limbs and head and neck affecting upper limb movement will require assistance with oral intake during the acute phase. It is important to consult with the medical team regarding positioning for oral intake, and the occupational therapist regarding assisted support for feeding. Following burn injury, positioning may be limited for the following reasons:
    - Patients tend to assume a position of comfort (similar to the fetal position where the arms, legs, and neck are flexed), especially where pain is uncontrolled. Patients feel more comfortable when the burned tissue is contracted and shortened rather that stretched and elongated. However, maintaining a position of comfort promotes formation of contractures that further impact upon positioning. Consequently, despite the discomfort, patients may need to be maintained in a position of extension in order to prevent contracture formation. Individuals with significant total body burns may be required to remain in a position with arms and legs extended for prolonged periods of time.

- Extensive bulky dressings, such as those providing compression forces to entice grafted skin to take, can further limit ROM.
- Decreased levels of alertness due to pain medication and surgical anesthesia can impact upon the patient's ability to actively maintain appropriate positioning (Buchholz, 1995; Johnson et al., 1981; Jones, 2002; Muir, Barclay, & Settle, 1987; Palmer & Collier, 1999; Pankhurst & Pochkhanawala, 2002).
- For patients with head and neck burns, a reduced ability to flex, extend, or rotate the neck may occur due to contracture and hypertrophic scar formation in the later stages of recovery.

- Oral sensation. Oral sensation should be evaluated for the patient with significant facial and inhalation injury. Significant oral inhalation injury can lead to nerve destruction, thus reducing the patient's ability to gauge the myriad of sensory stimuli that is provided upon the acceptance of a bolus into the oral cavity. The patient's lack of awareness of light touch on the lips, tongue, buccal mucosa, and faucial arches may suggest reduced sensation. If oral sensation is reduced, there may also be concomitant pharyngeal and laryngeal sensory impairments. The possibility of impaired sensation will impact on decisions regarding the presentation of food and drink during the clinical exam.
- Taste impairment. Intraoral burns may result in trauma to the taste buds, with patients potentially experiencing disorders of taste called hypogeusia (Clayton & Kennedy, 2007). Furthermore, altered zinc metabolism that follows burn injury has also been associated with altered perceptions of flavor (Cohen, Schecter, & Henkin, 1973).
- Neurological involvement. The presence of abnormal oral and pharyngeal reflexes should be noted. Presentation of atypical reflexive patterns is not anticipated in the burn patient, yet concomitant injuries sustained at the time of the burn may lead to neurological impairment. It is important to recognize the potential for patients with burn injury to present with neurological deficits as a result of exposure to a smoke-filled environment causing subsequent hypoxic injury, as part of a multitrauma presentation, or subsequent to an electrical current passing through the body.
- Laryngeal impairment. Assessment of vocal function should involve the patient phonating on sustained vowels at various intensity levels in order in investigate respiratory and laryngeal control. The presence of hoarse voice is indicative of respiratory burn or post-operative damage to the laryngeal structures from endotracheal intubation. This profile may be associated with reduced glottic closure during the swallow. If the patient has not been formally reviewed by an otorhinolaryngologist (ENT) for the presence of airway damage post-burn injury, but has noticed a change in their own vocal quality, otolaryngologic investigation of laryngeal pathology is warranted.

To establish whether a patient with dysphagia is tolerating a prescribed diet, clinicians may use information including change in chest status, change in temperature (temperature spike), and nursing reports of clinical indicators of aspiration. In relation to the patient with burn injury, however, it is critical to note that little or no emphasis should be placed on the clinical symptom of temperature spiking in association with aspiration. As discussed earlier, the patient with burn injury has very poor temperature regulation and may be prone to temperature spikes as a result of a "septic shower." As a result, the occurrence of a temperature spike may be associated with other factors and will often not be related to aspiration.

Instrumental Swallow Examination

An endoscopic swallowing examination (ESE) may be the procedure of choice during the acute phase following burn and inhalation injury, for the following reasons:

- ESE can be performed at the bedside when positioning and patient mobility are limited, or when the patient has not yet reached medical stability.
- ESE allows direct visualization of the pharyngeal and laryngeal structures, enabling assessment of the following:
    - Edema, erythema, and ulceration following inhalation injury
    - Sensory impairment
    - Vocal fold integrity and function following endotracheal intubation for airway protection during the swallow
    - Management of secretions
    - Post-swallow residue of food/drink
    - Penetration or aspiration of food/drink
    - Effectiveness of compensatory strategies to prevent residue and penetration/aspiration.
- ESE can easily be repeated within 24 to 48 hours to allow frequent monitoring of status.

Videofluoroscopic swallowing examination (VFSE) may not be feasible for some burns patients for the following reasons:

- Patient may not be medically stable for transport to radiology.
- Optimal positioning in the radiology suite may not be possible, precluding the ability to obtain a clear image of the pharyngeal and laryngeal structures during the swallow. As discussed earlier in this section, numerous factors including the burn injury, head and neck contractures, and wound dressings can alter the optimal positioning of the head and neck and make it difficult to acquire an unobstructed view.
- Frequent repetition of the procedure is not advisable due to unnecessary radiation exposure risk.

Where the above issues can be overcome, a VFSE may be sought during the acute phase when assessment of the following is desired:

- Coordination of the oral and pharyngeal phase of swallow
- Oromotor function during oral preparation of the bolus
- Latency of the swallow response
- Laryngeal elevation
- Pharyngeal pooling

- Upper esophageal sphincter function
- The esophageal phase

Characteristics of Dysphagia Post-Burn Injury

Patients with dysphagia after burn injury may present with multifaceted swallowing deficits, encompassing difficulties with oral and pharyngeal movements, an inability to self-feed, and decreased levels of alertness secondary to pain management. A discussion of the known clinical and physiological features of swallowing behavior post-burn injury, as well as factors that may contribute to the dysphagia presentation in this population, are outlined below.

Intubation and Ventilation

Existing studies in the current literature that have described dysphagia following thermal injury have reported a high prevalence of intubation and ventilation in their populations (Edelman et al., 2008; McKinnon DuBose et al., 2005; Ward et al., 2001; see Table 4–5). Individuals with higher TBSA and inhalation injury were reported to have undergone lengthy periods of ventilation, between 3 and 6 weeks. As associated with long periods of ventilation, the prevalence of patients requiring tracheostomy was high, ranging from 70 to 100%. Conversion from endotracheal (ETT) intubation to tracheostomy was reported to occur within 1 to 2 weeks following admission.

Increased duration of ETT intubation, ventilation, and the presence of a tracheostomy may impact negatively on swallowing function. Considering the protracted period of intubation reported in the current literature, this may be one of the likely possible variables placing a patient at risk for dysphagia.

Impact of Pain

Both pain and the physiological consequences of its management may contribute to the patient being at an ongoing risk of aspiration, necessitating longer periods of alternative feeding. Odynophagia (pain on swallowing) in patients with oropharyngeal and facial burns has been found to be correlated with a reduced ability to consume food and fluid orally (Clayton & Kennedy, 2007; Muir et al., 1987). Pain in these areas can cause considerable distress, and patients may wish to cease oral feeding even if they are capable of maintaining a diet orally. Topical anesthesia may be administered in an attempt to alleviate this discomfort. In addition to the possible generalized systemic effects of pain medication previously discussed, the application of topical anesthetics to ease pain manifesting from burns in and around the oropharynx may lead to reduced oropharyngeal sensation and a reduced ability to generate a strong cough (Broniatowski et al., 1999). The need for further investigation into the use of topical anesthetics as a treatment for odynophagia and its effect on facilitating nutritional intake has been highlighted (Clayton & Kennedy, 2007).

Possible side effects of medications utilized for pain management in this population present a barrier to dysphagia management. As discussed earlier in this chapter, pain medications can have a considerable impact on the patient's ability to safely manage oral intake. The SLP's clinical judgement will be used to determine a patient's suitability for oral intake within the context of current pain management medications.

Clinical Characteristics of the Swallow Post-Burn Injury

Dysphagia assessment in this population can be challenging due to the rapid physical changes that occur during the early stages of treatment. The process of dysphagia examination is similar to that currently used for other clinical populations, yet there are factors specific to patients with burns that should be closely observed. Clinical features of swallow behavior post-burn injury are outlined in Table 4–7.

Oral Phase. Swallowing function of a patient with burn damage in the orofacial region, even in the absence of inhalation burns, may be significantly impaired by the presence of edema in the acute stages of recovery. In order to accept, chew, manipulate, and propel a food or fluid bolus through the oropharynx, the anatomy and physiology of structures underpinning these skills must be relatively intact. Restricted oral motor abilities due to the presence of edema, alongside dehydration and tenderness of the facial skin, can therefore potentially limit or inhibit nutritional intake in the acute phase post-injury (Pankhurst & Pochkhanawala, 2002).

Additional complications brought about by the early inflammatory process include hindrance of the patient's ability to extend the neck, open the mouth, and efficiently manage oral secretions (Boardman, 1991; Clark, 1992b). Authors have acknowledged that neck position has major effects on swallowing (Logemann, 1993; Palmer, DuChane, & Donner, 1991; Siebens & Linden, 1985) and that eschar on the neck can accentuate pharyngeal edema, drawing the neck into flexion and compressing the airway (Edlich et al., 1984).

Burns to the face, particularly those around and inside the oral cavity, can be functionally distressing and debilitating. The skin may begin to contract after inflammation has subsided, further reducing ROM ability (Figure 4–5) and resulting in impaired lateral lip and cheek movement and jaw opening. Scar tissue around the oral cavity forms around the border of the lip vermillion; the tendency is for burns of the upper lip to lead to inward contraction, whereas injury to the lower lip tends to result in outward contraction. Such alterations to the lips may impinge upon the patient's ability to form an adequate lip seal, resulting in oral incompetence with subsequent anterior loss of secretions and fluid/food boluses.

The development of microstomia due to circumoral contracture may occur if the burn covers the lateral borders of the mouth (Johnson et al., 1981). Patients will prefer to keep the lips closed to minimize pain during wound healing. Consequently, mouth opening can become limited (Figure 4–6). Reduced ability to access and manipulate the oral cavity may adversely affect the patient's ability to communicate via speech, use of facial expression to convey the suprasegmental aspects of conversation, provision of oral and dental care, administration of general anesthesia via oral endotracheal intubation without hazard, and the ability to successfully eat and drink (Bahnof, 2000; Daugherty & Carr-Collins, 1994; Dougherty & Warden, 2003; Shikowitz et al., 1996). Additionally, microstomia may impede utensil access to the mouth and may hinder the patient from accepting larger boluses (Clayton & Kennedy, 2007). Patients with partial and full thickness burns to the head and neck will often have a protracted length of stay in intensive care.

Table 4–7. Observations from CBE and Instrumental Assessment

		Instrumental	
	Clinical Swallow Examination	***ESE***	***VFSE***
Oral Phase	• Odynophagia due to burns/edema/erythema • Reduced strength and range of movement of the lips, tongue, and jaw (secondary to edema, tightening of the skin as it heals, disuse atrophy) • Poor ability to contain, manipulate, and propel the bolus in the oral cavity (secondary to altered sensation as a result of oral burns, edema, reduced movement of oromusculature due to pain or contracture formation) • Increased oral transit time	Unable to objectively assess this phase using this instrumental tool.	• Altered anatomical positioning due to contracture formation • Reduced bolus preparation • Reduced ability to form a cohesive bolus • Reduced base of tongue to posterior pharyngeal wall contact • Reduced bolus control • Timeliness of bolus propulsion
Pharyngeal Phase	• Delayed swallow initiation • Decreased/incoordinated hyolaryngeal excursion • Possible pharyngeal residue and possible penetration/aspiration as indicated through wet/gurgly vocal quality, and frequent coughing/throat clearing; note: decreased pharyngeal sensation may lead to a higher incidence of silent aspiration and undetected pharyngeal residue in this clinical population • Odynophagia due to burns/edema/erythema/NGT	• Edema/erythema • Decreased ability to manage secretions • Reduced pharyngeal sensation (may tolerate scoping for an extended period of time, even in absence of topical anesthesia) • Delayed swallow initiation • Poor base of tongue to posterior pharyngeal wall contact as indicated by an incomplete whiteout during the swallow • Pharyngeal pooling/residue • Laryngeal penetration/aspiration	• Altered anatomical positioning and function due to contracture formation • Laryngeal or pharyngeal stricture formation (injuries resulting from chemical ingestion or significant airway damage) • Delayed swallow initiation • Decreased hyolaryngeal excursion • Decreased epiglottic deflection • Decreased cricopharyngeal opening • Poor pharyngeal contraction resulting in pharyngeal pooling/residue • Laryngeal penetration/aspiration
Other	• Level of alertness and medical stability • Degree and impact of pain • Impact and extent of fatigue • Feeding and positioning restrictions	• Assessment of vocal cord function • Mucosal integrity of the upper airway • Extent and damage of burn to upper airway	• Examination of the esophageal phase of the swallow to assess stricture formation

NGT = nasogastric tube.

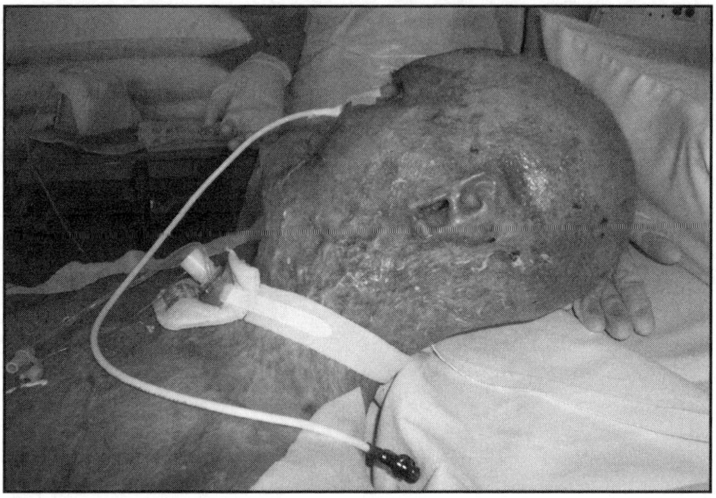

Figure 4–5. Maximum head extension.

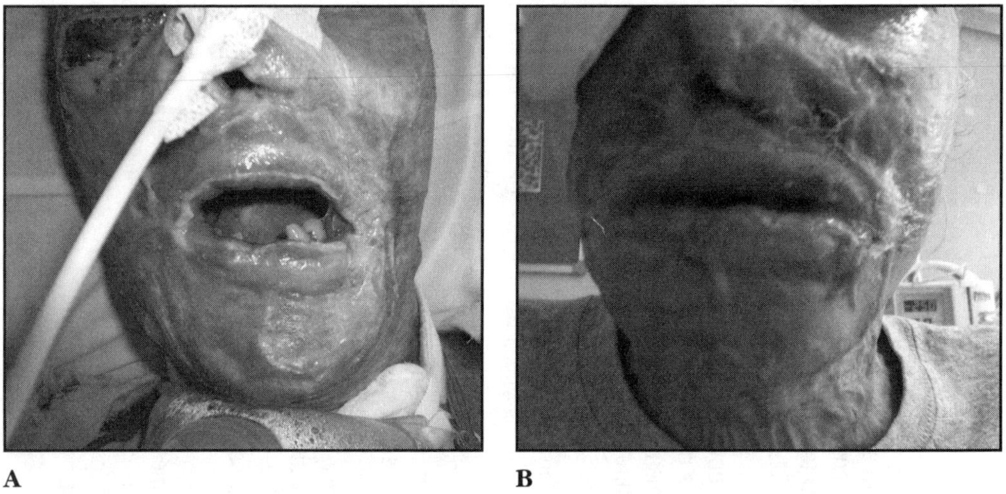

Figure 4–6. Examples of maximal mouth opening (~15 mm) (**A**) and maximum lateral spread (~55 mm) (**B**) achieved after Z-plasty.

As a result, they may already have oral contracture by the time of first SLP contact if splinting regimens have not been initiated early in the admission.

Pharyngeal Phase. A range of pharyngeal stage deficits may be suspected in patients with burn injury, including delayed swallow initiation and decreased and/or uncoordinated hyolaryngeal excursion (see Table 4-7). As the patient may require neck dressings or splints, it is often difficult to palpate laryngeal movement or use cervical auscultation as a clinical adjunct to determine swallowing efficiency. In the event of bulky dressings or neck scarring, an alternative approach to determining swallowing efficiency may be cheek auscultation. Contracture formation on the neck may alter normal anatomical positioning and hinder the movement of pharyngeal structures. This is particularly the case where adhesions occur between the scarred tissue and underlying cartilaginous or bony structures.

Mucosal damage from oropharyngeal burns can result in increased mucosal sloughing and a reduction in cilia function that may contribute to the patient's inability to manage oral secretions (Cohen & Guzzardi, 1983; Gaissert et al., 1993). A wet, gurgly vocal quality may indicate the presence of pharyngeal pooling or residue, penetration into the laryngeal inlet, and possibly aspiration. It is important to remember that these individuals may be more susceptible to reduced laryngopharyngeal sensation, and subsequently a reduced cough reflex, following burns to the airway and prolonged periods of ventilation, possibly leading to a higher incidence of silent aspiration.

Physiological Characteristics of Dysphagia Post-Burn Injury

There is currently a lack of published evidence regarding the physiological deficits contributing to dysphagia following burn injury. Edelman et al. (2008) reported that an abnormal clinical swallow examination was predictive (10 of 11 = 91%) of an abnormal VFSE for patients with thermal burn injury, with 64%, 82%, and 18% of patients presenting with oral, pharyngeal, and esophageal dysphagia, respectively. Unfortunately, no further data were provided in this study regarding the specific physiological deficits present in each phase of the swallow. Similarly, Muehlberger et al. (1998) reported minimal information regarding the results of VFSE assessments conducted with 11 patients with clinical symptoms consistent with dysphagia, stating only that 36% ($n = 4$) had swallowing deficits including mild pharyngeal pooling and delayed swallow initiation. From our own clinical experience, instrumental assessment reveals a number of deficits in the oral and pharyngeal phases of the swallow. A summary of possible anticipated physiological characteristics evident on instrumental examination of this population have been outlined in Table 4–7.

Natural History and Prognosis of Dysphagia

Considering the nonuniform, highly localized, and systemic changes after burn injury, it is not surprising that dysphagia recovery can show variable outcomes. There are a number of factors that can influence rate of recovery and resolution of dysphagia in this population. These include:

- The severity of burns to the head/neck, oral cavity, pharynx, and larynx
- General medical condition, including episodes of sepsis
- Number of occasions the patient is required to return to the operating room for grafting procedures
- Delay in decannulation due to surgery
- Contracture formation and its management (surgical or nonsurgical)
- Presence of pharyngoesophageal strictures
- Airway patency
- Patient motivation for rehabilitation

Current literature suggests that initial SLP assessment occurs between 20 and

54 days after admission, with resumption of oral intake achieved by 30 to 63 days after admission (see Table 4-5). Clinically, however, this may vary between burn units, depending upon referral practices and the role of SLP in orofacial contracture management in that facility. The majority of patients referred to SLP require some form of diet modifications when commencing oral intake after burn injury (73-100%; Edelman et al., 2008; McKinnon DuBose et al., 2005; Ward et al., 2001). Only a small proportion of patients (0-9%) are able to commence oral intake on a normal consistency diet (i.e., without restriction of food or fluid consistencies; Edelman et al., 2008; McKinnon DuBose et al., 2005; Ward et al., 2001). At discharge, a proportion of patients were reported to remain nil by mouth on alternative feeding (10-55%). Most patients, however, were safely managing a normal oral diet at discharge (39-90%).

Management of Dysphagia Post-Burn Injury

Reestablishing safe oral intake is an important early rehabilitation goal to facilitate healing, minimize respiratory complications, and enhance psychological wellbeing. This goal can be significantly hindered for those patients who present with dysphagia. During the early phase, alternative (non-oral) nutritional approaches allow the sedated, mechanically-ventilated, and/or severely injured burn patient to achieve the high caloric intake required. Alternative feeding helps reconstitute the metabolic system and promotes healing during this early phase of recovery, yet long-term nutrition by these means is unsuitable. Burn recovery is often divided into two phases: the early (acute) phase and the late (rehabilitation) phase. Management of dysphagia during these phases will require different strategies depending on the severity of the burns and the need for surgical management of the burn wounds.

Early Phase (Acute Stage)

This encompasses the time from admission until a large amount of the burn wounds are closed. This stage may be characterized by reduced alertness and cognition as a side effect of analgesics used to control pain following surgical procedures, daily wound cleansing, dressing changes, and physical therapy. The patient's medical state is typically fluctuating at this stage, influenced by the need for repeated surgical procedures and grafts. These factors impact the patient's ability to participate in specific swallowing exercises and/or comply with techniques and maneuvers to improve swallowing function and prevent aspiration. Consequently, the primary goals of swallowing intervention during the early stage of recovery are to: (a) prevent medical complications from aspiration, (b) facilitate decannulation, and (c) prevent further deterioration due to a lack of use of the swallowing mechanism. These goals can be achieved by:

- Use of compensatory strategies, including positioning, altering bolus size, taste and temperature variation, and modification of oral consistencies (see Chapter 1), to facilitate oral intake with minimal aspiration risk.
- Exploring use of alternate tracheostomy tubes such as a Suctionaid tracheostomy tube (Smiths Medical, http://www.suctionaid.com) that allow for close monitoring of the

patient's ability to manage secretions. Trials of a speaking valve can also help facilitate weaning from tracheostomy and dysphagia management. Specifically, a one-way speaking valve enhances voicing, coughing, and achievement of supraglottic pressures during swallowing. The valve may also aid in restoration of laryngopharyngeal sensation, assisting in secretion management. When indicated, consultation by an ENT should be sought to determine patient suitability for the commencement of speaking valve use.

- Encouraging frequent, small amounts of oral intake as tolerated to promote swallowing, avoid disuse atrophy, improve secretion management, and enhance endurance for oral intake.
- Beginning oromotor and swallowing exercises (see Chapter 1) to improve strength, speed, endurance, and coordination of movement. If the patient has undergone any facial or neck grafts, ROM and stretching are contraindicated until day 5 after grafting, or until approval is granted by the surgical team.
- Managing level of oral and pharyngeal pain to promote increased oral intake.
- Implementing anticontracture positioning (discussed further below) to assist in minimizing the effect of contracture on positioning and oromotor function.

Late Stage (Rehabilitation Phase)

This stage involves the period from completed wound closure to maturation of scarring. At this stage, cognition and alertness have improved as use of pain medications has reduced. The majority of large wounds have now closed and patients are typically able to participate in more aggressive rehabilitation. This stage involves aggressive splinting and ROM exercises to minimize or prevent contracture formation now that wounds are healed. Introduction of specific swallowing exercise programs to improve strength and coordination of swallowing is now appropriate.

Non-Oral Supplementation

As previously mentioned, the need for nutritional support via non-oral means for the burn patient is largely due to the hypermetabolic state induced following burn injury, not solely because of aspiration risk. If the increased nutrition and energy requirements associated with burn injury are not met, the risk of reduced outcomes due to infection and poor wound healing is increased. Consequently, even for those patients who are determined to be safe to resume oral intake, many other factors such as frequent trips to surgery, pain, pain-induced fatigue, and positioning issues make it impossible to meet the increased nutritional requirements via oral intake alone. Enteral nutrition is therefore critical to allow the provision of the nutritional support necessary to reduce caloric deficits and promote wound healing. Enteral feeding will continue until the medical and dietetic team members determine that the patient's nutritional needs can be met fully and consistently via oral intake.

Considering the exceptional nutritional demands of patients with dysphagia associated with burn injury, it is surprising that between 90 and 100% of all patients studied to date have received periods of supplementary feeding, largely by means of orogastric or nasogastric

(NG) feeding (see Table 4-5). The average duration of supplementary feeding for this group is reported to be quite long, approximately 50 days. Even following initiation of oral intake, supplementary feeding has been reported to continue for a period of almost 3 weeks (Ward et al., 2001).

Enteral nutrition (see Chapter 1), typically via NG or nasoduodenal (ND) tube, is the most common mode of supplementary feeding for this patient group. The use of parenteral nutrition (PN; see Chapter 1) with burn patients is less preferable, as it has been shown to increase mortality threefold and is associated with diminished tolerance for enteral calories (Herndon et al., 1989b; Herndon, Stein, Rutan, Abston, & Linares, 1987). Parenteral nutrition should only be considered the route of choice in patients with total enteral failure, and therefore it is very rarely used in burn patients.

Enteral nutrition is preferred to nonenteral feeding as it promotes gastric mucosal integrity and the release of intestinal and growth hormones (Magnotti & Deitch, 2005; Saffle & Graves, 2007). Even in the presence of severe facial burns involving both nostrils, NG tubes can be secured in a manner that avoids friction against the burn wounds. Patients who develop gastric stasis may require nasojejunal feeding. The clinician should be aware of patient discomfort and erosion of the nasopharyngeal mucosa in this case, however, because of the need to pass larger gauge tubes in the nasopharynx to compensate for gastric stasis (Kreis, Middelkoop, Vloemans, & Kreis, 2002).

Current literature reports minimal use of gastrostomy (PEG) feeding, despite the protracted duration of supplemental feeding. One factor limiting the use of PEG feeding in this patient group is the presence of burn injury to the upper body/chest. Burns to the abdomen will prevent surgical placement of a PEG tube, especially during the acute phase of recovery. Skin grafting to the burn sites on the abdomen must be performed and wounds healed prior to PEG tube placement being considered.

Management of Oral Phase Deficits

Long-term oral stage deficits are largely the result of limited lip and jaw movement due to contracture formation. Management should involve trying to minimize contracture formation throughout both the acute and rehabilitation phases of treatment and should commence as early as possible before the wounds have healed. A proposed flowchart for determining nonsurgical management of patients at risk for orofacial contractures is illustrated in Figure 4-7 and an example of possible management is detailed in Table 4-8. Without contracture management, direct and indirect methods of swallowing rehabilitation may provide minimal functional gains.

A wide range of protocols for oral contracture prevention and management have been developed. These include oromotor stretching and/or splinting (detailed below) in addition to surgical release (detailed previously in this chapter). Depending on the severity of the burn injury, a combination of techniques may be required.

Range of Movement Exercises. These are active, active-assisted, and passive stretches. The aim of ROM exercises is to preserve and restore movement and improve the patient's physiologic and functional status. ROM/stretching exercises help to reduce edema, maintain joint mobility, and prevent contractures.

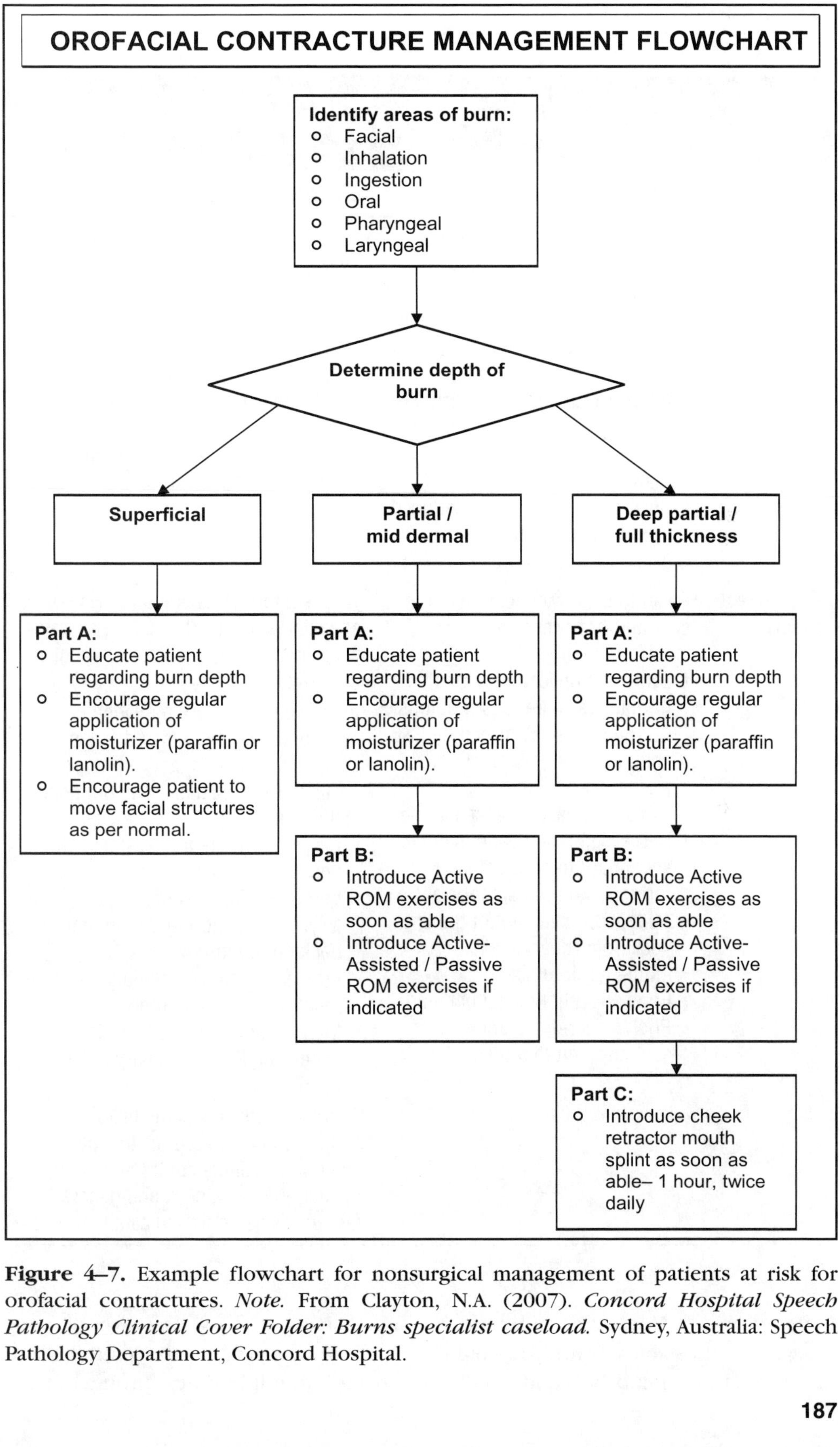

Figure 4–7. Example flowchart for nonsurgical management of patients at risk for orofacial contractures. *Note.* From Clayton, N.A. (2007). *Concord Hospital Speech Pathology Clinical Cover Folder: Burns specialist caseload.* Sydney, Australia: Speech Pathology Department, Concord Hospital.

Table 4–8. An Example of an Individualized Treatment Program for Oral Contractures and Swallowing Dysfunction for a Patient with Severe Thermal Burn Injury

	Deficits	*Treatment Prescribed*
Oral Stage	Patient presents with severe partial thickness facial burns: • Deficits: Severely restricted movement of lips, jaw, and face (tongue strength and ROM within normal limits). Presents with 35 mm vertical mouth opening. Surgical intervention not required for contracture management. • Swallow implications: Reduced mouth opening, reduced lip seal and anterior loss of saliva.	Active and passive assisted ROM exercises of the lips and jaw. Exercise program repeated 2–3 times daily; individual exercises (e.g., lip rounding, lip spread) repeated 10 times each session. Sufficient mouth opening allows use of commercial mouth splint. Splinting performed three times a day for 1 hour duration each time.
Pharyngeal Stage	Patient has a tracheostomy in situ, and has presence of inhalation injury • Swallow implications: Unable to manage secretions (copious secretions as confirmed by ESE and suctioning via Suctionaid tracheostomy tube) • Reduced pharyngeal sensation • Decreased laryngeal movement secondary to contracture formation on the anterior neck • Reduced movement of the left vocal fold (query initial intubation trauma) • Poor cricopharyngeal opening • Pooled secretions and aspiration on thin fluids	Tracheostomy management: Use of speaking valve (SV) to assist airway secretion management and laryngeal sensation. Initial compensatory management with modified textures and fluids. Once decannulated, active pharyngeal swallow rehabilitation can commence including: • Laryngeal adduction exercises for vocal fold deficit • Laryngeal ROM exercises for laryngeal anchoring due to anterior neck contractures • Effortful swallow technique for poor pharyngeal muscle tone • Mendelsohn maneuver for laryngeal anchoring and cricopharyngeal opening *Note:* Exercises such as head lift cannot be prescribed for this patient as circumferential contracture formation on the neck and general fatigue levels contraindicate their use.

ROM exercises should be commenced as early as possible (prior to wound healing). They should be conducted as aggressively as possible (without causing further harm to the patient) and repeated multiple times throughout the day. Stretching may be achieved by the following:

- Active ROM. Active stretching is where the person actively and independently assumes a position to maximize tissue stretch potential with no assistance. Figure 4–8 illustrates possible active range of movement regimes. Active ROM is the preferred type of exercise as it works to prevent contracture, assists in edema reduction and promotes circulation. Functional exercises promote the goal of physical independence and serve to increase self-esteem and/or personal satisfaction when the patient can accomplish ADLs.
- Active-assisted ROM. Active-assisted stretching is achieved through performing the usually active stretch position. Either the patient or therapist then assists in providing an additional stretch in the same direction in order to maximize the stretch potential (e.g., using gloved fingers to assist lateral lip spread). Stretches should be gentle but firm, with the patient holding each stretch for at least 10 seconds. Indications for use include: limited ROM, scar contracture, skin graft adherence, increased physiologic demands, and decreased strength due to prolonged hospitalization.
- Passive ROM. Passive stretching is achieved purely through manual assistance. Passive stretching maintains ROM, assesses joint motion, elongates tissues, and requires little energy expenditure by the patient. This technique is often used in the comatose patient or in intensive

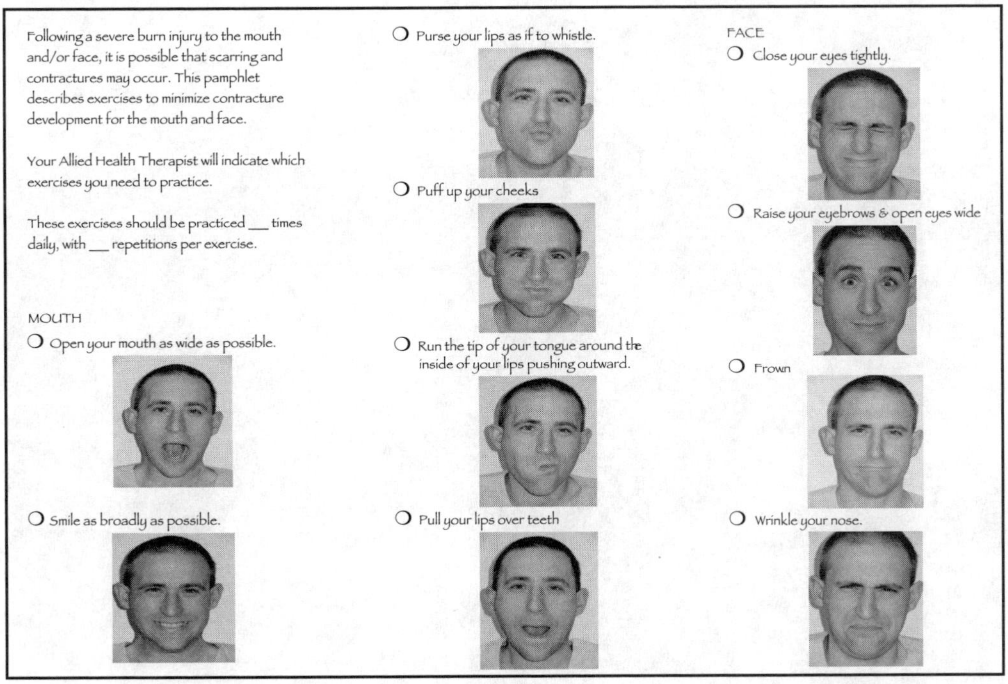

Figure 4–8. An example of an active range of motion exercise sheet provided to patients.

care. Scar tissue responds well to a passive force when applied steadily, controlled, and over a prolonged period. This may be achieved through direct manipulation of the lips and oral cavity by the therapist, patient, or an appliance. Stretches should be gentle but firm, holding for at least 10 seconds. Although originally designed as a rehabilitation device for trismus, the commercially available Therabite device (Atos Medical, http://www.atosmedical.com; Figure 4–9) can be used to achieve a passive vertical mouth stretch for the burn patient. For those patients

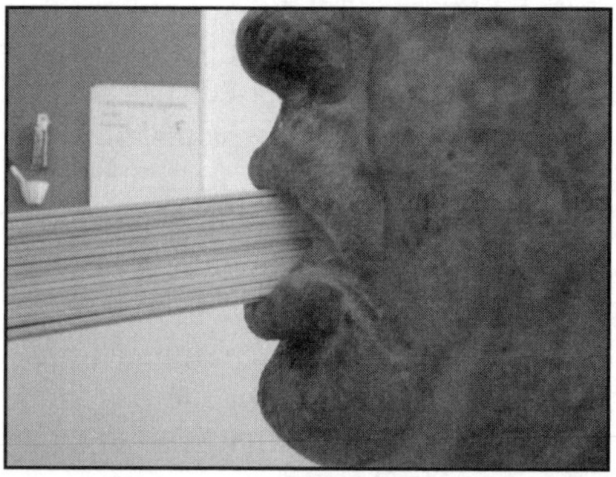

A

Figure 4–9. Stacks of tongue depressors (**A**) or commercially available devices such as the Therabite (**B**) can be useful for passive stretching. Courtesy of Atos Medical (http://www.atosmedical.com).

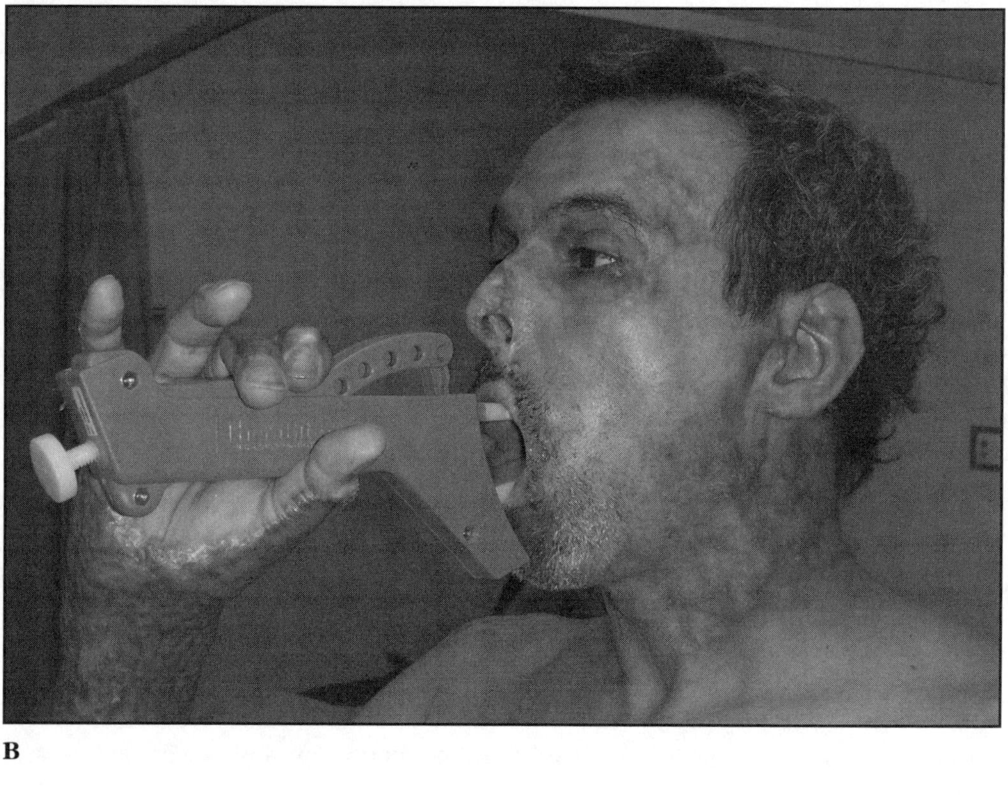

B

with dramatically reduced mouth opening preventing insertion of the Therabite mouth trays, stacks of tongue depressors (see Figure 4-9) can be used to assist passive stretching until mouth/jaw opening is sufficient to enable use of the Therabite.

Splinting. In addition to ROM exercises, severe burn injury patients may require splinting that provides a static stretch over a longer period of time. The objective of splinting is to maintain the patient's range of motion and prevent further loss of motion. Splints are used to obtain the best position and prevent the movement of an otherwise mobile body part to promote healing of grafts, prevent contracture formation, and restore joint ROM. Although splinting is necessary for patients with deep partial or full thickness burns (see Figure 4-7), less extensive burns may also benefit. A commercial or an individually fabricated oral splint (Figure 4-10) may be used in accordance with the patient's needs and abilities. Consideration must be given to the patient's wound status when selecting the type of splint and the duration of application so as to prevent pressure areas or wound breakdown.

Different approaches to managing orofacial contractures are well discussed within the literature and references to seminal papers are provided in the Further Reading section of this chapter. Generally, nonsurgical management of contracture formation is a collaborative approach between the SLP, occupational therapy, and physiotherapy disciplines. Consultation with the occupational therapist, maxillofacial surgeons, and dental technicians may be required if an individualized splint is the preferred method of treatment.

Management of Pharyngeal Phase Deficits

There are a number of reasons why a patient with burn injury may present with pharyngeal swallowing deficits, whether it be damage directly resulting from the burn (inhalation injury, contracture formation) or subsequent effects from medical

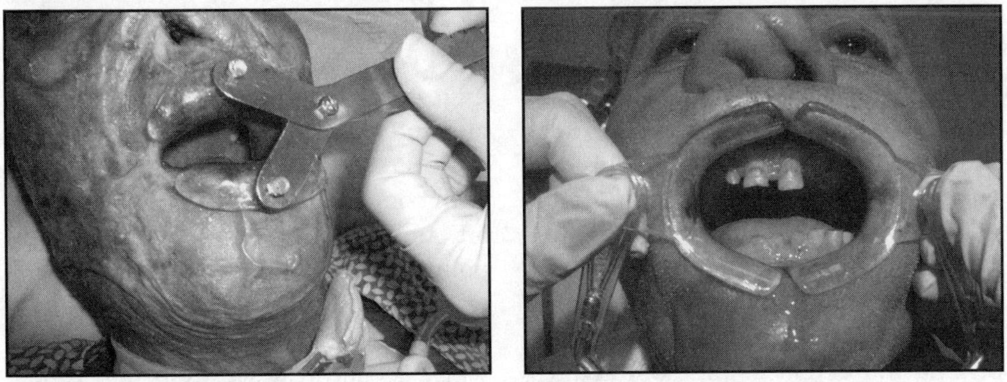

A B

Figure 4–10. Examples of an individually fabricated dynamic splinting device (**A**) and a commercial device (**B**), the Free Access II Cheek retractor, used to minimize oral contractures. Courtesy of J. Morita USA Inc. (http://www.jmoritausa.com/consumables.asp).

management (intubation, tracheostomy). Common to this population is reduced pharyngeal sensation. Pharyngeal sensation may spontaneously resolve as the pharyngeal mucosa heals over a relatively short period of time. Alternatively, some individuals may require further intervention depending on whether inhalation injury is present and the period of intubation and ventilation experienced. Swallowing trials using different bolus types (hot, cold, and carbonated) may aid in increasing pharyngeal sensation during the height of the swallow if the person is considered safe for oral intake. Improvement of sensation in tracheostomized individuals may be aided by the use of either a speaking valve or a Suctionaid tracheostomy tube with an air source attached to the side port to allow air to pass through the upper airway.

Although the patient may not present with any anatomical deficits on instrumental examination, altered physiological functioning is not uncommon due to the alterations in skin tissue properties. Burns to the neck can result in restrictions to both head movement and hyolaryngeal excursion. The most commonly anticipated deformity associated with burns on the anterior aspect of the neck is a flexion contracture, as this position is most comfortable and ADLs, including eating and drinking, encourage neck flexion (Johnson et al., 1981). This contracture type can result in significantly limited ability to put the neck into extension and an inability to close the mouth when the head is elevated to a neutral position (Johnson et al., 1981). To avoid or limit the extent of the contractures, the patient must be positioned with the neck extended. This can be accomplished by eliminating the use of normal pillows, and using a neck extension pillow and/or soft neck collar. Splints should be worn throughout the day, except during therapeutic activities and ADLs. Neck splints may need to be removed when eating or drinking if the patient requires specific head positions (e.g., a chin tuck or head turn posture) to help prevent aspiration. If the posterior neck sustains burns, the patient will prefer to extend the neck back, leaving the head in a hyperextended position. In this case, the patient should be positioned so that the head is flexed.

To help compensate for restricted movement secondary to laryngeal anchoring by contracture formation, exercises targeting increased hyolaryngeal movement may be prescribed (see Table 4-8). These may include but are not limited to: laryngeal adduction and abduction, laryngeal squeeze, supraglottic swallow, super-supraglottic swallow, Mendelsohn maneuver, and head lift (detailed in Chapter 1). Pharyngeal deficits not attributable to contracture formation such as poor airway protection, cricopharyngeal opening, and pharyngeal pooling are also treated using traditional swallow rehabilitation techniques. Compensatory strategies such as a chin tuck or head turn may be beneficial to assist bolus clearance through the pharynx. It is important, however, to be aware of potential contraindications for the use of certain strategies and exercises in this population. For example, physical strain is associated with some maneuvers, such as the head lift. As fatigue is an issue with the burn population, and although muscle strengthening may occur from these exercise regimens, immediate effects may present with a decline in swallow function. Patient motivation, education, and premorbid or comorbid deficits may also impact on what treatment regimen can be prescribed, as the patient may be unable to perform these tasks independently from instruction. Furthermore, consultation with the physiotherapist may be beneficial before beginning some rehabilitation exercises, as certain activities may serve as dual targets (e.g., neck stretching exercise and the Shaker maneuver) so that the patient can be performing simultaneous treatment targets within one session, thus minimizing fatigue for these muscles over the day.

Overall, the main consideration is the individual patient's presenting deficits when developing swallowing rehabilitation regimens for the population with burn injury. Diet modification may be the most successful management option in the acute phase, with individualized and intensive swallow rehabilitation commencing once medical stability has been achieved.

OTHER SPEECH AND VOICE COMORBIDITIES

SLP intervention may also be required to manage voice and speech disorders after burn trauma. It is not uncommon for those individuals who have sustained inhalation injury, or those who have been intubated and ventilated for a period of time, to present with some degree of dysphonia. Causes for dysphonia in the burn patient are similar to those for patients who have been intubated for a protracted period of time. In addition, the patient with inhalation burn injury is at increased risk for scarring and stenosis in the posterior cricoid region or heterotopic ossification of the cricoarytenoid joint, resulting in poor adduction and abduction of the vocal folds. Furthermore, a presence of aphonia/dysphonia due to a conversion reaction to trauma may be a further factor for consideration if ENT examination does not identify deficits that are consistent with the presenting difficulty (i.e., vocal cords are anatomically and physiologically normal).

Speech disorders may occur for the patient with burns resulting in a loss of structure or function to any part of the anatomy that is usually required for articulation. This may occur in the case of severe burn injury that results in loss or partial loss of the lips, tongue, or even the facial nerve. If radical reconstructive surgery is required, articulation if often affected. Preoperative planning is essential and post-operative rehabilitation targets the speech sounds that are directly affected by the altered anatomy. For example, lip reconstruction will require therapy for bilabial speech sounds.

CONCLUSION

Burn injury is an insult that has deleterious effects on the physiological functioning of many of the body's systems. Indeed, such fast-acting and dramatic systemic alterations can manifest as significant obstacles to patient recovery for the medical and allied health treatment teams. Changes to the structures involved in the swallow mechanism are directly related to the extent and location of injury. Thus, each patient must be individually considered, with no two presenting with the same anatomical and physiological damage.

FURTHER READING

Barone, C. M., Hulnick, S. J., Grigsby de Linde, L., Sauer, J. B., & Mitra, A. (1994). Evaluation of treatment modalities in perioral electrical burns. *Journal of Burn Care and Rehabilitation*, *15*(4), 335–340.

Clark, W. R., & McDade, G. O. (1980). Microstomia in burn victims: A new appliance for prevention and treatment and literature review. *Journal of Burn Care and Rehabilitation*, *1*(2), 33-36.

Donelan, M. B. (2007). Reconstruction of the head and neck. In D. N. Herndon (Ed.), *Total Burn Care* (3rd ed., pp. 701-718). Edinburgh, UK: Elsevier Saunders.

Fraulin, F. O. G., Illmayer, S. J., & Tredget, E. E. (1996). Assessment of cosmetic and functional results of conservative versus surgical management of facial burns. *Journal of Burn Care and Rehabilitation*, *17*(1), 19-29.

Heinle, J. A., Kealey, G. P., Cram, A. E., & Hartford, C. E. (1988). The microstomia prevention appliance: 14 years of clinical experience. *Journal of Burn Care and Rehabilitation*, *9*(1), 90-91.

Johnson, J., Candia, J., La Trenta, G., Madden, M. R., Goodwin, C. W., & Finkelstein, J. (1992). A nasal trumpet orthosis to maintain nares openings and respiratory function for patients with facial burns: A case report. *Journal of Burn Care and Rehabilitation*, *13*(6), 677-679.

Macmillan, A. R. G., Oliver, A. J., Richardson, L., & Reade, P. C. (1991). An intraoral splint for the prevention of microstomia from facial burns. *Burns*, *17*, 72-74.

McGowan, R. H. (1980). Prevention of microstomia following facial burns. *British Dental Journal*, *149*(3), 83-84.

Ridgway, C. L., & Warden, G. D. (1995). Evaluation of a vertical mouth stretching orthosis: Two case reports. *Journal of Burn Care and Rehabilitation*, *16*(1), 74-78.

Silverglade, D., & Ruberg, R. L. (1986). Nonsurgical management of burns to the lips and commissures. *Advances in Burn Care*, *13*, 87-94.

Sykes, L. (1996). Scar traction appliance for a patient with microstomia: A clinical report. *Journal of Prosthetic Dentistry*, *76*(5), 464-465.

Taylor, L. B., & Walker, J. (1997). A review of selected microstomia prevention appliances. *Pediatric Dentistry*, *19*, 413-418.

Wust, K. J. (2006). A modified dynamic mouth splint for burn patients. *Journal of Burn Care and Research*, *27*(1), 86-92.

REFERENCES

Abdi, S., & Zhou, Y. (2002). Management of pain after burn injury. *Current Opinion in Anaesthesiology*, *15*(5), 563-567.

American College of Surgeons. (2006). Guidelines for the Operation of Burn Centers. In *Resources for Optimal Care of the Injured Patient 2006*. Retrieved February 5, 2008, from http://www.ameriburn.org/BurnCenterReferralCriteria.pdf

Atiyeh, B. S., Gunn, S. W., & Dibo, S. A. (2008). Metabolic implications of severe burn injuries and their management: A systematic review of the literature. *World Journal of Surgery*, *32*(8), 1857-1869.

Australian and New Zealand Burn Association [ANZBA]. (2004). *Burn injuries requiring transfer to a burns unit*. Retrieved July 9, 2008, from http://www.anzba.org.au/

Australian and New Zealand Burn Association [ANZBA]. (2008). *Emergency management of severe burns [EMSB] Course manual*. Brisbane, Australia: The Education Committee of the Australian and New Zealand Burn Association Limited.

Bahnof, R. (2000). Intra-oral burns: Rehabilitation of severe restriction of mouth opening. *Physiotherapy*, *86*(5), 263-266.

Bailie, F., & Wilson, D. (2002). Early wound excision and grafting. In C. Bosworth Bousfield (Ed.), *Burn trauma: Management and nursing care* (2nd ed, pp. 142-157). London: Whurr.

Barret, J. P., Desai, M. H., & Herndon, D. N. (2000). Effects of tracheostomies on infection and airway complications in pediatric burns patients. *Burns*, *26*(2), 190-193.

Barrow, R. E., & Herndon, D. N. (2007). History of treatments of burns. In D. N. Herndon (Ed.), *Total burn care* (3rd ed., pp. 1-8). Edinburgh, UK: Elsevier Saunders.

Bayat, A., McGrouther, D. A., & Ferguson, M. W. (2003). Skin scarring. *British Medical Journal, 326*(7380), 88-92.

Bayley, E. W. (1991). Care of the burn patient with an inhalation injury. In R. B. Trofino (Ed.), *Nursing care of the burn-injured patient* (pp. 325-348). Philadelphia: F. A. Davis.

Bessey, P. Q. (2007). Wound care. In D. N. Herndon (Ed.), *Total burn care* (3rd ed., pp. 127-135). Edinburgh, UK: Elsevier Saunders.

Blakeney, P., & Meyer, W. (1994). Psychological aspects of burn care. *Trauma Quarterly, 11*(2), 166-179.

Boardman, S. (1991). Treatment of respiratory problems. In A. Leverage (Ed.), *Therapy for the burn patient* (pp. 29-33). London: Chapman and Hall.

Broniatowski, M., Sonies, B. C., Rubin, J. S., Bradshaw, C. R., Spiegel, J. R., Bastian, R. W., et al. (1999). Current evaluation and treatment of patients with swallowing disorders. *Otolaryngology-Head and Neck Surgery, 120*(4), 464-473.

Brooks, J., & Hammond, J. S. (1986). Nonverbal communication: Role of the speech pathologist on the burn team. *Journal of Burn Care and Rehabilitation, 7*(1), 42-44.

Buchholz, D. W. (1995). Oropharyngeal dysphagia due to iatrogenic neurological dysfunction. *Dysphagia, 10*(4), 248-254.

Calhoun, K. H., Deskin, R. W., Garza, C., McCracken, M. M., Nichols, R. J., Jr., Hokanson, J. A., et al. (1988). Long-term airway sequelae in a pediatric burn population. *Laryngoscope, 98*(7), 721-725.

Choiniere, M., Melzack, R., Rondeau, J., Girard, N., & Paquin, M. J. (1989). The pain of burns: Characteristics and correlates. *Journal of Trauma, 29*(11), 1531-1539.

Clark, W. R. (1992). Inhalation injury. In L. T. A. Rylah (Ed.), *Critical care of the burned patient* (pp. 59-77). Wiltshire, UK: Cambridge University Press.

Clark, W. R. (1992). Smoke inhalation: Diagnosis and treatment. *World Journal of Surgery, 16*(1), 24-29.

Clayton, N. A. (2007). *Concord Hospital Speech Pathology Clinical Cover Folder: Burns specialist caseload.* Sydney, Australia: Speech Pathology Department, Concord Hospital.

Clayton, N. A. (September, 2006). *The effect of endotracheal tube size and duration of intubation on voice and swallow function*. Paper presented at ANZBA ASM 2006, SPA Conference 2007.

Clayton, N. A., Ledgard, J. P., Haertsch, P., Kennedy, P. J., & Maitz, P. K. M. (May & September 2008a). *Rehabilitation of speech and swallowing following burns reconstructive surgery of the lips and nose.* Paper presented at RACS Conference 2008, IBSI Conference 2008, ANZBA ASM 2008.

Clayton, N. A., & Kennedy, P. J. (2007). Management of firecracker induced oropharyngeal burns: A case report. *International Journal of Speech-Language Pathology, 9*(3), 265-270.

Clayton, N. A., Kennedy, P. J., & Maitz, P. K. M. (September, 2008b). *The severe burns patient with tracheostomy: Implications for management of dysphagia, dysphonia and laryngotracheal pathology.* Paper presented at ISBI Conference 2008, ANZBA ASM 2008.

Clayton, N. A., Whitney, S., O'Loughlin, G., Crouch, A., & Patterson, M. (2005). Speech pathology. In D. Edgar (Ed.), *Burn survivor rehabilitation: Principles and guidelines for the allied health professional* (pp. 74-88). Brisbane, Australia: Australian and New Zealand Burn Association.

Cohen, M. A., & Guzzardi, L. J. (1983). Inhalation of products of combustion. *Annals of Emergency Medicine, 12*(10), 628-632.

Cohen, I. K., Schechter, P. J., & Henkin, R. I. (1973). Hypogeusia, anorexia, and altered zinc metabolism following thermal burn. *Journal of the American Medical Association, 223*(8), 914-916.

Coln, C. E., Purdue, G. F., & Hunt, J. L. (1998). Tracheostomy in the young pediatric burn patient. *Archives of Surgery, 133*(5), 537-539.

Cook, D. (2002a). Classification of burn trauma. In C. Bosworth Bousfield (Ed.),

Burn trauma: Management and nursing care (2nd ed., pp. 13–29). London: Whurr.

Cook, D. (2002b). Pathophysiology of burns. In C. Bosworth Bousfield (Ed.), *Burn trauma: Management and nursing care* (2nd ed., pp. 1–12). London: Whurr.

Cromes, G. F., Holavanahalli, R., Kowalske, K., & Helm, P. (2002). Predictors of quality of life as measured by the Burn Specific Health Scale in persons with major burn injury. *Journal of Burn Care and Rehabilitation, 23*(3), 229–234.

Daugherty, M. B., & Carr-Collins, J. A. (1994). Splinting techniques for the burn patient. In R. L. Richard & M. J. Staley (Eds.), *Burn care and rehabilitation: Principles and practice* (pp. 242–323). Philadelphia: F. A. Davis.

Demling, R. H. (2005). The burn edema process: Current concepts. *Journal of Burn Care and Rehabilitation, 26*(3), 207–227.

Demling, R., & Seigne, P. (2000). Metabolic management of patients with severe burns. *World Journal of Surgery, 24*(6), 673–680.

Dougherty, M. E., & Warden, G. D. (2003). A 30-year review of oral appliances used to manage microstomia, 1972–2002. *Journal of Burn Care and Rehabilitation, 24*(6), 418–431.

Duggan, D., & Quine, S. (1995). Burn injuries and characteristics of burn patients in New South Wales, Australia. *Burns, 21*(2), 83–89.

Dyer, C. (1988). Burn wound management: An update. *Plastic Surgical Nursing, 8*(1), 6–13.

Dyer, C., & Roberts, D. (1990). Thermal trauma. *Nursing Clinics of North America, 25*(1), 85–117.

Eckhauser, F. E., Billote, J., Burke, J. F., & Quinby, W. C. (1974). Tracheostomy complicating massive burn injury: A plea for conservatism. *American Journal of Surgery, 127*(4), 418–423.

Edelman, D. A., Sheehy-Deardorff, D. A., & White, M. T. (2008). Bedside assessment of swallowing is predictive of an abnormal barium swallow examination. *Journal of Burn Care and Rehabilitation, 29*(1), 89–96.

Edlich, R. F., Nichter, L. S., Morgan, R. F., Persing, J. A., Van Meter, C. H., & Kenney, J. G. (1984). Burns of the head and neck. *Otolaryngologic Clinics of North America, 17*(2), 361–388.

Ehde, D. M., Patterson, D. R., Wiechman, S. A., & Wilson, L. G. (1999). Post-traumatic stress symptoms and distress following acute burn injury. *Burns, 25*(7), 587–592.

Ehde, D. M., Patterson, D. R., Wiechman, S. A., & Wilson, L. G. (2000). Post-traumatic stress symptoms and distress 1 year after burn injury. *Journal of Burn Care and Rehabilitation, 21*(2), 105–111.

Esselman, P. C. (2007). Burn rehabilitation: An overview. *Archives of Physical Medicine and Rehabilitation, 88*(12 Suppl. 2), S3–S6.

Faucher, L. D. (2003). Modern pain management in burn care. *Problems in General Surgery, 20*(1), 80–87.

Faucher, L., & Furukawa, K. (2006). Practical guidelines for the management of pain. *Journal of Burn Care & Research, 27*(5), 659–668.

Fauerbach, J. A, Heinberg, L. J., Lawrence, J. W., Munster, A. M., Palombo, D. A., Richter, D., et al. (2000). Effect of early body image dissatisfaction on subsequent psychological and physical adjustment after disfiguring injury. *Psychosomatic Medicine, 62*(4), 576–582.

Gaissert, H. A., Lofgren, R. H., & Grillo, H. C. (1993). Upper airway compromise after inhalation injury: Complex strictures of the larynx and trachea and their management. *Annals of Surgery, 218*(5), 672–678.

Gallagher, G., Rae, C. P., & Kinsella, J. (2000). Treatment of pain in severe burns. *American Journal of Clinical Dermatology, 1*(6), 329–335.

Grunwald, T. B., & Garner, W. L. (2008). Acute burns. *Plastic and Reconstructive Surgery, 121*(5), 311e–319e.

Hart, D. W., Wolf, S. E., Chinkes, D. L., Beauford, R. B., Mlcak, R. P., Heggers, J. P., et al. (2003). Effects of early excision and aggressive enteral feeding on hypermetabolism, catabolism, and sepsis after severe burn. *Journal of Trauma, 54*(4), 755–761.

Hart, D. W., Wolf, S. E., Chinkes, D. L., Gore, D. C., Mlcak, R. P., Beauford, R. B., et al. (2000). Determinants of skeletal muscle catabolism after severe burn. *Annals of Surgery, 232*(4), 455-465.

Hartford, C. E., & Kealey, G. P. (2007). Care of outpatient burns. In D. N. Herndon (Ed.), *Total burn care* (3rd ed., pp. 67-80). Edinburgh, UK: Elsevier Saunders.

Herndon, D. N., Barrow, R. E., Rutan, R. L., Rutan, T. C., Desai, M. H., & Abston, S. (1989). A comparison of conservative versus early excision. *Annals of Surgery, 209*(5), 552-553.

Herndon, D. N., Barrow, R. E., Stein, M., Linares, H., Rutan, T. C., Rutan, R., et al. (1989). Increased mortality with intravenous supplemental feeding in severely burned patients. *Journal of Burn Care and Rehabilitation, 10*(4), 309-313.

Herndon, D. N., Stein, M. D., Rutan, T. C., Abston, S., & Linares, H. (1987). Failure of TPN supplementation to improve liver function, immunity, and mortality in thermally injured patients. *Journal of Trauma, 27*(2), 195-204.

Hoseok, I., Shim, Y. M., Son, Y .I., Kim, K., & Choi, Y. S. (2006). Pharyngo-colostomy with supraglottic partial laryngectomy in caustic oropharyngeal stricture. *Annals of Thoracic Surgery, 81*(2), 712-714.

Hunt, J. L., Arnoldo, B. D., & Purdue, G. F. (2007). Prevention of burn injuries. In D. N. Herndon (Ed.), *Total burn care* (3rd ed., pp. 33-42). Edinburgh, UK: Elsevier Saunders.

Johnson, C. L., O'Shaughnessy, E. J., & Ostergren, G. (1981). *Burn management.* New York: Raven Press.

Jones, O. (2002). Management of pain for an individual following burn trauma. In C. Bosworth Bousfield (Ed.), *Burn trauma: Management and nursing care* (2nd ed., pp. 121-140). London: Whurr.

Jones, W. G., Madden, M., Finkelstein, J., Yurt, R. W., & Goodwin, C. W. (1989). Tracheostomies in burn patients. *Annals of Surgery, 209*(4), 471-474.

Klaus, H. J. (2004). *History of burns.* Rotterdam, The Netherlands: Erasmus.

Knights, D. (2002). Management of the patient with an inhalation injury. In C. Bosworth Bousfield (Ed.), *Burn trauma: Management and nursing care* (2nd ed., pp. 109-120). London: Whurr.

Kreis, B. E., Middelkoop, E., Vloemans, A. F. P. M., & Kreis, R. W. (2002). The use of a PEG tube in a burn centre. *Burns, 28*(2), 191-197.

Locke, J., Rossignol, A., & Burke, J. (1990). Socioeconomic factors and the incidence of hospitalised burn injuries in New England USA. *Burns, 16*(4), 273-277.

Logemann, J. A. (1993). *Manual for the videofluorographic study of swallowing* (2nd ed.). Austin, TX: Pro-Ed.

Lund, C. C., & Browder, N. C. (1944). Estimation of areas of burns. *Surgery, Gynecology and Obstetrics, 79*, 352-358.

Luterman, A., & Curreri, P. (1990). Chemical burn injury. In M. Jurkiewcz, T. Krizek, & S. Mathes (Eds.), *Plastic surgery: Principles and practice* (pp. 1355-1440). St. Louis, MO: CV Mosby.

MacLeod, A. (1970). Adult burns in Melbourne. *Medical Journal of Australia, 2*, 772-777.

Madnani, D. D., Steele, N. P., & de Vries, E. (2006). Factors that predict the need for intubation in patients with smoke inhalation injury. *Ear, Nose & Throat Journal, 85*(4), 278-280.

Magnotti, L. J., & Deitch, E. A. (2005). Burns, bacterial translocation, gut barrier function and failure. *Journal of Burn Care and Rehabilitation, 26*(5), 383-391.

Masterton, J., Pressley, T., & Ramsay, G. (1979). A survey of adults with flame burns at a Melbourne hospital. *Medical Journal of Australia, 1*, 332-334.

McCall, J. E., & Cahill, T. J. (2005). Respiratory care of the burn patient. *Journal of Burn Care and Rehabilitation, 26*(3), 200-206.

McKinnon DuBose, C., Groher, Carnaby Mann, G. S., & Mozingo, D. W. (2005). Pattern of dysphagia recovery after thermal burn injury. *Journal of Burn Care and Rehabilitation, 26*(3), 233-237.

Medicine Australia. (2006). *Burns Management*. Retrieved January 9, 2008, from http://www.medicineau.net.au

Meyer, W. J., III, Patterson, D. R., Jaco, M., Woodson, L., & Thomas, C. (2007). Management of pain and other discomforts in burned patients. In D. N. Herndon (Ed.), *Total burn care* (3rd ed., pp. 797-818). Edinburgh, UK: Elsevier Saunders.

Mlcak, R. P., & Buffalo, M. C. (2007). Prehospital management, transportation, and emergency care. In D. N. Herndon (Ed.), *Total burn care* (3rd ed., pp. 81-92). Edinburgh, UK: Elsevier Saunders.

Muehlberger, T., Kunar, D., Munster, A., & Couch, M. (1998). Efficacy of fiberoptic laryngoscopy in the diagnosis of inhalation injuries. *Archives of Otolaryngology-Head and Neck Surgery, 124*(9), 1003-1007.

Muir, I. F. K., Barclay, T. L., & Settle, J. A. D. (1987). *Burns and their treatment* (3rd ed.). London: Butterworths.

Muller, M., Gahankari, D., & Herndon, D. N. (2007). Operative wound management. In D. N. Herndon. (Ed.), *Total burn care* (3rd ed., pp. 177-195). Edinburgh, UK: Elsevier Saunders.

Muller, M. J., Pegg, S. P., & Rule, M. R. (2001). Determinants of death following burn injury. *British Journal of Surgery, 88*(4), 583-587.

Nawar, E. W., Niska, R. W., & Xu, J. (2007). National Hospital Ambulatory Medical Care Survey: 2005 Emergency Department Summary. *Advance Data for Vital and Health Statistics, 386*, 1-32.

Nicol, J., & Rudd, M. (2004). *Royal Brisbane and Women's Hospital Burns Unit: 1972-2004 Mortality and determinants of death*. Brisbane, Australia: RBWH Burns Unit, University of Queensland.

Norbury, W. B., & Herndon, D. N. (2007). Modulation of the hypermetabolic response after burn injury. In D. N. Herndon. (Ed.), *Total burn care* (3rd ed., pp. 420-433). Edinburgh, UK: Elsevier Saunders.

Palmer, J. B., DuChane, A. S., & Donner, M. W. (1991). The role of radiology in the rehabilitation of swallowing. In B. Jones & M. W. Donner (Eds.), *Normal and abnormal swallowing: Imaging in diagnosis and therapy* (pp. 215-225). New York: Springer-Verlag.

Palmer, M., & Collier, S. (1999). Continuing care of burn-injured patients. *Nursing Times, 95*(37), 44-46.

Palmieri, T. L., Jackson, W., & Greenhalgh, D. G. (2002). Benefits of early tracheostomy in severely burned children. *Critical Care Medicine, 30*(4), 922-924.

Pankhurst, S., & Pochkhanawala, T. (2002). Wound care. In C. Bosworth Bousfield (Ed.), *Burn trauma: Management and nursing care* (2nd ed., pp. 81-108). London: Whurr.

Patterson, D. R., Tininenko, J., & Ptacek, J. T. (2006). Pain during burn hospitalization predicts long-term outcome. *Journal of Burn Care & Research, 27*(5), 719-726.

Pereira, C. T., Murphy, K. D., & Herndon, D. N. (2005). Altering metabolism. *Journal of Burn Care and Rehabilitation, 26*(3), 194-199.

Pham, T. N., Gibran, N. S., & Heimbach, D. M. (2007). Evaluation of the burn wound: Management decisions. In D. N. Herndon (Ed.), *Total burn care* (3rd ed., pp. 119-126). Edinburgh, UK: Elsevier Saunders.

Prater, M. E., & Deskin, R. W. (1998). Bronchoscopy and laryngoscopy findings as indications for tracheotomy in the burned child. *Archives of Otolaryngology-Head and Neck Surgery, 124*(10), 1115-1117.

Pruitt, B. A., Jr., Wolf, S. E., & Mason, A. D., Jr. (2007). Epidemiological, demographic, and outcome characteristics of burn injury. In D. N. Herndon (Ed.), *Total burn care* (3rd ed., pp. 14-32). Edinburgh, UK: Elsevier Saunders.

Purdue, G. F., Arnoldo, B. D., & Hunt, J. L. (2007). Electrical injuries. In D. N. Herndon (Ed.), *Total burn care* (3rd ed., pp. 513-520). Edinburgh, UK: Elsevier Saunders.

Rose, D. D., & Jordan, E. B. (1999). Perioperative management of burn patients. *Association of periOperative Registered Nurses Journal, 69*(6), 1211-1222.

Saffle, J. R., & Graves, C. (2007). Nutritional support of the burned patient. In D. N.

Herndon (Ed.), *Total burn care* (3rd ed., pp. 398-419). Edinburgh, UK: Elsevier Saunders.

Saffle, J. R., Morris, S. E., & Edelman, L. (2002). Early tracheostomy does not improve outcome in burn patients. *Journal of Burn Care & Rehabilitation*, *23*(6), 431-438.

Sanford, A. P. (2007). Chemical burns. In D. N. Herndon (Ed.), *Total burn care* (3rd ed., pp. 536-541). Edinburgh, UK: Elsevier Saunders.

Sheridan, R. L., Hinson, M. I., Liang, M. H., Nackal, A. F., Schoenfeld, D. A., Ryan, C. M., et al. (2000). Long-term outcome of children surviving massive burns. *Journal of the American Medical Association*, *283*(1), 69-73.

Shikowitz, M. J., Levy, J., Villano, D., Graver, M. L., & Pochaczevsky, R. (1996). Speech and swallowing rehabilitation following devastating caustic ingestion: Techniques and indicators for success. *Laryngoscope*, *106*(2), 1-12.

Siebens, A. A., & Linden, P. L. (1985). Dynamic imaging for swallowing reeducation. *Gastrointestinal Radiology*, *10*, 251-253.

Snyder, C., & Ubben, P. (2003). Use of speech pathology services in the burn unit. *Journal of Burn Care and Rehabilitation*, *24*(4), 217-222.

Sologub, V. K., Zaets, T. L., Tarasov, A. V., Mordkovitch, M. R., & Yu Yashin, A. (1992). Enteral hyperalimentation of burned patients: The possibility of correcting metabolic disorders by early administration of prolonged high calorie evenly distributed tube feeds. *Burns*, *18*(3), 245-249.

Tejero-Trujeque, R. (2000). How effective is the abbreviated Burn Severity Index in predicting patient mortality? *Journal of Wound Care*, *9*(10), 475-478.

Trofino, R. B., & Braun, A. E. (1991). Pathophysiology of burns. In R. B. Trofino (Ed.), *Nursing care of the burn-injured patient* (pp. 13-27). Philadelphia: F. A. Davis.

Valdez, T. A., Desai, U., Ruhl, C. M., & Nigri, P. T. (2006). Early laryngeal inhalation injury and its correlation with late sequelae. *Laryngoscope*, *116*(2), 283-287.

van Rijn, O., Bouter, L., & Meertens, R. (1989). The aetiology of burns in developed countries: Review of the literature. *Burns*, *15*(4), 217-221.

Vyrostek, S. B., Annest, J. L., & Ryan, G. W. (2004). Surveillance for fatal and non-fatal injuries—United States, 2001. *Morbidity and Mortality Weekly Report*, *53*(SS07), 1-57.

Wallace, A. B. (1951). The exposure treatment of burns. *Lancet*, *1*(9), 501-504.

Ward, E. C., Uriarte, M., & Conroy, A.-L. (2001). Duration of dysphagic symptoms and swallowing outcomes after thermal burn injury. *Journal of Burn Care and Rehabilitation*, *22*(6), 441-453.

Wiechman, S. A., Ptacek, J. T., Patterson, D. R., Gibran, N. S., Engrav, L. E., & Heimbach, D. M. (2001). Rates, trends, and severity of depression after burn injuries. *Journal of Burn Care and Rehabilitation*, *22*(6), 417-424.

Williams, A. I., & Baker, B. M. (1992). Advances in burn care management: Role of the speech-language pathologist. *Journal of Burn Care and Rehabilitation*, *13*(6), 642-649.

Wilmore, D. W., Long, J. M., Mason, A. D., Skreen, R. W., & Pruitt, B. A. (1974). Catecholamines: Mediator of the hypermetabolic response to thermal injury. *Annals of Surgery*, *180*(4), 653-669.

Yu, B. H., & Dimsdale, J. E. (1999). Posttraumatic stress disorder in patients with burn injuries. *Journal of Burn Care and Rehabilitation*, *20*(5), 426-433.

5 Multitrauma and Iatrogenic Trauma

JANE M. CROMBIE, ANN-LOUISE SPURGIN, AND ELIZABETH C. WARD

INTRODUCTION

Multitrauma is a term used to define the event of physical injuries occurring simultaneously in several parts of the body. These simultaneous injuries may include orthopedic injury, brain and spinal cord injury, soft tissue wounds, and burn injury. Clinical management of the multitrauma patient is therefore complex, as each of the simultaneously occurring physical injuries may have its own specific impact on swallowing function. For instance, a multitrauma patient who has experienced both a traumatic brain injury (TBI) and midfacial fracture in a motor vehicle accident will have both neurological impairment (from the TBI) and structural damage (from the midfacial fracture and its management). Both of these injuries may impact on swallowing function and may have different influences on the course of rehabilitation.

Whereas multitrauma occurs following an injurious event, *iatrogenic trauma* refers to trauma inflicted inadvertently on a patient by a medical or surgical intervention or diagnostic procedure. This may occur following an isolated surgical event, such as a carotid endarterectomy for carotid stenosis, or as part of post-injury trauma management, such as anterior cervical spinal fusion surgery following spinal cord injury. Although the mechanisms of injury for multitrauma and iatrogenic trauma may differ, both may impact significantly on swallowing function, particularly when the trauma or surgery is in the head and neck region. Multitrauma and iatrogenic trauma may co-occur, such as in a patient with injuries from a high fall (climbing incident) who presents with multitrauma involving spinal injury, mandibular fracture, and thoracic injury, as well as iatrogenic laryngeal trauma from intubation.

In the previous chapters on TBI, traumatic spinal cord injury (TSCI), and burns, reference has been made to the potential for patients to have suffered additional trauma (multitrauma) at the time of injury, and possible iatrogenic trauma during acute care management, further complicating dysphagia assessment and management. It is the intent of the current chapter to discuss these other types of injury (e.g., facial fractures, thoracic injury, etc.) that frequently co-occur in the multitrauma patient in more detail. Further, some of the common causes of iatrogenic trauma will be discussed. Consequently, unlike the previous chapters, the present chapter will discuss a number of different injury types and surgical procedures. Each form of injury is discussed separately in relation to the damage that can occur and its potential impact on swallow function. However, the reader should remain cognizant that there is great potential for these injuries to coexist. In the following sections, key information is presented that is specific to the impact of a certain injury or surgical procedure on swallowing, providing the clinician with information on how this may alter standard practice for the assessment and the management of dysphagia.

MULTITRAUMA

Trauma is the leading cause of death in people under 44 years of age and accounts for 63% of all deaths in the 15–24 year age group (Rance, 2000). Males are twice as likely to suffer fatal traumatic injuries as females (Conn & Petrovik, 2004; Rance, 2000). In no particular order, the most common causes of multitrauma are motor vehicle accidents, sporting injuries, suicide attempts, assault, work-related injuries, risk-taking behaviors, and falls.

The most frequently occurring trauma etiologies also vary between different age groups. In adults over 75 years of age, 82% of traumatic injuries requiring hospital treatment occur as a result of falls, whereas falls are the cause of only 20% of traumatic injuries in young adults (Rance, 2000). Studies have shown that young adult males are at increased risk for experiencing traumatic injuries. This has been attributed to the greater prevalence of risk taking behavior and attempts at suicide displayed by this age group.

Mechanisms of Multitrauma

The mechanisms of injury that cause multitrauma can be grouped under two main classifications: (a) chemical/thermal injury, such as in the case of burn injury (see Chapter 4) and (b) kinetic injury. Kinetic injuries result from the energy of motion and can be subclassified into either blunt force injury or penetrating injury:

- Blunt force injury. This term describes physical trauma that results from the kinetic energy of an impact, such as in the case of motor vehicle accidents, sporting accidents, assault, falls, or explosions. Specific types of trauma may occur as a result of blunt force trauma, including factures, contusions, or abrasions. Blunt force trauma is by far the most common cause of injury.
- Penetrating injury. Penetrating injury is caused by an object passing into or through tissue, such as in the case of a stab wound. The extent and severity of the injury is largely determined by the velocity of the penetrating object. Low-velocity projectiles such as knives typically cause damage to the region in immediate proximity to the object. In contrast, projectiles of medium to high velocity, such as bullets, damage those tissues they come into contact with, as well as causing a cavitation injury resulting from the pressure wave of the entering projectile.

Subsequent to the initial blunt force or penetrating injury, various other types of specific injury can result, including:

- Fracture. Fractures occur when greater forces are exerted to bone than it can withstand. There are many different types of bone fractures that may occur, dependent upon the nature of the force. More details regarding specific types of fractures are outlined below in the section covering Hard Tissue Trauma (see also Chapter 3 for types of spinal fractures).

- Crush injury. When a body part is compressed between two objects it is referred to as a crush injury. A crush injury can cause injury to both hard and soft tissue as well as neural and vascular tissues.
- Compression injury. This type of injury occurs when pressure or crushing under the area of impact causes damage to the underlying tissues and internal organs.
- Blast injury. Primary blast injury is caused by the pressure wave generated by the blast from an explosion as it strikes the body. It creates a pressure differential at the air-tissue interface, causing tissue contusion, edema, and hemorrhage. Secondary blast injuries refer to injuries sustained from objects set in motion by the explosion that make impact with the patient.
- Shear injury. This form of injury is caused by rapid acceleration or deceleration. Soft tissue and vascular tissue become damaged when the tensile strength of the tissue is exceeded, causing tearing or rupture.
- Lacerations. Lacerations are full thickness wounds of the skin, created by the tearing of soft tissue against bone or a blunt object. These injuries often result in an irregular or jagged wound.
- Punctures. As opposed to a laceration injury, a puncture injury is more contained to the tissues immediately surrounding the penetrating object. Puncture wounds may appear to close up when the penetrating object is removed.
- Abrasions. An abrasion is a superficial wound that does not penetrate the dermis. Deeper abrasions often involve foreign bodies such as gravel, dirt, and wood splinters.
- Contusions. Commonly known as bruising, contusions occur as a result of subcutaneous bleeding due to blunt trauma.
- Avulsions. Sections of tissue torn from the body that include all three layers of skin are known as avulsions. An avulsion is less extensive than an amputation. These injuries are commonly caused by animal bites, industrial equipment, or motor vehicle accident.

Classifying the Severity of Multitrauma

A number of scales have been outlined in the previous chapters for classifying the severity of specific injury, such as the Glasgow Coma Scale (GCS) for coma severity (Chapter 2, Traumatic Brain Injury) and the Lund and Browder charts (Lund & Browder, 1944; Chapter 4, Burn Injury) for calculating extent of burn injury. More general trauma severity scales also exist, as used by paramedical and medical teams to help convey severity of injury and to provide an indication of prognosis. Such information may be used to triage patients, although many centers rely more heavily on the clinical experience of the trauma team rather than calculated severity scores. Systems such as the injury severity score (ISS) can be used to document overall trauma severity. Scoring ranges from 0 to 75, with 75 being the most severe. To calculate injury severity, all injuries located in each of six body regions (head and neck, face, chest, abdomen, extremity, external) are first assigned an abbreviated injury scale (AIS) score of 1to 6 (where 6 is an unsurvivable injury; any region receiving an AIS of 6 results in an immediate ISS score of 75). Where multiple injuries occur in any region, only the highest AIS score is used. Finally, the three most severely injured regions have their scores squared and added together to produce the ISS score. An example of an ISS calculation can be found in Table 5-1.

Impact of Multitrauma Management

Multitrauma patients usually require an extended stay in the intensive care setting in order to stabilize and treat their injuries. Sedation, intubation, and ventilation are necessary in the initial stages of injury management, yet these interventions have been found to have adverse effects on the patient's swallowing ability. The high risk of infection and the development of sepsis can further complicate recovery and necessitate cautious implementation of oral intake during this critical phase. Patients are also at risk for developing critical illness polyneuropathy (CIP) due to the protracted duration in critical care. The following sections provide a summary of these issues.

Sedation

Pharmaceutical sedation is frequently used to facilitate intubation, ventilation, and optimal intensive care management of the multitrauma patient. Neuromuscular blocking agents (NMBAs) are required to keep the patient comfortable, to prevent agitation, and to improve pulmonary compliance. Sedation may adversely affect the patient's cognition and level of alertness, impairing airway protection and therefore placing the patient at increased risk of aspiration. A strong correlation has been found between the use of NMBAs and the development of CIP

Table 5–1. A Worked Example of an Injury Severity Score (ISS) Calculation

Region	*Injury Description*	*Abbreviated Injury Scale (AIS) Score*	*Square of Top Three AIS Scores*
Head and Neck	Base of skull fracture	3	9
Face	Fractured mandible	2	4
Chest	Pneumothorax	3	9
Abdomen	No injury	0	—
Extremity	Fractured radius	1	—
External	No injury	0	—
		Injury Severity Score	**22**

(discussed below) in intensive care patients. CIP presents as a neuromuscular weakness and is thought to be a contributing factor in long-term intensive care patients who present with dysphagia with no known etiology.

Intubation and Ventilation

Many multitrauma patients will require intubation to maintain a patent airway and to provide a means for mechanical ventilation. An endotracheal tube (ETT) is the most common means of intubation. It is documented that patients who have had an ETT in situ for more than 7 to 10 days are at risk of dysphagia due to the increased risk of laryngeal injury (Conlan & Kopec, 2000). Laryngeal injury may occur as the tube is being inserted, or may be result as a complication of prolonged intubation. Possible complications during insertion of the tube include damage to laryngeal and tracheal epithelium and hematoma of the vocal fold (particularly of the left vocal fold). Reported laryngeal trauma, as a result of prolonged intubation, includes vocal fold paralysis or edema, mucosal ulceration, formation of granulation tissue, subglottic stenosis, and a "crushed" epiglottis. An overinflated ETT cuff has been associated with neurapraxia of the recurrent laryngeal nerve, causing unilateral vocal fold paralysis. These complications may cause impaired airway protection, impaired laryngeal sensation, and pain on swallowing. It is reported that most laryngeal symptoms resolve within 4 to 8 weeks; however, some injuries may be more permanent (McHardy & Chung, 1999).

For patients requiring longer term ventilation, or where head and neck injuries or swelling prevents an ETT being inserted, a tracheostomy may be performed. Many tracheostomized individuals are able to resume oral intake, yet the potential for swallowing dysfunction is heightened by the presence of the tracheostomy tube.

Dikeman and Kazandjian (2003) outline the interrelationship between tracheostomy, ventilator dependence, and swallowing, highlighting that the presence of a tracheostomy tube may impact upon a number of laryngeal processes, including: decreased laryngeal excursion due to anchoring of the tube to the surrounding musculature and/or additional difficulty arising from an inflated tracheostomy cuff; impaired coordination of the glottic closure response secondary to long-term diversion of air; and blunting of the cough reflex secondary to reduced laryngeal sensation due to lack of laryngeal airflow. Even once the tracheostomized individual is able to resume normal respiratory functioning and the tube is removed, the initial surgical incision performed for tube placement may have caused muscle and nerve damage, causing compromised laryngeal elevation and vocal cord functioning, increasing the risk of laryngeal penetration or aspiration (Hauck, 1999). In addition to the potential negative impact on swallow function, potential complications caused by the presence of a tracheostomy tube include injury to the recurrent laryngeal nerve, tracheoesophageal fistula, and stenosis (ischemia induced by cuffed tracheostomy tube); however, such negative effects can be offset to some degree by ensuring the use of appropriately sized tracheostomy tubes and avoiding overinflation of the cuff.

Patients receiving prolonged mechanical ventilation (more than 21 days) have been found to have a high incidence of dysphagia (80%), even in the absence of a neurological disorder (Tolep, Getch, &

Criner, 1996). Features of dysphagia associated with prolonged mechanical ventilation include: reduced lingual control of the bolus, reduced laryngeal elevation, and aspiration (Tolep et al., 1996). It is unclear whether dysphagia occurs solely due to the implications of intubation or critical illness neuropathy (see section below) or whether mechanical ventilation alone has the potential to cause dysphagia. One theory is that the absence of airflow through the glottis may cause reduced laryngeal sensation. It is also proposed that prolonged mechanical ventilation is a marker of severe illness rather than a causative factor of dysphagia (Tolep et al., 1996).

Sepsis

Sepsis is a systemic inflammatory response syndrome (SIRS) resulting from a bacterial, viral, fungal, or parasitic infection. Critically ill trauma patients are predisposed to developing severe sepsis. SIRS may lead to multiple organ dysfunction and often necessitates extended periods of ventilation and intensive care admission. CIP occurs in 70% of septic patients (Bolton, 1996), causing neuromuscular weakness that may potentially include dysphagia. Clinical manifestations of SIRS include: a body temperature of more than 38°C, increased heart rate, and an increased respiratory rate (more than 20 breaths/minute) that may impact on the dysphagia assessment (de Letter et al., 2001). Spikes in body temperature will not be a reliable clinical indicator of an aspiration-related chest infection in septic patients. An increased respiratory rate has the potential to adversely affect breath-swallow coordination by reducing the apneic period during the swallow. Due to the systemic nature of the illness, a reduced level of alertness is common in patients with sepsis, and may further impair a patient's ability to swallow safely.

Critical Illness Polyneuropathy

CIP is the most common type of critical illness neuromuscular abnormality. The disorder is defined as a predominantly motor axonal dysfunction of unknown etiology that causes neuromuscular weakness in the critically ill population. The incidence rate ranges from 50 to 80% of all critical care patients (Garnacho-Montero et al., 2001). In a systematic review of prospective clinical studies of neuromuscular abnormalities in the intensive care unit (ICU), 46 of the 242 patients (19%) were identified as trauma patients (De Jonghe et al., 1998).

CIP is diagnosed by clinical presentation (difficulty in weaning from the ventilator and limb weakness) and electrophysiologic findings (nerve conduction and needle electromyography [EMG]). It occurs frequently in septic patients who develop multiple organ dysfunction syndrome. It is not limited to septic patients, however, and multitrauma patients who require an extended ICU admission are also at risk of developing CIP. Aminoglycosides (a group of antibiotics that are effective against certain types of bacteria), corticosteroids, and neuromuscular blockers have been suspected to cause or contribute to CIP (De Jonghe et al., 1998).

CIP involves primary axonal degeneration of motor and sensory fibers and subsequent muscle denervation and degeneration. This leads to generalized muscle weakness and atrophy and decreased deep tendon reflexes. Muscle weakness may persist for as long as 12 months. CIP has also been associated with longer periods of mechanical ventilation and increased mortality. The causes of CIP are unknown but malnutrition and drugs (neuromuscular blocking agents in particular) have been hypothesized as contributing factors. Aside from supportive care and rehabilitation, there is no effective treatment reported for CIP.

CIP is often thought to be the cause of persistent dysphagia following a prolonged ICU admission where there is no other significant neurological history. Dysphagia associated with CIP often presents as a generalized weakness of the oral and pharyngeal musculature, consistent with other neurological disorders such as stroke or traumatic brain injury. It may result in poor bolus control, pharyngeal residue, and laryngeal penetration or aspiration of saliva, food, or fluid. Clinical experience has found that these patients are often slow to have their tracheostomy tube removed due to their swallowing impairment and reduced airway protection.

Assessment of dysphagia for a person with CIP should involve a thorough clinical examination to determine the strength of the oral and facial musculature. An endoscopic swallowing examination (ESE) or videofluoroscopic swallowing examination (VFSE) assessment is necessary to determine the impact of CIP on the pharyngeal phase. In relation to treatment, as soon as the patient is alert, oromotor exercises and pharyngeal exercises (e.g., the Shaker exercise and laryngeal excursion exercises) should be commenced. These exercises may help to minimize atrophy and strengthen the muscles of swallowing. Specific management of the dysphagia is based on the findings of the instrumental assessment. Compensatory and rehabilitation strategies (see Chapter 1) should be individualized dependent upon the presenting clinical features of a particular patient.

Neurological Trauma

Multitrauma can cause both neurological and structural damage. Neurotrauma (damage to the central nervous system) and the mechanisms that cause it have been covered in detail in Chapter 2 (Traumatic Brain Injury) and Chapter 3 (Spinal Cord Injury) and so will not be covered further here. The reader is referred to those chapters for more detailed information regarding neurotrauma and its impact on dysphagia. In the sections below on structural trauma, potential injury to the cranial nerves and any peripheral nerves that may accompany structural damage will be discussed.

Structural Trauma

In addition to neurological injury, patients who suffer multitrauma can present with extensive structural damage caused by trauma to hard and soft tissue. Specific types of structural damage to the hard and soft tissue structures of the head and neck and injury to the chest (thorax) will be discussed further below in relation to their impact on the assessment and management of dysphagia. Although it is recognized that multiple structures may be impaired or disrupted simultaneously in the multitrauma patient, the following sections will outline how each injury type, and its subsequent management, may in turn impact on swallowing physiology, and the ensuing assessment and management process.

Hard Tissue Trauma

Hard tissue trauma involves a fracture of a bony or cartilaginous structure of the body. Fractures can be referred to as either open or closed. An open (compound) fracture is a broken bone that penetrates the skin. Closed fractures do not penetrate the skin and are classified further as either simple or comminuted. Simple fractures occur along one line, splitting the bone into two pieces. A comminuted fracture occurs when the bone is broken into more than two fragments. If the fragments are in normal alignment, it is called an undisplaced fracture. Conversely, displaced fractures describe those where there is a large gap between the bone fragments.

The management of fractures involves supporting reunion of the bones and promoting soft tissue healing, in order to restore normal function. Management may be surgical or conservative (nonsurgical), but the principles of treatment are the same:

- *To reduce* the fracture (restore normal anatomy)
- And *to stabilize* the fracture

Restoration of the bony segments to their proper anatomic location can be achieved via *open reduction* or *closed reduction*. In closed reduction, the surgeon manipulates the bone into place without directly visualizing the fracture. An example of closed reduction is manipulation of a broken arm prior to casting. Open reduction, which is most commonly used in head and neck fractures, requires surgical access to enable the surgeon to directly visualize the bony fragments.

Stabilization (also referred to as fixation) creates optimal conditions for the production of callus, which is responsible for bone healing. Stabilization of the fracture may be achieved through *external fixation* or *internal fixation*. External fixation involves stabilizing the area using techniques such as splinting or casting, which are applied externally. Internal fixation involves surgery to stabilize and join the ends of fractured bones using wires, plates, pins, and screws to support the bone directly. Open reduction internal fixation (ORIF) using surgically placed titanium plates, screws, and wires is the most common management for fractures in the head and neck area.

The following is a list of different types of bony fractures that may occur in the head and neck region. The impact and subsequent management of fractures is usually determined by the type of fracture.

Base of Skull Injury. Base of skull fractures occur in 24% of blunt head injuries and may involve damage to cranial nerves, the internal carotid arteries, and the cavernous sinus. They also have the potential to cause a cerebrospinal fluid (CSF) fistula, that is, a breech of the arachnoid and dura mater (the skull bone and its underlying mucosa). Base of skull fractures are often associated with a TBI. Temporal bone fractures are the most common type of skull base fractures, and 25% of these are associated with facial nerve injury. Base of skull fractures are usually managed conservatively (i.e., nonsurgically). If there is temporal bone fracture, cranial nerve damage, meningitis or a CSF fistula, however, surgical management is indicated.

Implications for Assessment and Management. Given that they arise from the brainstem immediately adjacent to the skull base, the cranial nerves are frequently damaged following skull base injury. Damage to the trigeminal, facial, glossopharyngeal, vagus, and hypoglossal nerves, in particular, will impact on swallowing (see Chapter 1). Dysphagia may be transient if it is purely the result of bruising or edema around the brainstem. In more severe cases, nerves can be severed, causing permanent impairment to the patient's swallowing mechanism.

Clinical assessment involves a thorough assessment of cranial nerve function with specific attention to the trigeminal, facial, glossopharyngeal, vagus, and hypoglossal nerves. VFSE is the only objective assessment technique that should be used to supplement clinical assessment and advise management. ESE should be avoided for this patient group due to the risk of the endoscope being misdirected and entering the skull at the site of the fracture.

Specific issues to consider in the management of dysphagia following skull base damage include:

- Damage to the cranial nerves has the potential to cause impairments to both the oral and pharyngeal phases of the swallow. Compensatory and rehabilitation techniques (see Chapter 1) targeting the presenting physiological deficits identified through clinical and instrumental assessment should be implemented as warranted.
- If the patient is experiencing CSF leak, he may be unable to sit upright for oral intake. Texture modification of diet or assistive equipment (e.g., dysphagia cup, straw) may be required if the patient is restricted from upright positioning for oral intake.
- If the patient's dysphagia is compromising nutritional intake and alternative feeding is required, this should only be provided via an orogastric tube or percutaneous gastrostomy tube (PEG). Insertion of nasogastric tubes in these patients has been known to lead to misdirection of the tube intracranially.

Mandibular Fractures. Mandibular fractures are one of the most common fractures in the human body due to the prominent, isolated position of this bone. Sites of mandibular fracture include the symphysis, parasymphysis, body, angle, ramus, coronoid, and condyle (Figure 5–1).

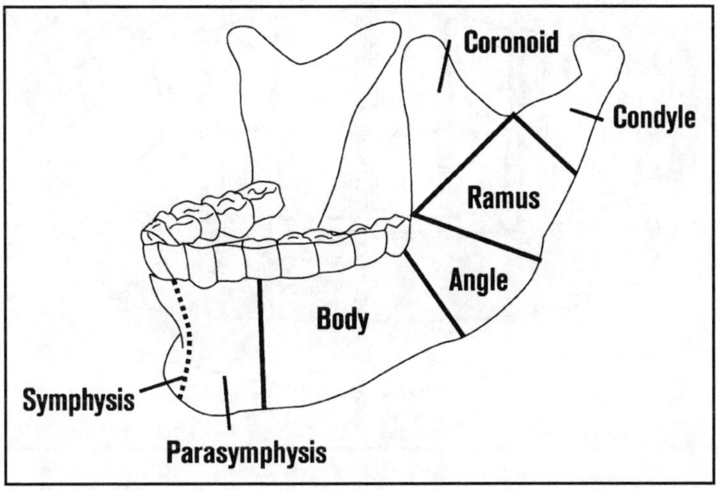

Figure 5–1. Common sites of mandibular fractures (symphysis, parasymphysis, body, angle, ramus, condyle, and coronoid).

The management of a mandibular fracture can be via surgical or nonsurgical management. Nonsurgical management for undisplaced fractures involves analgesia and a puree diet for a period of 6 weeks. The puree diet minimizes the risk of occlusal force (bite force), which may place the bony fragments out of alignment. Operative management varies depending on the type of fracture and the surgeon's preference, but it typically involves ORIF, which is open surgery to reduce the fragments and fixate them with screws or plates in order to enable healing.

Historically, mandibular fractures were treated with long periods of intermaxillary fixation. Intermaxillary fixation, or maxillo-mandibular fixation, establishes a proper bite by wiring the teeth together. This means that the jaw is fixed in a closed position using arch bars, intermaxillary fixation screws, or eyelet wiring, with wires or function-guided elastics holding the occlusion together for a period of 2 to 6 weeks. Fixation may be rigid (using wires or heavy elastics; Figure 5–2) or semirigid. Semirigid fixation is achieved with function-guided elastics, which allow guided opening of the jaws. Unfortunately, this prolonged period of fixation has the potential to cause trismus (reduced jaw opening), ankylosis (stiffness) of the condyles, and significant weight loss. Today, the management of fractures has been greatly improved with the advent of plates and screws for internal fixation (Figure 5–3). Internal fixation allows earlier return to function as the jaw can be opened.

Implications for Assessment and Management. Mandibular fractures are likely to only affect the oral phase of the

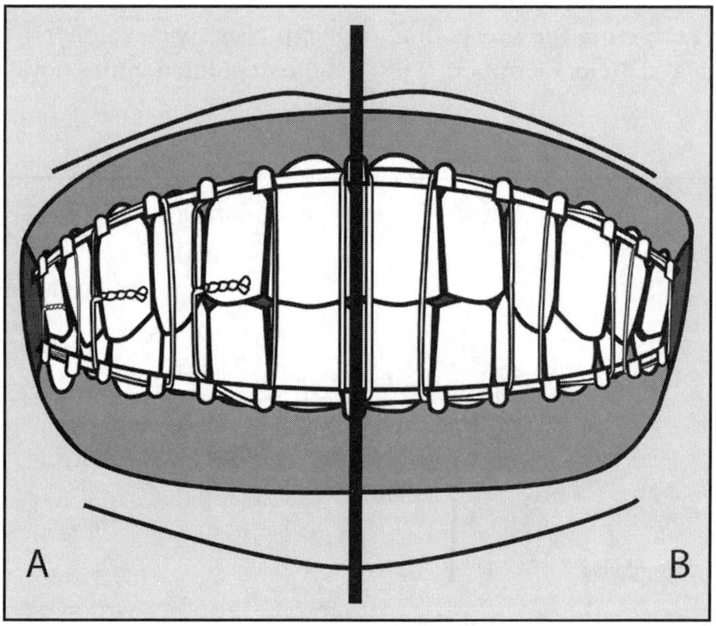

Figure 5–2. Stylistic representation of a mouth with arch bars with wires **(A)** and arch bars with elastics **(B)**.

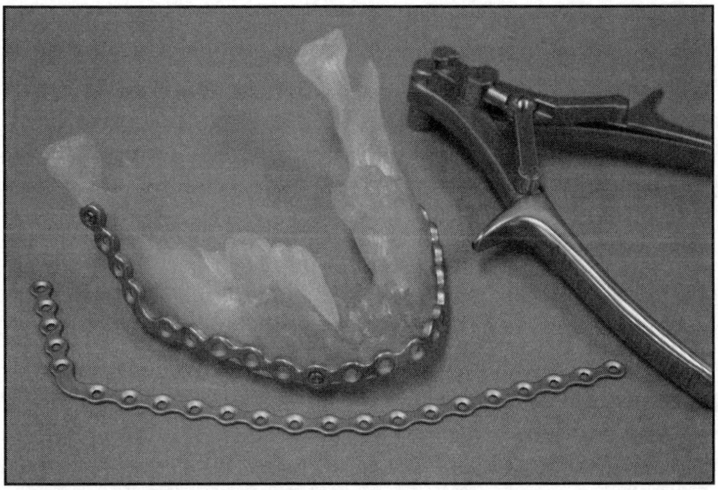

Figure 5–3. Example of plating system for internal fixation of a mandible. Photo courtesy of Anatomics (http://www.anatomics.com).

swallow. If the jaw is fixed by wires, a clinical oromotor exam and clinical assessment of the oral phase of the swallow will be impossible. If there is suspicion of dysphagia, a VFSE is the best objective assessment of oral preparation, control, and transfer of the bolus.

Potential factors that may impact on the oral stage of the swallow include post-injury swelling, potential iatrogenic damage from internal fixation surgery, and long-term issues with mastication and jaw opening. Due to the highly vascular nature of the mandibular region, there is likely to be significant swelling post-injury. The swelling usually peaks 3 days after the injury and then resolves within 1 to 2 weeks. Pain and muscle spasm from the injury or from surgery may also contribute to reduced mouth opening. Again, this should resolve within 1 to 2 weeks of the injury.

A potential iatrogenic complication for this population is damage (stretched or severed) to the inferior alveolar nerve (mandibular branch of the trigeminal nerve). This may reduce sensation in the lower lip for many months, or even permanently. Reduced lip sensation may lead to drooling of saliva and/or anterior spillage of food or fluid from the lips. Damage to the lingual nerve may also be observed post-surgery. This may cause impaired sensation and taste on the affected side. The impairment is usually temporary, resolving within 6 to 12 months; however, some patients have permanently impaired sensation and taste.

Following the 6-week healing period, studies have shown some patients have a chronic reduction in efficiency in mastication, yet this has not been found to have any significant functional impact on eating (Throckmorton, Ellis, & Hayasaki, 2003). Trismus (reduced mouth opening) is also a common complication of mandibular fractures or their management; thus, jaw opening should also be evaluated. A degree of mouth opening (maximal interincisor measurement) of less than or equal to 35 mm is a functional definition of trismus (Dijkstra, Huisman, & Roodenburg, 2006).

Management of oral intake during the period of recovery typically involves the following strategies:

- For 6 weeks post-trauma, the patient must remain on a puree diet or high-energy free fluids as prescribed by the surgeon. This diet modification serves to minimize the load or pressure placed on the fracture, thus optimizing conditions for bone healing. Following this 6-week healing period and the surgeon's approval, the patient may resume a normal textured diet as tolerated.
- For patients with intermaxillary fixation, a straw or large syringe needs to be used to deliver high-energy free fluids into the oral cavity. If there are any comorbidities affecting neurological status, cognition, or level of alertness, a clinical assessment should be conducted to assess the patient's ability to safely swallow this consistency with a modified method of bolus delivery.
- If the patient is experiencing mandibular hypomobility, or trismus, after the period of fixation and healing, passive jaw stretches are recommended. Research literature has reported that the Therabite Jaw Motion System by Atos Medical (http://www.atosmedical.com; Figure 5–4) and performing stretches using stacks of tongue depressors are effective treatments for reduced jaw opening (Dijkstra, Kalk, & Roodenburg, 2004). It is essential to seek approval from the treating surgeon before commencing these exercises. An outline of these therapeutic regimes for improving jaw opening has been provided in Table 5–2.

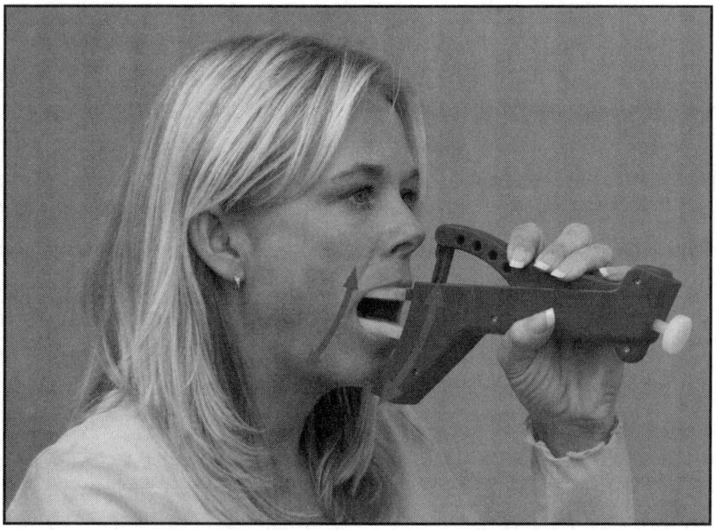

Figure 5–4. Therabite. Photo courtesy of Atos Medical (http://www.atosmedical.com).

Table 5–2. Example of Treatment Programs for Trismus

Treatment Type	*Unassisted Exercises*	*Treatment Device Exercises*
Tongue blade therapy	Daily regime includes: • Open mouth as wide as possible without pain. Hold for 5 seconds. • Move your jaw as far as possible to the left, then right, and then protrude it. • Repeat each exercise five times. Exercises must be completed five times per day.	Daily regime includes: • Place the required number of stacked tongue depressors between teeth. Allow tongue depressors to stretch your jaw for 30 seconds, working within pain limitations, and then rest for 10 seconds. • Repeat five times per day. • Place another tongue depressor in the stack to increase the stretch over time.
Therabite Jaw Motion Rehabilitation System	Daily regime includes: • Open mouth as wide as possible without pain. Hold for 5 seconds. • Move your jaw as far as possible to the left, then right, and then protrude it. • Repeat each exercise five times. Exercises must be completed five times per day.	Daily regime includes: • Use the Therabite system to achieve and sustain maximum comfortable stretch (to a predetermined MIO distance). • Hold for 30 seconds, and then rest for 10 seconds. • Repeat five times per day. • Increase the MIO distance on the Therabite to increase the stretch over time.

Note. Regardless of treatment type (tongue blades or Therabite), patients complete both unassisted and device-specific exercises daily.

Midfacial Fractures. The middle third of the face consists of 18 bones in total, made up of a number of single and paired bones: the vomer, ethmoid, maxillae, zygomas, zygomatic processes of the temporal bones, palatine bones, lacrimal bones, nasal bones, pterygoid plates of the sphenoids, and the inferior conchae. Fractures to the midface usually result from a significant blunt force to the face. Midfacial fractures fall broadly into three categories: Le Fort I, Le Fort II, and Le Fort III. These injuries may occur in isolation or in combination. Descriptions of these classifications have been outlined in Table 5-3 and are illustrated in Figure 5-5.

An important consideration in the management of the patient with a midfacial fracture is maintaining an open airway. The midface skeleton supports the upper airway (i.e., nasopharynx and oropharynx), and subsequently, patients with significant midfacial trauma may require intubation. Commonly, management of midfacial fractures involves ORIF of the bones involved. When the midfacial fracture involves the maxilla, management may also include intermaxillary

Table 5–3. Description of Le Fort Categories

Category	*Description*
Le Fort I	Separation of the inferior portion of the maxilla in a horizontal fashion extending from the pyriform aperture of the nose to the pterygoid maxillary suture area.
Le Fort II	Separation of the maxilla and nasal complex from the cranial base, the zygomatic orbital rim area, and the pterygoid maxillary suture area.
Le Fort III	Complete separation of the midface at the level of the naso-orbital ethmoid complex and zygomatico-frontal suture area. The fracture also extends through the orbits bilaterally.

Note. Adapted from *Contemporary Oral and Maxillofacial Surgery* (pp. 596–597), by L. J. Peterson, E. Ellis, J. Hupp, and M. Tucker, 1998, St. Louis, MO: Mosby.

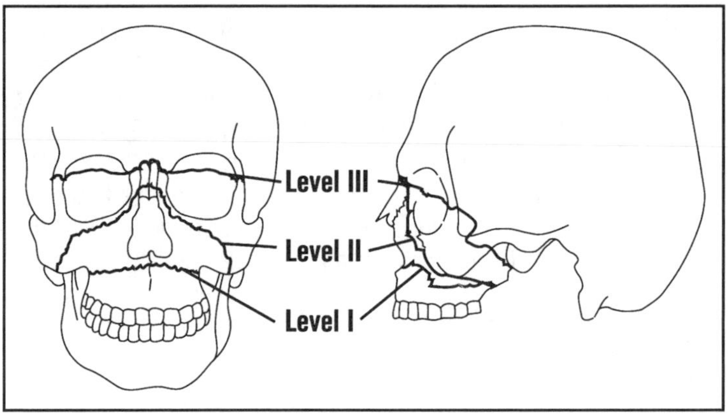

Figure 5–5. Diagrammatic representation of the three Le Fort classifications.

fixation (refer to Mandibular Fractures section) if the occlusal relationship of the teeth (the bite) needs to be reestablished.

Implications for Assessment and Management. Midfacial fractures commonly co-occur with multitrauma and traumatic brain injury: etiologies that often require intensive care management with intubation and alternative feeding. If the patient does need intubation, the endotracheal tube or tracheostomy tube has the potential to adversely affect the patient's swallowing ability. If the patient requires alternative feeding, the presence of an orogastric tube will impair the patient's ability to commence oral intake.

When it is appropriate to initiate the swallowing assessment, thorough evaluation of the oral stage of the swallow is required. Midfacial fractures have the potential to lead to infraorbital nerve (maxillary branch of the trigeminal nerve) damage. As the infraorbital nerve provides sensation to the upper lip and teeth, damage may impair mastication efficiency and oral control and preparation of the bolus. In most cases, the oral phase of the swallow will be adequately assessed with a clinical swallowing examination (CSE). If required, further instrumental assessment should be conducted using a VFSE, as this is the most appropriate instrumental assessment method for assessing the oral phase of the swallow.

Dysphagia management for this population involves the following specific considerations:

- With the orogastric tube in situ, the patient will be unable to achieve lip seal, tongue mobility will be limited, and complete base of tongue to posterior pharyngeal wall contact will not be achieved. Commencing oral intake is not ideal while the orogastric tube remains in situ; however, the medical team may request that small amounts of oral intake be allowed for patient comfort and quality of life. The CSE must consider limitations to the oral phase caused by the presence of the orogastric tube.
- For optimal assessment, the speech-language pathologist (SLP) should liaise with the medical team to remove the orogastric tube prior to conducting the swallowing assessment. Prior to removal of the orogastric tube, however, it must be agreed with the medical team that the orogastric tube will be reinserted if adequate, safe oral intake cannot be maintained.
- For patients with intermaxillary fixation, a straw or large syringe should be used to deliver high-energy free fluids into the oral cavity. If there are any comorbidities affecting neurological status, cognition, or level of alertness, a clinical assessment should be conducted to assess the patient's ability to safely swallow this consistency with a modified method of bolus delivery.

Laryngeal Cartilage Injury. Trauma to the laryngeal skeleton may involve damage to the epiglottis, arytenoids, thyroid cartilages, and/or cricoid cartilages. The low incidence of this injury is likely due to the flexibility of the laryngeal cartilage and the protected location of the larynx, which is surrounded by the bony structures of the mandible, sternum, and cervical spine. When injury occurs, the mechanism of injury may be either blunt or penetrating trauma. Blunt trauma, where the larynx is compressed against the cervical spine, can cause a vertical fracture of the thyroid and/or the cricoid cartilage. Penetrating injuries usually involve soft tissue injury as well as damage to the cartilage.

Trauma to the laryngeal cartilage may lead to life-threatening airway obstruction, requiring intubation. As endotracheal intubation may cause further laryngeal damage, tracheostomy and cricothyroidotomy (incision through the skin and cricothyroid membrane to secure a patient's airway) are more commonly performed. Arytenoid cartilage dislocation and recurrent laryngeal nerve injury are potential complications of laryngeal trauma. Paresis of the external branch of the superior laryngeal nerve has also been reported (Schroeder, Motzko, Wittekindt, & Eckel, 2003).

Nondisplaced thyroid cartilage injuries may be managed conservatively with airway observation, voice rest, humidification, and antireflux medications to minimize risk of granulation. Treatment of displaced thyroid cartilage fractures involves ORIF with titanium miniplates or wiring. Dislocated arytenoid cartilages are managed by surgical reduction and repair of the overlying mucosa. Patients with comminuted laryngeal fractures or damage to the anterior commissure will usually require insertion of a stent (a tube inserted as a mechanical scaffold to keep the airway open) to provide support during healing and to prevent webbing or adhesions developing in the airway.

Implications for Assessment and Management. Recurrent laryngeal nerve or superior laryngeal nerve injury and dislocation of the arytenoid cartilages may result in impaired vocal fold function. This is likely to compromise airway protection during the swallow and may lead to laryngeal penetration and aspiration of oral intake. In addition to the laryngeal trauma, further swallowing complications may arise from intubation (tracheostomy or cricothyroidotomy). However, surprisingly, the incidence of dysphagia following laryngeal trauma appears to be low, with a study involving 37 patients with laryngeal fractures reporting that all patients were decannulated and resumed a normal diet following treatment and only two patients reported subjective dysphagia (Verschueren, Bell, Bagheri, Diercks, & Potter, 2006).

Prior to clinical assessment, the SLP should note any information from the laryngoscopic assessments regarding extent of laryngeal injury, paying particular attention to the operation notes if surgical exploration of the injury was conducted. It is also critical that the SLP consult with the surgical team as to whether any soft tissue injuries are suspected prior to undertaking any oral trials. A contrast swallow may be needed to rule out fistulae prior to trials of any oral intake.

Laryngeal edema may make it difficult to palpate the neck to feel for movement of the thyroid cartilage (i.e., to subjectively examine laryngeal excursion) during the CSE. Consequently, instrumental assessments are strongly recommended in this patient group. ESE is the optimal instrumental assessment method for investigation of trauma to the larynx in most cases. Endoscopic assessment affords a view of edema, anatomical changes to the pharynx and larynx, vocal cord mobility, and their impact on the swallowing mechanism. Severe edema, however, may limit visibility in this exam. VFSE may be a useful supplement to ESE, potentially providing further information on the patient's airway protection during the swallow. If penetrating soft tissue injuries exist or are suspected, however, consultation is required with the radiologist as to the appropriate contrast to be used.

Key issues for consideration when managing dysphagia for this population include:

- Airway protection is likely to be the primary concern for these patients. Vocal fold adduction exercises and airway protection strategies (see Chapter 1) are typical components of rehabilitation. Laryngeal excursion exercises may also be useful to prevent reduced range of hyolaryngeal excursion due to fibrosis. It is important that the SLP consult with the surgical team prior to commencing any exercises.
- If active rehabilitation has been unsuccessful in assisting vocal fold adduction, surgical intervention may be warranted. Surgical repair of the

recurrent laryngeal nerve is controversial. It is unlikely to improve vocal fold movement, but it may help to maintain vocal cord bulk and assist with vocal cord approximation. Teflon or autologous fat injections of the affected cord and medialization thyroplasty are other surgical options to improve vocal fold approximation and airway protection.

Soft Tissue Trauma

Soft tissue injury may be the result of motor vehicle accidents, assault, gunshot wounds, or animal bites, and may frequently co-occur with hard tissue trauma. Types of soft tissue trauma include contusions, abrasions, lacerations, and avulsions (described earlier in the present chapter). Many injuries will result in a combination of these types of trauma. For example, bite wounds may inflict a combination of penetration, contusion, and avulsion trauma. Soft tissue injury, particularly bite wounds, carry a high risk of infection.

Facial Tissue and Oral Cavity Trauma. Soft tissue injuries to the face and oral cavity have the potential to impact significantly on function and appearance. Soft tissue trauma to the face may involve the skin, muscles, blood supply, and nerves of the face. Successful management and repair of these injuries aims to restore premorbid function (e.g., chewing, speech, vision) as well as optimal esthetics.

Management of soft tissue facial injury depends on the type of trauma. Contusions and abrasions are usually quite superficial, with minimal impact on function. Bite wounds, due to the high risk of infection, are treated with irrigation (cleaning by flushing with water) of the wound, debridement, primary closure, and broad-spectrum antibiotics. Management of abrasions involves debridement and primary closure of the wound. Larger lacerations and avulsion injury require surgical repair with the use of a skin graft or flap to fill the defect. Floor of mouth lacerations are usually not repaired, as suturing may damage the lingual nerve or the submandibular salivary ducts. An exception is "through and through" wounds (i.e., where the penetrating object comes into and out of the body part of penetration, commonly the result of a gunshot wound), which require suturing in layers to prevent the formation of fistulae.

Implications for Assessment and Management. Soft tissue injuries to the lips or cheeks and intraoral injuries to the palate, floor of mouth, buccal cavity, or tongue may have an impact on chewing and swallowing. This impact may be acute due to pain and restricted movement while wound healing occurs, or may be a chronic consequence of the injury and its repair.

Prior to conducting a clinical assessment, it is important to review the medical notes paying particular attention to the surgical repair of the injury, as this is likely to indicate any potential restriction to the range of movement of the structures involved. As mentioned above, laceration and avulsion injuries are repaired surgically with either a primary closure or, for larger deficits, with a skin graft or a pedicled or free tissue flap. These interventions may result in fibrotic scar tissue or reduced mobility of tissues. For example, repaired lip trauma may result in impaired lip seal and microstomia.

Following review of the medical history, a thorough examination of facial nerve damage should be undertaken as part of the clinical assessment. Blunt trauma or penetrating injuries to the lateral face and temporal area can cause injury to branches of the facial nerve (Figure 5–6). Blunt injury to the facial nerve is managed conservatively and regeneration should begin to occur within 3 months. Severed branches of the facial nerve may be surgically repaired. If not repaired, however, facial nerve trauma may cause either: (a) damage to the buccal branch (which innervates the buccinator and muscles of the upper lip) that may result in difficulty chewing and paralysis of the upper lip, or (b) injury to the mandibular branch (which innervates the lower lip) that may impair lip seal by causing paralysis of the lower lip.

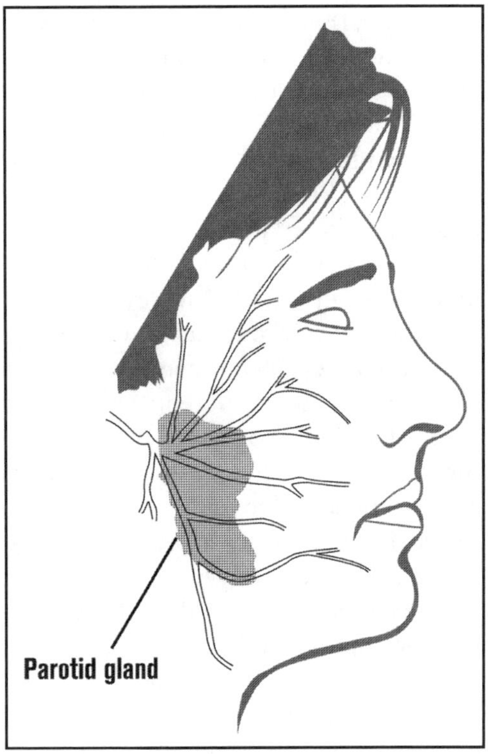

Figure 5–6. Schematic representation of the branches of facial nerve and relative positioning of the parotid gland.

In most cases, the oral phase of the swallow will be adequately assessed with a CSE. If instrumental assessment is warranted, ESE is contraindicated, as it cannot provide detailed information on the oral stage of the swallow. VFSE is therefore the preferred assessment in order to provide further information on the function of the intraoral structures for bolus manipulation and control.

Dysphagia management largely consists of improving mobility and strength of the articulators, with strategies including:

- If impaired mobility of structures is diagnosed, management includes range of motion exercises for the affected area (e.g., lip or jaw), passive stretching regimens (for example, oral splinting for reduced lip range of movement), and use of assistive devices for bolus delivery such as a dysphagia cup, straw, or teaspoon.
- If muscle weakness is present due to facial nerve damage, management includes active muscular exercises once reinnervation has occurred. These exercises should first focus on achieving facial symmetry at rest and avoiding overrecruitment of muscles on the nonaffected side. Range of motion exercises should be employed to improve movements for facial expression.

Pharynx, Larynx, and Esophagus. Soft tissue trauma to the pharynx, larynx, and esophagus is often the result of penetrating or blunt trauma. Penetrating injuries to this area are uncommon but are potentially fatal, as they may involve injury to the adjacent vascular structures in the mediastinum. They are most commonly inflicted by gunshot or stabbing wounds. Blunt trauma to this area is usually a consequence of assault or a motor vehicle accident that may cause the neck to impact against the steering wheel or dashboard or may cause compression of the laryngeal cartilages against the vertebrae in acceleration-deceleration injuries.

Injuries to the upper aerodigestive tract and laryngeal injuries often lead to airway obstruction requiring intubation with an endotracheal tube or, more commonly, a tracheostomy tube. Penetrating injuries in this highly vascular area may lead to localized edema, hemorrhage, or hematoma. Long-term consequences of these injuries include dysphagia, dysphonia, and prolonged tracheostomy (Bumpous, Whitt, Ganzel, & McClane, 2000). Penetrating injuries can also involve recurrent laryngeal nerve damage.

Contrast (gastrograffin or barium) swallows and fiberoptic endoscopy or rigid esophagoscopy are used to identify the injury and to evaluate healing and repair. A standard barium swallow has been found to detect injury with 89% sensitivity and 100% specificity, whereas esophagoscopy reportedly has 89% specificity and 95% specificity (Weigelt et al., 1987). A combination of both tests provides 94% accuracy in identifying esophageal injuries (Weigelt et al., 1987).

Treatment of penetrating injuries may be conservative or involve surgical repair of the defect. Historically, surgical exploration and repair was the most common method of management. Recent management trends are nonoperative and include intravenous antibiotics, nil by mouth status, enteral nutrition, and antireflux medication to reduce the formation of granulation tissue.

Implications for Assessment and Management. Tracheoesophageal fistula (see below), aspiration, bilateral hypoglossal nerve palsy, and vocal cord paralysis are reported complications of surgical repair of soft tissue injury to the pharynx, larynx, and esophagus (Goudy, Miller, & Bumpous, 2002; Kylachkin, Rohmiller, Charash, Sloan, & Kearney, 1997). The literature reports that 19 to 21% of patients with penetrating injuries to the neck experience dysphagia; however, it is suspected that this is underreported, as most studies are single-facility surgical audits with little detail of functional outcomes (Bumpous et al., 2000; Goudy et al., 2002).

Tracheoesophageal fistula is a communication between the trachea and the esophagus that can lead to aspiration of oral intake and life-threatening aspiration pneumonia. It is treated surgically with the placement of a stent in the patent area. Prior to commencing oral intake, a contrast swallow must be performed to assess for any leaks at the site of the repair.

The CSE should include a thorough investigation of the structures innervated by the recurrent laryngeal nerve (vocal cords) and the hypoglossal nerve (muscles of the tongue). The hypoglossal nerve provides the motor supply to the muscles of the tongue. Bilateral hypoglossal nerve palsy will severely impair tongue movement bilaterally and will cause very limited bolus control and transfer.

Damage to the recurrent laryngeal nerve (Figure 5-7) results in reduced vocal fold movement on the affected side. Depending on how the affected cord is positioned (abducted, adducted, or paramedian), it can cause impaired laryngeal closure and airway protection during swallowing.

If a VFSE is to be performed, it is important that the SLP discusses which contrast is most appropriate for the patient with the radiologist prior to the assessment. Barium can cause infection and inflammation if it enters the mediastinum or an open wound. Water-soluble contrast, however, can cause severe

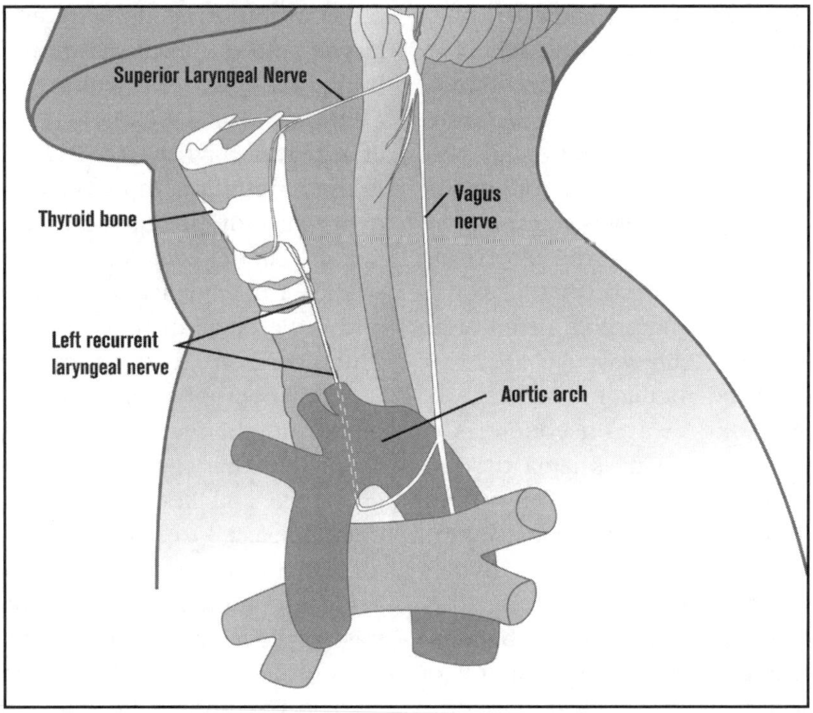

Figure 5–7. Schematic representation of the branches of the vagus nerve, including the pathway of the recurrent laryngeal nerve.

pneumonia if aspirated. Through coordination with the medical team, it may be possible to conduct the VFSE assessment after the contrast swallow evaluation, enabling both assessments to be performed in one trip to radiology. Similarly, if the patient is scheduled for a fiberoptic endoscopy, it may be possible to extend this examination into an ESE for evaluation of swallowing safety and to trial compensatory strategies.

Specific management considerations for this population include:

- Patients who are treated conservatively are to remain nil by mouth for at least 7 days post-injury (Goudy et al., 2002). Similarly, patients with a tracheoesophageal fistula need to remain nil by mouth until a stent is inserted.
- Patients with recurrent laryngeal nerve damage will benefit from airway protection exercises and strategies (see Chapter 1).
- Tongue range of movement and tongue strengthening exercises should be prescribed if the hypoglossal nerves are damaged.

Thoracic Trauma

In addition to structural damage to the hard and soft tissues of the head and neck, thoracic trauma may also co-occur in the multitrauma patient. The term thoracic trauma is used to signify serious injury to the chest, with the primary injury type being blunt force to the chest caused by motor vehicle accident. The combination of both chest wall and intrathoracic visceral injury following thoracic trauma contribute to potentially life-threatening complications and high patient morbidity (Wanek & Mayberry, 2004). Patients with diminished pulmonary reserve and the elderly are most at risk for pulmonary deterioration and require close monitoring. Thoracic injury is largely managed by simple tube thoracostomy (incision of the chest wall, with maintenance of the opening for drainage), mechanical ventilation, aggressive pain control, and other supporting care (Wanek & Mayberry, 2004). Surgery may be required when penetrating injuries are sustained. Recovery following penetration injury is typically faster than following blunt force injury.

There are a number of specific chest injuries that can result from thoracic trauma. The most common of these injuries include:

- Pulmonary contusion. Patients that have sustained a significant high-energy blunt chest impact should be thoroughly investigated for pulmonary contusion. Focal or diffuse opacification on chest x-ray is the main form of diagnosis. Pulmonary contusion is not always immediately present on x-ray and may take anywhere from 6 to 48 hours to become apparent (Wanek & Mayberry, 2004). The principal treatment for pulmonary contusion is supportive care, with the focus directed toward treating the respiratory dysfunction that it produces.
- Fractures. Forces exerted on the chest can cause fractures of the ribs, sternum, clavicle, and shoulder girdle. Rib fractures in particular are a source of significant respiratory pain. It is common for ribs to break only at one point; however, when at least two ribs are broken in at least two places, this can result in part of the chest wall moving independently from the rest of the structure and is a condition known as *flail chest*. A significant impact is required to cause the rib to break in two or more places. During respiration, the "flail segment" moves in paradoxical (opposite) motion to the rest of the chest wall, creating pain, increased work of breathing and fatigue. If left untreated, the broken edges of the ribs can puncture the pleural sac and lung and cause pneumothorax.
- Pneumothorax. A pneumothorax is caused by the accumulation of air in the pleural cavity. Typically, it is due to a penetrating chest wound, but can also be from other chronic lung pathologies (e.g., emphysema) or infections. Pneumothorax can be classified as either *tension* or *nontension*. A tension pneumothorax is a medical emergency, which can lead to death within minutes. In this condition, air accumulates in the plural space with each breath, causing increased intrathoracic pressure and compression of the intrathoracic vessels. Nontension pneumothorax is less severe as there is no increasing accumulation of air. Small pneumothoraces may require no treatment other than providing the patient with oxygen. Management of larger pneumothoraces may require chest tube placement that is removed once the pneumothorax is resolved.
- Hemothorax. A hemothorax is the accumulation of blood in the thoracic cavity. When this occurs in conjunction with pneumothorax, it creates a hemopneumothorax. The resulting condition can be serious

and may interfere with breathing as blood and air fill the pleural space, putting pressure on the lung. The placement of thoracostomy tubes to relieve the hemopneumothorax is the primary form of treatment for this injury. Surgery may also be needed to close off the injuries that caused the blood and air to enter the pleural cavity.

- Injury to thoracoabdominal muscles and organs. Damage to the liver and spleen are common in blunt force injuries to the thorax. Other injuries may include tracheobronchial injury, which is caused by physical trauma to the tracheobronchial tree. Some people with this injury die before receiving emergency care as a result of injuries to vital organs, profuse bleeding and insufficient airway, myocardial contusion, traumatic aortic rupture, esophageal perforation, and diaphragmatic injury.

Implications for Assessment and Management. Swallowing function can be affected in patients who have sustained chest injuries following thoracic trauma, and indeed many of the multitrauma patients referred for swallow assessment and management in the intensive care setting are likely to have some form of chest injury.

Patients that have a flail chest will have a disruption of their chest wall mechanics, decreasing tidal volume and reducing the effectiveness of their cough. This may impact on a patient's ability to protect the airway on food and fluid trials, particularly if the patient is unable to be positioned optimally for eating, or if the condition is in combination with a neurological swallowing problem. These patients will often be predisposed to sputum retention, atelectasis (collapse of all or part of the lung), and pneumonia. This predisposition to pneumonia can create a challenge to the SLP managing the patient's swallowing function, as it may be difficult to determine whether the poor chest status is due to an aspiration event from food and fluid trials, or whether it is due to the underlying thoracic injuries.

Patients who have sustained chest injuries from thoracic trauma are also likely to have poor respiratory patterns, which may impact on their swallow-respiratory cycle during eating and drinking. Morton, Minford, Ellis, and Pinnington (2002) investigated a group of patients with dysphagia who also had poor respiratory control. They found that aspiration results from an interaction between the time the bolus is held in the pharynx, the time spent in inspiration, and the abnormality of the respiratory rhythm. Patients who have sustained chest injuries may therefore be at higher risk of aspiration due to their impaired respiratory pattern, which may impact on their swallow function and overall airway protection.

In addition to impaired respiratory patterns, the resting respiratory rate should also be considered when assessing dysphagia in a patient who has sustained thoracic trauma. In a study by Leslie, Drinnan, Ford, and Wilson (2002) it was suggested that there may be higher risk of a patient developing chest infections if he has an abnormal resting respiratory rate due to the suspected lack of swallow-respiratory coordination. The normal respiratory rate in adults is between 16 and 24 breaths per minute. A patient is thought to have an elevated respiratory rate if the rate exceeds 24 breaths per minute, and therefore, a clinical decision may be made to delay swallow assessment if the respiratory rate exceeds this level in order to reduce aspiration risk.

Close liaison within a multidisciplinary team is essential in managing dysphagia in patients with thoracic trauma. It is not uncommon within an intensive care setting for the SLP to perform initial dysphagia assessments with the physiotherapist in attendance so that respiratory function can be monitored simultaneously. These patients will often have oxygen support via either nasal prongs or an oxygen mask. It is difficult to do a thorough CSE when the patient is dependent on the oxygen mask; however, some patients' oxygen requirements are so high that changing to nasal prongs is not appropriate. Discussion with the treating team will be essential prior to assessment, in order to determine appropriate oxygen support methods during assessment.

Respiratory rate should be monitored before, during, and after the swallow assessment. Clinical assessment of aspiration risk may also be assisted through the use of pulse oximetry (Lim et al., 2001). It has been found that reflex bronchoconstriction occurs after aspiration and may result in a subsequent ventilation perfusion mismatch, hypoxia, and oxygen desaturation (O'Brien, Zarro, Gelb, Bhargava, & Ludwig, 2005). Swallow and respiratory fatigue should also be monitored closely during the swallow assessment and any signs of aspiration for a period of time after the assessment due to post-swallow aspiration from pooled material in the pharynx.

Further evaluation of swallowing including VFSE and ESE may be indicated for this patient population in order to provide information on anatomy and physiology of the swallow, sensory deficits, and vocal cord movement. ESE may be the assessment of choice for this patient population, particularly those patients who are immobile, in an intensive care setting, or unable to be positioned upright, as this assessment is portable and can be carried out at the patient's bedside.

Specific dysphagia management issues to consider for the patient with thoracic injury include:

- Optimal positioning for eating and drinking will be a common challenge with patients who have sustained a thoracic injury. It is recommended that the SLP works closely with the physiotherapist and nursing staff to achieve the best possible position for facilitating safe swallowing at mealtimes.
- Patients with elevated respiratory rates or respiratory-swallowing incoordination will commonly find a texture modified diet easier, such as pureed or minced, as this helps reduce the oral preparatory phase of the swallow.
- The person assisting with feeding should also be aware of the timing of the respiratory phase. In particular, sufficient time should be allowed for the patient to swallow and regain respiration before the next bolus is presented.
- Smaller bolus size may also be useful in reducing the amount of post-swallow residue. The clinician should also be cognizant, however, that the bolus must be large enough to trigger a sensory response. Given their potential for swallowing fatigue, patients with poor respiratory control and reserve may also be better served by having small, regular meals throughout the day rather than three large meals.

IATROGENIC TRAUMA

As mentioned at the beginning of this chapter, iatrogenic trauma refers to trauma that may be inadvertently caused by a medical or surgical treatment or diagnostic procedure. There are a number of surgical procedures that may result in dysphagia, and often these procedures are related to trauma to the cranial nerves or other structures of the head and neck region that are integral to normal swallowing. For many of the procedures discussed below, their impact on swallowing tends to be transient in nature, with more long-term severe dysphagia cited in only a small percentage of patients undergoing these procedures. In addition to the dysphagia resulting from the iatrogenic trauma itself, many of the patients undergoing the procedures discussed may present with premorbid swallowing disorders.

Neurosurgery

There is a wide variety of neurosurgical procedures that may alter a patient's neurological status, and depending on the specific site of damage and location of surgery, these procedures may have a significant impact on swallowing function. Some of these procedures commonly include:

- Tumor debulking or removal
- Aneurysm clipping
- Arteriovenous malformation removal
- Craniotomy
- Subdural hematoma evacuation
- Temporal lobectomy
- Ventriculostomy
- Ventriculoperitoneal (VP) shunt insertion or revision

A common feature of many patients undergoing neurosurgical procedures may be a reduced level of alertness and fluctuating neurological state. For instance, a patient who has experienced an intracranial hemorrhage may have a collection of blood in the ventricles that prevents drainage of the cerebrospinal fluid (CSF) and results in a buildup of the CSF. As this CSF accumulates, it will often lead to a gradual deterioration in the patient's neurological function and overall level of consciousness and thereby impact on swallowing function. The acute neurosurgical management for this will commonly be the insertion of a VP shunt to reduce the increased intracranial pressure and thereby improve neurological function. Close assessment and monitoring of swallowing function during this period will be essential to enable the patient to continue on oral intake for as long as possible and to minimize the risk of aspiration.

It may also be common for patients who have undergone extensive neurosurgical procedures to require a tracheostomy due to the risk of aspiration on their secretions. The SLP should play an integral role within the multidisciplinary team to assess and manage the patient's safety on saliva prior to periods of tracheostomy cuff deflation, and the process of tracheostomy decannulation may take weeks or months depending on the extent of swallowing impairment.

Implications for Assessment and Management

Due to the diverse range of neurosurgical procedures, there is an equally diverse range of potential swallowing implications. Wherever possible, the SLP should be involved prior to neurosurgical procedures to enable a baseline of swallowing function to be taken. One example of this may be in a patient who is undergoing neural debulking or removal of a brain tumor. A thorough review of the surgical notes and close dialogue with the treating surgical team will be essential to better understand the expected neurological damage following the procedure. Where possible, instrumental assessment of swallowing (VFSE/ESE) preoperatively may be worthwhile in order to more objectively assess swallowing function and to more promptly manage the swallowing difficulties that may arise postoperatively. Postoperative management will be directed by the surgical notes regarding the location and extent of the procedure.

Anterior Cervical Spinal Surgery

Anterior cervical spine surgery is performed in order to stabilize the cervical spine following fracture (see Chapter 3) or for the removal of pathologic lesions or cervical osteophytes. Cervical osteophytes are bony growths on the anterior cervical spine that occasionally push against the posterior pharynx, causing difficulty in swallowing. Some of the main surgical techniques that may use the anterior approach in treating patients with cervical spine injury include:

- Corpectomy. This procedure involves the removal of the vertebral bodies as well as the intervertebral disks at either end of the vertebra to decompress the vertebral canal. One or more vertebral bodies may be removed and this defect must be restored with another material, that is, a graft. The risks from this procedure include spinal cord injury, bleeding, infection, spinal nerve damage, and graft damage.
- Spinal fusion. This procedure is undertaken to restore intervertebral stability following surgical removal of vertebral structures. Stability is achieved through the addition of a bone graft to the vertebrae (often from the iliac crest of the hip if the patient is the donor or an allograft from the facility bone bank).

Various surgical approaches to expose the cervical spine have been well documented in the literature, and controversy remains as to which is the best approach as far as reducing the risks of cranial nerve damage (Park et al., 2007). The procedure generally begins with either a longitudinal or transverse incision in the lower front of the neck. The underlying musculature of the neck is carefully dissected in order to expose the anterior cervical spine. The esophagus and trachea are retracted toward the midline and the carotid artery and associated structures are moved laterally. Muscles and membranes overlying the cervical spine are dissected and retractors are placed to protect the soft tissues of the neck as the operation proceeds.

In cases where a high anterior cervical approach to the upper cervical spine is necessary, for instance cervical vertebrae one to four, a higher neck incision just below the mandible is required. This procedure poses risks to significant structures, such as injury to the hypoglossal and superior laryngeal nerves, the marginal mandibular branch of the facial nerve, and the submandibular glands

(Park et al., 2007). Incision of the left neck is commonly reported in the literature in order to avoid the recurrent laryngeal nerve (see Figure 5–7). On this side, the recurrent laryngeal nerve is vertical and ascends to the tracheoesophageal groove and is therefore less susceptible to stretching than the right nerve.

Implications for Assessment and Management

Dysphagia following anterior cervical spine surgery has been reported to occur in nearly 50% of patients (Smith-Hammond et al., 2004). Proposed mechanisms include esophageal edema secondary to stretch injury to nerves used in the swallowing mechanism (Smith-Hammond et al., 2004). In cases where a high anterior cervical approach to the upper cervical spine is necessary, several increased risks have been well documented, such as injury to the hypoglossal and superior laryngeal nerves, the marginal mandibular branch of the facial nerve, and the submandibular gland (Park et al., 2007). The presence of the endotracheal tube and the associated cuff pressure has also been postulated to impact on compression of the recurrent laryngeal nerve, thereby causing vocal cord paralysis after anterior cervical spine surgery. Monitoring of endotracheal tube cuff pressure and release after retractor placement during the surgery, however, has been found to prevent injury to the recurrent laryngeal nerve (Apfelbaum, Kriskovich, & Haller, 2000).

Patients with cervical osteophytes that undergo cervical spine surgery will often have a threefold risk of presenting with dysphagia. In addition to the dysphagia commonly reported following anterior cervical spine surgery, cervical osteophytes have been found in approximately 20 to 30% of elderly patients and swallowing dysfunction is already common in this group due to diseases such as stroke, Parkinson's disease, and dementia (Kissel & Youmans, 1992). In addition, patients who have large osteophytes that protrude from the anterior edge of the cervical vertebrae can impinge on the pharynx and upper esophagus and may also cause dysphagia, odynophagia, and globus symptoms (Strasser et al., 2000). A study by Strasser et al. (2000) reported that 75% of the 55 patients who had cervical osteophytes larger than 10 mm were found to aspirate when assessed using VFSE.

Although dysphagia is a common early finding following anterior cervical spine surgery, studies have found that the incidence decreases significantly over time. An investigation by Bazaz, Lee, and Yoo (2002) reported on 249 patients assessed for dysphagia at 1, 2, 6, and 12 months after anterior cervical spine surgery. Dysphagia incidences of 50.2%, 32.2%, 17.8%, and 12.5% at 1, 2, 6, and 12 months, respectively, were reported. Of the patients experiencing dysphagia at 6 months postoperatively, 4.8% of those patients were classified as moderate to severe. Whereas the etiology of the dysphagia in most patients was unknown, 1.3% of the patients at the 12-month assessment were found to have a vocal cord paresis indicating long-term damage to the vagus nerve. A study by Smith-Hammond et al. (2004) reported that 47% of the cohort of 38 patients undergoing anterior cervical spine surgery demonstrated dysphagia on postoperative VFSE. Interestingly, however, over 70% of these patients were managing a regular diet at 2 months and only 23% required some level of compensatory swallow behavior such as throat clearing and head turning to reduce the risk of aspiration up to 10 months following surgery.

Patients who have undergone anterior cervical spine surgery are generally able to commence an oral diet within hours of emergence from the general anesthetic; however, the likelihood of postoperative swelling of the pharynx and upper esophagus needs to be considered during initial assessment. Early assessment and intervention of the swallow may assist in preventing aspiration in those patients already at risk of aspiration prior to the surgery and allow compensatory and rehabilitation swallowing techniques to be implemented immediately postoperatively as required (O'Brien et al., 2005).

Dysphagia management for this population also involves consideration of a number of specific issues, as outlined below:

- Management may include the use of techniques such as head positioning, diet alterations, double swallowing, and the Mendelsohn maneuver. The rehabilitation exercise program is dependent on the specific cranial nerves affected and may focus on oral preparatory stimuli and oromotor exercises to restore impaired function. Exercises chosen may include those that promote tongue mobility and laryngeal closure pending potential damage to the hypoglossal and recurrent laryngeal nerves. If the superior laryngeal nerve is involved, the supraglottic swallow technique to voluntarily close the airway during the swallow should be taught, as the patient may be at higher risk of silent aspiration.
- If a rehabilitation exercise program is not effective, long-term management of recurrent laryngeal nerve damage may include potential fat or Teflon injection into the affected vocal cord(s) to increase tension. If the glottis is narrowed in the case of paralysis of one or both of the cords in the paramedian position, then the excision of an arytenoid cartilage (arytenoidectomy) to increase laryngeal opening may be appropriate.

Carotid Endarterectomy

Carotid endarterectomy (CEA) may be defined as a surgical procedure that removes blockages such as plaque or a blood clot from the carotid artery to restore blood flow to the brain. This procedure has become the treatment of choice for patients with stenosis of the extracranial portion of the carotid arteries and represents one of the most commonly performed peripheral vascular procedures (Monini et al., 2005). CEA is now widely recognized as the most effective method of treatment for stroke prevention in the presence of carotid artery stenosis, and the risks associated with this procedure in terms of neurological morbidity and mortality have reduced significantly over time to occur in less than 2% of cases (Holloway et al., 1998). There are, however, other postoperative complications involving the peripheral neural structures such as the cranial nerves that are located in close proximity to the carotid vessels. Damage to cranial nerves has been postulated to occur due to normal intraoperative manipulation, traction, and mobilization of the nerves needed to gain good vascular exposure of the carotid artery, especially in patients with high carotid bifurcation (Masiero, Previato, Addante, Grego, & Armani, 2007)

The incidence of cranial and/or cervical nerve injuries after primary CEA has been reported at approximately 11% in a number of studies (AbuRahma & Choueiri, 2000; Aldoori & Baird, 1988; Ballota et al., 1999). However, in a study where the assessment was carried out by dedicated specialists such as SLPs and ENT surgeons using fiberoptic laryngoscopy, cranial nerve deficit following CEA was found to reach 35% (Evans, Mendelovitz, & Liapis, 1982). Whereas some studies have reported these complications to be "minor," in a very small percentage of patients the long-term side effects such as dysphagia may be significant and greatly impact on the patient's quality of life.

Implications for Assessment and Management

Studies examining the impact of CEA on cranial nerve damage have reported on a range of findings in terms of the frequency of specific cranial nerve injury. In literature reviewed by Masiero et al. (2007), they report that the hypoglossal nerve is the most commonly affected nerve during CEA. Hypoglossal nerve damage was reported in approximately 5 to 20% of cases, followed by the vagus nerve (in particular the recurrent laryngeal nerve), that was involved in about 4 to 6% of cases (Masiero et al., 2007). The mandibular branch of the facial nerve is reported to be involved less frequently, and the glossopharyngeal nerve is not usually exposed in the surgical wound. In other studies (AbuRahma & Choueiri, 2000; Schauber, Fontonelle, Somolomon, & Hanson, 1997), the vagus nerve has been reported to be more frequently affected, followed in order of frequency by the hypoglossal, marginal mandibular, greater auricular, and glossopharyngeal nerves.

In most cases, the functional deficit arising from cranial nerve involvement is transient and does not need any particular form of treatment. In a study by Monini et al. (2005), 59% of 98 patients showed a cranial nerve deficit at 3 days after surgery; however, none of the deficits were classified as "severe," and in particular nasogastric tube feeding was not necessary in any of the patients with swallowing disorders. When the same patients were reassessed at 60 days postoperatively, only four had vagus nerve involvement, two had hypoglossal nerve damage, and one patient showed glossopharyngeal deficits. Of these patients, only two patients required rehabilitation of their swallow function.

A further study by Maseiro et al. (2007) examined the recovery of 19 dysphagic patients following CEA. Fifteen of the patients presented with dysphagia for liquids and solids and four patients for solid food only. Twelve of the patients had sensory-motor tongue impairment, and eight had a weak reflex and voluntary cough. ESE revealed aspiration in six patients. Ten patients recovered complete swallowing function within 1 month, and six patients showed recovery between 2 to 3 months and were able to return to their preoperative diet, whereas the remaining three patients did not complete the follow-up assessment. On the 3-month ESE follow-up, only one patient who underwent the procedure was found to have bronchial aspiration.

Many studies investigating cranial nerve damage following CEA do not report on a systematic assessment battery required to adequately assess for the presence of dysphagia, nor do they report on set protocols regarding the optimal timing for performance of dysphagia assessment postoperatively. An exception to this is the study by Masiero et al. (2007) in which SLPs performed both a CSE and an ESE assessment at 5 days and 3 months after the operation. The results of this study suggested that patients undergoing CEA should have a careful evaluation of their swallowing by a SLP, and early rehabilitation may be advisable for some patients. Patients that present with dysphagia following CEA are typically managed using clinical assessment alone; however, if the signs and symptoms warrant further examination, a VFSE may be beneficial as an alternative or in addition to ESE, to more completely assess swallow function.

Management of dysphagia following CEA should:

- Be based on an early rehabilitation intervention approach that may include texture modification of diet and fluids where necessary, and compensatory swallowing strategies to facilitate bolus flow and minimize aspiration risk. Trialing different bolus sizes of various tastes and temperatures may also be beneficial.
- Include a rehabilitation exercise program dependent on the specific cranial nerves affected. This may include exercises focused on tongue range of movement and resistance, base of tongue retraction, soft palate closure, laryngeal adduction, and exercises to promote relaxation of the cricopharyngeus such as laryngeal excursion maneuvers.

Cardiac Surgery

Dysphagia may be present following cardiac surgery, and some of the common mechanisms for this can be cerebral injury and recurrent laryngeal nerve damage associated with the cardiac procedure. It is recognized that cerebral injury is a frequent complication of cardiac surgery. The cerebral injury that results may include ischemic stroke (and less commonly hemorrhagic stroke) in 1.5 to 5.2% of patients, encephalopathy affecting 8.4 to 32% of patients, and neurocognitive impairment affecting 20 to 30% of patients 1 month after surgery (Hogue, Gottesman, & Stearns, 2008). There are a number of possible mechanisms for this cerebral injury including cerebral embolism, cerebral hypoperfusion, atherosclerosis of the aorta, lipid embolism from pericardial suction aspirate, cerebral hyperthermia, hyperglycemia, perioperative anemia, atrial fibrillation, and genetic disposition (for further reading, see Hogue et al., 2008).

Recurrent laryngeal nerve damage may also occur following cardiac surgery, although it is relatively uncommon, with the frequency of vocal cord dysfunction in adult coronary artery bypass graft (CABG) patients ranging anywhere from approximately 2 to 8% (Kawahito, Kitahata, Kimura, Tanaka, & Oshita, 1999; Shafei, El-Kholy, Azmy, Ebrahim, & Al-Ebrahim, 1997). As can be seen in Figure 5-7, the left recurrent laryngeal nerve lies very close to the parietal pleura in the upper and posterior part of the thoracic cavity as it circles around the arch of the aorta, whereas the right branch loops around the right subclavian artery. If the pleura is opened during internal mammary artery dissection and ice slush is placed in the pleural cavity, the left recurrent laryngeal nerve can suffer hypothermic nueropathy (Tewari & Aggarwal, 1996). Sharma, Parmley,Sreeram, and Grocott (2000) discuss several other causes of recurrent laryngeal nerve damage during cardiac surgery, including: endotracheal intubation, central venous catheter placement, surgical dissection, and a malpositioned or overinflated endotracheal tube balloon that may lie against the vocal cords. In patients who develop respiratory insufficiency, an ineffective cough, and a hoarse voice quality after extubation, recurrent laryngeal nerve damage and thus swallowing impairment should be suspected.

Implications for Assessment and Management

Cerebral injury following cardiac surgery may have a significant impact on swallowing function depending on the site and extent of the injury to the cerebral cortex. Upper motor neuron damage to cranial nerves V, VII, IX, X, and XII may all impact on swallowing function (see Chapter 1 for more details), and the recovery from this damage can range from mild, transient effects to permanent, long-term dysphagia.

Damage to the recurrent laryngeal nerve can also impact on swallowing function. This nerve innervates the only abductor of the vocal cords, the posterior cricoarytenoid muscles. It also innervates the muscles that adduct the vocal cords. Because the recurrent laryngeal nerve has a dual function of abducting and adducting the vocal cords, palsy of this nerve causes the vocal cords to assume a paramedian position. The recurrent laryngeal nerve also provides sensation below the level of the cords. Palsy of one or both of the recurrent laryngeal nerves may impact on laryngeal closure and airway protection during swallowing. If material is aspirated, the reflexive cough response may also be affected leaving the patient at higher risk of silent aspiration. A study by Shafei et al. (1997) found that unilateral vocal cord neuropathy usually takes 8 to 12 months to resolve, and most patients can be treated conservatively. In other studies reporting on more severe cases, patients may require reintubation and tracheostomy due to airway compromise.

For patients with cerebral injury or laryngeal damage following cardiac surgery, it is imperative that a thorough swallow assessment is carried out by a SLP as soon as possible postoperatively. In addition to preventing aspiration risk, this proactive approach to dysphagia management may also assist in preventing the patient from developing generalized deconditioning of the swallowing musculature. The swallowing examination should include a thorough clinical assessment of swallowing. Where laryngeal trauma has been identified, ESE and VFSE are warranted in order to provide a dynamic study of the anatomical and physiological function of the swallowing mechanism and to determine aspiration risk.

The management of dysphagia related to cerebral injury, laryngeal damage, or generalized muscle deconditioning following cardiac surgery will be dependent upon the site and extent of the injury. However, specific issues to consider include:

- Management may include techniques such as head positioning, diet alterations, and various other maneuvers. Design of the rehabilitation exercise program is dependent on the cranial nerves affected and should focus on improving impaired function of the oropharyngeal musculature.
- For patients with recurrent laryngeal nerve damage, a rehabilitation program would be implemented to

improve adduction and/or abduction of the vocal cords. If an exercise program is not effective, long-term management of recurrent laryngeal nerve damage may include potential fat or Teflon injection into the affected vocal cord(s) to increase tension. If the glottis is narrowed in the case of paralysis of one or both of the cords in the paramedian position, then the excision of an arytenoid cartilage (arytenoidectomy) to increase laryngeal opening may be appropriate.

Thyroidectomy

Thyroid surgery is performed for a number of thyroid conditions including both cancerous and noncancerous thyroid nodules, overactive thyroid glands, and enlarged thyroid glands, otherwise known as goiters. The extent of surgery on the thyroid can be any of the following:

- A simple biopsy or lumpectomy, which involves removal of a small part of the thyroid gland
- A lobectomy, which involves removal of half of the thyroid gland
- A subtotal thyroidectomy, which leaves a small amount of tissue bilaterally
- A near total thyroidectomy, which leaves approximately one cm of thyroid tissue on one side only
- A total thyroidectomy, which removes all thyroid tissue identified

Several unique complications of thyroid surgery may occur because of its proximity to important neck base anatomy, with the main risk being damage to the recurrent and external laryngeal nerves (that control the vocal cords) and the parathyroid glands (that regulate calcium levels in the body). Additional complications include hypoparathyroidism and cervical hematomas (Pereira, Girvent, Sancho, Parada, & Sitges-Serra, 2003).

Implications for Assessment and Management

Dysphagia post-thyroidectomy has also been documented as a common problem occurring both pre- and post-thyroidectomy. Prior to thyroid surgery, reports of dysphagia in the literature can range anywhere from 41 to 49% (Rosato, Carlevato, Toma, & Avenia, 2005; Shen, Kebebew, Duh, & Clark, 2004; Wasserman, Sundaram, Alfonso, Rosenfeld, & Har-El, 2007). This potentially high prevalence of dysphagia demonstrates the need for patients undergoing thyroid surgery to have a thorough clinical and instrumental examination prior to this procedure to fully determine preoperative symptoms and better manage the postoperative sequelae. Reports of dysphagia postoperatively vary in the literature. In one study by Wasserman et al. (2007), 73% of the cohort of 33 patients complained of dysphagia postoperatively, whereas in another study by Pereira et al. (2003), only 15% of the 60 patients showed signs of impaired swallowing following bilateral thyroidectomy. In other studies, dysphagia is not reported as a postoperative complaint.

Different explanations have been postulated to account for the presence of dysphagia following thyroid surgery. These include injury to the larynx during intubation, surgical manipulation and traction, and damage to an extrinsic perithyroidal neural plexus (Pereira et al., 2003). Wasserman et al. (2007) conducted a study to determine whether the function of the internal branch of the superior laryngeal nerves (SLN) was at risk of being altered during thyroid surgery. The internal branch of the SLN provides sensation to the supraglottis and vocal cords, and damage to this branch has been known to cause dysphagia and aspiration. The conclusions of this study were that the sensory nerve to the laryngopharynx remains intact following thyroid surgery, and therefore postoperative dysphagia is not a result of iatrogenic damage to this nerve.

In many facilities the SLP is not routinely involved in the preoperative work-up of a patient and may only be referred if the patient presents with significant signs and symptoms of dysphagia such as coughing and choking on food and fluids. Given the common complaints of dysphonia and dysphagia following thyroid surgery in the literature, it is recommended that ideally all patients undergo baseline assessment of their swallow and voice function. These assessments should include a thorough case history and clinical assessment of swallowing. If the clinical assessment indicates that dysphagia is present, the patient may benefit from an instrumental assessment of swallowing using either a VFSE or ESE. A videostroboscopy and voice analysis should also be completed.

Management of the dysphagia postoperatively would commonly include:

- Exercises and strategies to improve adduction of the true vocal folds and therefore improve airway protection before, during, and after the swallow.
- Exercises to promote relaxation of the cricopharyngeus muscle (see Chapter 1).
- Diet and fluid texture modification that may enable some patients to safely continue oral intake.

Parotidectomy

In many facilities, tumors in the parotid gland are nearly all benign and constitute nearly 95% of all parotid neoplasms in adults (Fabian, 2007). Benign tumors of the parotid are usually less than 3 cm, are mobile, and are located in the body, tail, or posterior margin of the superficial lobe. The proportion of malignant neoplasms, however, may be higher in facilities that treat a large proportion of skin cancer, as this type of cancer tends to metastasize to the parotid gland.

As branches of the facial nerve are closely associated with the parotid gland (see Figure 5–6), parotidectomy involves removal of disease of the parotid gland while focusing on dissection of the facial nerve and where possible preservation of its function. A common operation is superficial parotidectomy. This procedure involves removal of the portion of the gland that is superficial to the plane of the facial nerve. In tumors that involve the whole parotid and are completely invading the facial nerve, a total radical parotidectomy will be performed. When the facial nerve cannot be preserved, the best functional results are achieved with direct facial nerve suture, interposition graft, or hypoglossal-facial nerve interposition jump anastomosis (Guntinas-Lichius, 2004). These procedures can be performed at the time of the parotidectomy. If this is not possible, grafting of the facial nerve should occur as close to the time of the nerve resection as possible and is not commonly recommended beyond 12 months following surgery due to atrophy of the muscles of the face. Patients are carefully selected for nerve grafting, and it is not routinely done on elderly patients due to suboptimal surgical outcomes.

Some of the possible complications of parotidectomy that need to be discussed with the patient preoperatively may include:

- Paresthesia of the earlobe and the lower half of the ear (due to damage or praxis of the greater auricular nerve). The sensation may take anywhere from 3 to 12 months to return to normal, or at times loss of sensation may be permanent.
- Temporary or permanent damage to the facial nerve resulting in partial or complete facial paralysis. If a facial nerve injury is sustained during the parotidectomy, it is usually a praxis, but in cases where the nerve needs to be resected and then grafted or the nerve resutured, it may take anywhere from 6 to 24 months for the injury to recover. It is possible for patients to have recovery of the facial nerve up to 3 to 4 years after the operation.
- Sweating associated with eating in the area of the resection of the parotid gland, otherwise known as Frei's syndrome. This may occur anywhere from 6 months to 2 to 3 years after the initial surgery and it may vary in its intensity.
- Salivary fistula, which is more common following a superficial parotidectomy and usually stops spontaneously.
- Hematoma or wound infection, which in some cases may require removal.

A total parotidectomy may be required for tumors involving the superficial and deep lobes of the parotid or in some cases a tumor of the parapharyngeal space. The problems that may arise from this procedure are more extensive than the superficial parotidectomy. Although very rare, the problems that may arise include damage to the vagus nerve leading to hoarseness, damage to the accessory nerve leading to shoulder droop or atrophy of the sternomastoid muscle, and finally damage to the hypoglossal nerve leading to impaired lingual movement, as this nerve is always at the inferior extent of the resection of the deep lobe of a parotid tumour.

Postoperative care of the patient who has undergone a total parotidectomy is similar to that for those who have undergone a superficial parotidectomy. The patient should, however, be encouraged to move the jaw in order to prevent problems with the temperomandibular joint due to spasm induced by dissection around the pterygoid and masseter muscles.

Implications for Assessment and Management

There is little evidence in the literature documenting the impact on swallowing following surgery to the parotid. Despite the sparseness of literature, damage to the facial nerve following parotidectomy may impact on swallowing function. The motor branches of the facial nerve innervate the muscles of the face used for facial expression and lip function, such as achieving and maintaining lip seal during eating. Damage to these branches may impact on mastication of solid foods, oral containment of the bolus, and clearance of food residue from the affected buccal cavity. Trismus can also develop postoperatively, and this can significantly impact on a patient's ability to maintain adequate mouth opening for eating and can cause pain around the temporomandibular joint during mastication of food and also at rest.

In a total parotidectomy, swallowing problems may also arise from damage to the vagus and hypoglossal nerve; however, damage to these nerves is rare. The vagus nerve is responsible for laryngeal closure during the swallow, providing sensation to the lower pharynx and larynx, and providing innervation to the cricopharyngeus. Damage to the vagus nerve may lead to aspiration with diminished or absent cough reflex, and impairment to the upper esophageal sphincter. The hypoglossal nerve is responsible for lingual movement, and therefore damage to this nerve may impact on the patient's ability to prepare, manipulate, and transfer a bolus within the oral cavity; there may also be reduced base of tongue contact with the posterior pharyngeal wall leading to post-swallow residue within the valleculae.

Assessment of swallowing function following surgery to the parotid should commence with a thorough oromotor examination to determine the extent of cranial nerve damage. Dialogue with the treating surgeon and examination of the operation notes will also provide important details of intraoperative nerve damage and indications for potential timelines for nerve recovery. A baseline measure of jaw opening within the first week postoperatively is a good way of assessing for the presence of trismus (maximal interincisor measurement of less than or equal to 35 mm; Dijkstra et al., 2006).

If damage to the vagus and hypoglossal nerves is suspected, the patient would benefit from instrumental assessment of their swallow using VFSE and/or ESE. This would determine the patient's risk of silent aspiration and would allow an opportunity to trial airway protection strategies and implementation of a focused swallowing rehabilitation program based on swallow physiology.

Key issues for the management of dysphagia for this population involve:

- Once the patient's drains have been removed and the surgeon is happy with wound healing, a gentle oromotor exercise program can be implemented. This may consist of gentle exercises focused on mobility of the jaw, lip, face, tongue, and larynx, dependent upon cranial nerve damage. These exercises may only be beneficial if there has been temporary nerve damage and the nerve has not been sacrificed. In the case of a patient with facial nerve bruising, exercises should first focus on achieving facial symmetry at rest and avoiding overrecruitment of muscles on the nonaffected side. Range of motion exercises should be employed to improve movements for facial expression.
- A swallow rehabilitation program should also commence, focusing on the specific areas of impairment. For example, a patient with vagus nerve damage would be given laryngeal adduction exercises and airway protection strategies such as the supraglottic swallow to be used during the swallow.
- Patients will commence an oral diet as directed by the surgical team as soon as possible following surgery. It is common for patients with facial nerve involvement to initially

commence on a pureed diet. Patients with a marked face or lip weakness or impaired tongue mobility may remain on a texture modified diet such as pureed/minced diet for some time, until mobility has improved or they have learned to compensate for their weakness.

- If trismus is present at approximately 2 to 3 weeks after the surgery, a trismus program should be commenced. This may utilize either the Therabite Jaw Motion System (http://www.atosmedical.com) (see Figure 5-4) or stretches using stacked tongue depressors as detailed in Table 5-2.

CONCLUSION

There is no set pattern of dysphagia common across this population; rather, the complications of surgery or the effects of multitrauma can adversely affect multiple aspects of swallowing function. Best practice management relies on the SLP's being an integral part of the health care team. The SLP should have specific knowledge of the patient's medical and surgical management and its impact on swallowing function. This will enable the implementation of an individualized and appropriate assessment battery. Further, it will also enhance the development of a swallowing rehabilitation program directed to achieve the best possible outcomes for a particular patient.

REFERENCES

AbuRahma, A. F., & Choueiri, M. A. (2000). Cranial and cervical nerve injuries after repeat carotid endarterectomy. *Journal of Vascular Surgery*, *32*(4), 649-654.

Aldoori, M. I., & Baird, R. N. (1988). Local neurological complication during carotid endarterectomy. *Journal of Cardiovascular Surgery*, *29*, 432-436.

Apfelbaum, R., Kriskovich, M., & Haller, J. (2000). On the incidence, cause, and prevention of recurrent laryngeal nerve palsies during anterior cervical spine surgery. *Spine*, *25*(22), 2906-2912.

Ballota, E., Da Giau, G., Renon, L., Narne, S., Saladini, M., Abbruzzese, E., et al. (1999). Cranial and cervical nerve injuries after carotid endarterectomy: A prospective study. *Surgery*, *125*, 85-91.

Bazaz, R., Lee, M., & Yoo, J. U. (2002). Incidence of dysphagia after anterior cervical spine surgery: A prospective study. *Spine*, *27*(22), 2453-2458.

Bolton, C. F. (1996). Sepsis and the systemic inflammatory response syndrome: Neuromuscular manifestations. *Critical Care Medicine*, *24*(8), 1408-1416.

Booth, P. W., Eppley, B. L., & Schmelzeisen, R. (2003). *Maxillofacial trauma and esthetic facial reconstruction*. Edinburgh, UK: Churchill Livingstone.

Bumpous, J. M., Whitt, P. D., Ganzel, T. M., & McClane, S. D. (2000). Penetrating injuries of the visceral compartment of the neck. *American Journal of Otolaryngology*, *21*(3), 190-194.

Conlan, A. A., & Kopec, S. E. (2000). Tracheostomy in ICU. *Journal of Intensive Care Medicine*, *15*(1), 1-13.

Conn, A., & Petrovik, L. S. (2004). Trauma systems and injury severity scoring. In R. L. Sheridan (Ed.), *The trauma handbook of the Massachusetts General Hospital* (pp. 10-28). Philadelphia: Lippincott Williams & Wilkins.

De Jonghe, B., Cook, D., Sharshar, T., Lefaucheur, J. P., Carlet, J, & Outin, H. (1998). Acquired neuromuscular disorders in critically ill patients: A systematic review. *Intensive Care Medicine*, *2*, 1242-1250.

de Letter, M. C. J., Schmitz, P. I. M., Visser, L. H., Verheul, F. A. M., Schellens, R. L. L. A.,

Op de Coul, D. A. W., et al. (2001). Risk factors for the development of polyneuropathy and myopathy in critically ill patients. *Critical Care Medicine, 29*(12), 2281-2286.

Dijkstra, P. U., Huisman, J. L. N., & Roodenburg, J. L. N. (2006). Criteria for trismus in head and neck oncology. *International Journal of Oral and Maxillofacial Surgery, 35*, 337-342.

Dijkstra, P. U., Kalk, W. W. I., & Roodenburg, J. L. N. (2004). Trismus in head and neck oncology: A systematic review. *Oral Oncology, 40*, 879-889.

Dikeman, K. J., & Kazandjian, M. S. (2003). *Communication and swallowing management of tracheostomized and ventilator-dependent adults* (2nd ed.). Clifton Park, NY: Thomson Delmar Learning.

Evans, W. E., Medelovitz, D. S., & Liapis, C. (1982). Motor speech deficit following carotid endarterectomy. *Annals of Surgery, 196*, 461-464.

Fabian, R. (2007). Surgery of the parotid gland. In K. J. Lee & E. H. Toh (Eds.), *Otolaryngology: A surgical notebook* (pp. 82-86). New York: Thieme Medical.

Garnacho-Montero, J., Madrazo-Osuna, J., Garcia-Garmendia, J. L., Ortiz-Leyba, C., Jimemez-Jimenez, F. J., Barrero-Almodovar, A., et al. (2001). Critical illness polyneuropathy: Risk factors and clinical consequences. A cohort study in septic patients. *Intensive Care Medicine, 27*, 1288-1296.

Goudy, S. L., Miller, F. B., & Bumpous, J. M. (2002). Neck crepitance: Evaluation and management of suspected upper aero digestive tract injury. *Laryngoscope, 112*, 791-795.

Guntinas-Lichius, O. (2004). The facial nerve in the presence of a head and neck neoplasm: Assessment and outcome after surgical management. *Current Opinions on Otolaryngology Head and Neck Surgery, 12*, 133-141.

Hauck, K. A. (1999). Communication and swallowing issues in tracheostomized/ventilator dependent geriatric patients. *Topics in Geriatric Rehabilitation, 15*(2), 56-70.

Hogue, C. W., Gottesman, R. F., & Stearns, J. (2008). Mechanisms of cerebral injury from cardiac surgery. *Critical Care Clinics, 24*, 83-98.

Holloway, R. G., Witter, D. M., Mushlin, A. I, Lawton, K. B., McDermott, M. P., & Samsa, G. P. (1998). Carotid endarterectomy trends in the patterns and outcomes of care at academic medical centres, 1990 through 1995. *Archives of Neurology, 55*, 25-32.

Kawahito, S., Kitahata, H., Kimura, H., Tanaka, K., & Oshita, S. (1999). Recurrent laryngeal nerve palsy after cardiovascular surgery: Relationship to the placement of a transoesophageal echocardiographic probe. *Journal of Cardiothoracic Vascular Anesthesia, 13*, 528-531.

Kissel, P., & Youmans, J. R. (1992). Posttraumatic anterior cervical osteophyte and dysphagia: Surgical report and literature review. *Journal of Spinal Disorders, 5*(1), 104-107.

Kylachkin, M. L., Rohmiller, M., Charash, W. E., Sloan, D. A., & Kearney, P. A. (1997). Penetrating injuries of the neck: Selective management evolving. *The American Surgeon, 63*(2), 189-194.

Leslie, P., Drinnan, M. J., Ford, G. A., & Wilson, J. A. (2002). Resting respiration in dysphagic patients following stroke. *Dysphagia, 17*, 208-213.

Lim, S. H. B., Lieu, P. K., Phua, S. Y., Seshadri, R., Venketasubramanian, N., Lee, S. H., et al. (2001). Accuracy of bedside clinical methods compared with fiberoptic endoscopic examination of swallowing (FEES) in determining the risk of aspiration in acute stroke patients. *Dysphagia, 16*, 1-6.

Lund, C. C., & Browder, N. C. (1944). Estimation of areas of burns. *Surgery, Gynecology and Obstetrics, 79*, 352-358.

Masiero, S., Previato, C., Addante, S., Grego, F., & Armani, M. (2007). Dysphagia in post-carotid endarterectomy: A prospective study. *Annals of Vascular Surgery, 21*, 318-320.

McHardy, F. E., & Chung, F. (1999). Postoperative sore throat: Cause, prevention and treatment. *Anaesthesia, 54*, 444-453.

Monini, S., Taurino, M., Barbara, M., Irace, L., Jabbour, J., Bandiera, G., et al. (2005). Laryngeal and cranial nerve involvement after carotid endarterectomy. *Acta Oto-Laryngologica, 125*, 298–402.

Morton, R., Minford, J., Ellis, R., & Pinnington, L. (2002). Aspiration with dysphagia: The interaction between oropharyngeal and respiratory impairments. *Dysphagia, 17*, 192–196.

O'Brien, J., Zarro, C., Gelb, D., Bhargava, A., & Ludwig, S. (2005). Dysphagia, aspiration, and dysphonia related to cervical surgery. *Current Opinion in Orthopaedics, 16*, 184–188.

Park, S. H., Sung, J. K., Lee, S. H., Park, J., Hwang, J. H., & Hwang, S. K. (2007). High anterior cervical approach to the upper cervical spine. *Surgical Neurology, 68*, 519–524.

Pereira, J. A., Girvent, M., Sancho, J. J., Parada, C., & Sitges-Serra, A. (2003). Prevalence of long-term upper aero-digestive symptoms after uncomplicated bilateral thyroidectomy. *Surgery, 133*, 318–322.

Peterson, L. J., Ellis, E., Hupp, J., & Tucker, M. (1998). *Contemporary oral and maxillofacial surgery.* St Louis, MO: Mosby.

Rance, K. (2000). The causes and effects of trauma—The young adult. In D. Langstaff & J. Christie (Eds.), *Trauma care: A team approach* (pp. 52–63). Oxford, UK: Butterworth-Heinemann.

Rosato, L., Carlevato, M. T., Toma, G. D., & Avenia, N. (2005). Recurrent laryngeal nerve damage and phonetic modifications after total thyroidectomy: Surgical malpractice only or predictable sequence? *World Journal of Surgery, 29*, 780–784.

Schauber, M. D., Fontonelle, L. J., Somolomon, J. W., & Hanson, T. L. (1997). Cranial/cervical vascular nerve dysfunction after carotid endarterectomy. *Journal of Vascular Surgery, 25*, 481–487.

Schroeder, U., Motzko, M., Wittekindt, C., & Eckel, H. E. (2003). Hoarseness after laryngeal blunt trauma: A differential diagnosis between an injury to the external branch of the superior laryngeal nerve and an arytenoid subluxation. A case report and literature review. *European Archives of Oto-rhino-laryngology, 260*(6), 304–307.

Shafei, H., El-Kholy, A., Azmy, S., Ebrahim, M., & Al-Ebrahim, K. (1997). Vocal cord dysfunction after cardiac surgery: An overlooked complication. *European Journal of Cardiothoracic Surgery, 11*, 564–566.

Sharma, A. D., Parmley, C. L., Sreeram, G., & Grocott, H. P. (2000). Peripheral nerve injuries during cardiac surgery: Risk factors, diagnosis, prognosis, and prevention. *Anesthesia & Analgesia, 91*, 1358–1369.

Shen, W. T., Kebebew, E., Duh, Q.-Y., & Clark, O. H. (2004). Predictors of airway complications after thyroidectomy for substernal goiter. *Archives of Surgery, 138*, 656–660.

Smith-Hammond, C. A., New, K. C., Pietrobon, R., Curtis, D. J., Scharver, C. H. & Turner, D. A. (2004). Prospective analysis of incidence and risk factors of dysphagia in spine surgery patients. *Spine, 29*(13), 1441–1446.

Strasser, G., Schima, W., Schober, E., Pokieser, P., Kaider, A., & Denk, D. M. (2000). Cervical osteophytes impinging on the pharynx: Importance of size and concurrent disorders for development of aspiration. *American Journal of Roentgenology, 174*, 449–453.

Tewari, P., & Aggarwal, S. K. (1996). Combined left-sided recurrent laryngeal and phrenic nerve palsy after coronary artery operation. *Annals of Thoracic Surgery, 61*, 1721–1722.

Throckmorton, G. S., Ellis, E., & Hayasaki, H. (2003). Jaw kinematics during mastication after unilateral fractures of the mandibular condylar process. *American Journal of Orthodontics and Dentofacial Orthopedics, 124*(6), 695–707.

Tolep, K., Getch, C. L., & Criner, G. J. (1996). Swallowing dysfunction in patients receiving prolonged mechanical ventilation. *Chest, 109*, 167–172.

Verschueren, D. S., Bell, R. B., Bagheri, S. C., Dierks, E. J., & Potter, B. E. (2006). Management of laryngo-tracheal injuries associated with craniomaxillofacial trauma. *Journal of Oral Maxillofacial Surgeons, 64*, 203–214.

Wanek, S., & Mayberry, J. C. (2004). Blunt thoracic trauma: Flail chest, pulmonary contusion, and blast injury. *Critical Care Clinics, 20*, 71-81.

Wasserman, J. M., Sundaram, K., Alfonso, A., Rosenfeld, R. M., & Har-El, G. (2007). Determination of the function of the internal branch of the superior laryngeal nerve after thyroidectomy. Retrieved on May 6, 2008, from http://www.interscience.wiley.com

Weigelt, J. A., Thal, E. R., Snyder, W. H., Fry, R. E., Meier, D. E., & Kilman, W. J. (1987). Diagnosis of penetrating cervical oesophageal injuries. *American Journal of Surgery, 154*, 619-622.

Index

Note: Page numbers in **bold** reference non-text material

C

D

E

F

G

H

I

J

K

L

M

N

O

P

T

U

V

W

Z